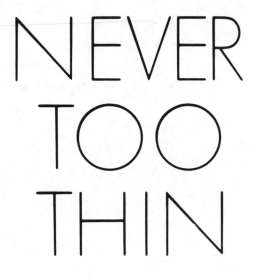

NEVER TOO THIN

Why Women Are at War with Their Bodies

ROBERTA POLLACK SEID

PRENTICE HALL PRESS

New York   London   Toronto   Sydney   Tokyo

Prentice Hall Press
Gulf+Western Building
One Gulf+Western Plaza
New York, New York 10023

Library of Congress Cataloging-in-Publication Data

Seid, Roberta Pollack, 1945–
    Never too thin : Why Women are at war with their bodies/
    Roberta Pollack Seid. — 1st ed.
    p. cm.
    Includes index.
    ISBN 0-13-925116-2 : $19.95
    1. Reducing—Social aspects—United States. 2. Women—Mental
health—United States. 3. Body image. 4. Women—Health and
hygiene—United States. 5. Obesity—Social aspects—United States.
I. Title.
RM222.2.S4   1988
305.4'8908—dc19   88-25537
                                                          CIP

Designed by Maggie Cullen

Manufactured in the United States of America

10 9 8 7 6 5 4 3 2 1

First Edition

To My Father,
Dr. Samuel Pollack
with love and gratitude

Acknowledgments

Although I am an historian, I wrote this book for a general audience, not for academics. I believe historians must participate in popular discourse, for history has been increasingly slighted in education and yet it is indispensable for understanding the present. This book is my own humble effort toward such participation. I saw that only a sweeping historical perspective could expose the peculiarity and destructiveness of our current beliefs about beauty and health, and I hope scholars will be tolerant of my forays into areas and eras that are not my specialty. In general, I tried to use the lay rather than the professional press for my data because I was most interested in the diffusion of popular ideas.

While working on this book, I was reminded time and again of how much an author's apparently solitary task is really a collaborative effort. I am particularly indebted to historians who thoroughly researched similar and related topics—Hillel Schwartz (*Never Satisfied*), Lois Banner (*American Beauty*), Valerie Steele (*Fashion and Eroticism*), Stephen Mennell (*All Manners of Food*), and Norbert Elias (*The Civilizing Process*)—and to those who trained me, Professors Natalie Davis and Richard Herr. I am equally indebted to those who boldly attacked our scientific distortions, particularly Hilde Bruch, Drs. Frederick Stare and Elizabeth Whelan, and Dr. William Bennett and Joel Gurin in *The Dieter's Dilemna*. My father, Dr. Samuel Pollack and my husband Dr. Arnold Seid, both physicians, helped me wrestle with the medical research. Of course, I bear sole responsibility for the ideas in this book.

A writer is also dependent on editors, and I was lucky to have Sarah Montague. The book would not have been what it is without her intelligence, sensitivity and wit. Michael Moore has been wonderfully helpful with the final editing stages.

Perhaps the most important collaborators were friends and family, those who had faith in me and in the project: Jurate Avizienis, Elizabeth Bailey,

Laurie Barre, Suzanne Borghei, Betsy Cohen, Danielle Corbell, Deborah Davis, Deborah Kraut, Carole Lord and my brother-in-law, Dr. Kenneth Seid. Special thanks must go to my colleague and dear friend, historian Michele Root-Bernstein who lent her expertise, time, and energy to several chapters and who ruminated with me about writing popular histories.

I especially want to thank my family. My in-laws, Jean and Irving Seid, were supportive and cheerfully helped me out whenever they came to visit. My parents, Samuel and Marjorie Pollack, my sister Miriam Richards and my brother Allan Pollack have all always been there for me. Above all, I must thank my immediate family, for they are the ones whose lives were most affected by a writing wife-mother. My husband Arnold spawned the idea for this book and helped me see the fallacies in medical and cultural conventions. My sons, Jamin and Michael, tolerantly shared their mother with her work—and somewhat less tolerantly, shared their computer. And finally, I want to acknowledge my late mother, Julia Goldschmidt Pollack, for I suddenly realized how much that her spirit animates this book.

Contents

NEVER
TOO
THIN

OUR PECULIAR
OBSESSION:
NEVER TOO THIN

1

The New American Creed: I Watch My Weight, Eat Right, and Exercise

The quest for a fit, fat-free body has become an American obsession. Webster's defines *obsession* as something that "occupies or troubles the mind to an excessive degree." The term is almost too mild to describe our current preoccupation with losing weight. Today it is held in almost as much esteem as that older American ideal, making money.

Evidence of this obsession is everywhere. A 1985 survey indicated that the vast majority of us—90 percent—think we weigh too much. On any day, 25 percent of us are on diets, with another 50 percent just finishing, breaking, or resolving to start one. We try pills, fasts, formulas, bizarre food combinations, psychotherapy, and even surgery to shed those stubborn pounds. In addition to trying desperately to keep food *out* of our mouths, we also agonize about what *does* go into our, or our loved ones', mouths. Not only diets, but diet, have become part of this complex obsession. We want natural, cholesterol-free, caffeine-free, fat-free, sugar-free, low-sodium, high-fiber, vitamin-rich foods that meet our new nutritional standards and that are, above all, not fattening. Our prehistoric ancestors, the fruit and nut gatherers, could serve as our culinary models. And we exercise. In 1985 more than 56 percent of adult Americans seemed gripped by a modern Saint Vitus's dance, impelled by the desire to burn fat and build muscle. We want the fat of the land to show everywhere but on our bodies.[1]

Most living Americans probably cannot remember a time when being overweight was not a problem. But in recent years, concern about it has both intensified and spread. Barely a decade ago we strove for thinness and health.

Today, swept up by the "wellness epidemic," we pant for fitness and super-health. This shift in emphasis has not changed our underlying goal—a fat-free body—but it has made that goal more complex, paramount, and insidious. It has also expanded the ranks of the fat fighters. Twenty-five years ago fear of fat primarily infected teenaged girls and women from the "comfortable" classes. Today it is spreading to less fortunate classes, to men, and to an ever-broader range of age groups. A 1986 study from the University of California in San Francisco reported that 50 percent of fourth-grade girls—that is, nine-year-olds—and close to 80 percent of ten- and eleven-year-old girls surveyed in San Francisco had put themselves on diets because they thought they were "too fat." The modest prescription, "Watch your weight, eat right, and exercise" has become a national compulsion and a national creed.[2]

The obsession has spawned a multibillion-dollar, recession-proof industry that continues to expand yearly, and it has infiltrated countless other industries. It has triggered an upheaval in America's life-style and affects our social relationships, our festivities, and our leisure activities. It has altered our attitudes about our bodies and has seduced us into letting these body attitudes profoundly affect both our judgments about our characters and our emotional and psychological reality. It is a compulsion that has totally disrupted that private and formerly very pleasurable necessity—eating.

To document its manifestations is to describe a familiar landscape. Diet books clutter bookstore shelves. And there is no confusion about what *diet* means. Though the term literally refers to *any* habitual pattern of eating, today it usually refers specifically to a weight-reducing program. In 1986 there were 313 diet books in print. They are purchased avidly.One or more of them hits the best-seller lists each season. In fact, sales of diet books outrank sales of all other books on the market, except for the Bible. One precursor of this now-common phenomenon, *Dr. Atkins' Diet Revolution,* made publishing history when in 1972—its first year in print—1,100,000 hardback copies were snatched off bookstore shelves. No other hardback book had ever sold so well. In 1979 Herman Tarnower's *The Complete Scarsdale Medical Diet* stayed on the *New York Times* best-seller list for forty-four weeks. *Jane Fonda's Workout Book,* with its 1980s blend of diet and exercise prescriptions, enjoyed a similar success.

This plethora of books is only the tip of the dieting iceberg. Magazines, especially the women's press, peddle endless diets and diet advice. Most of the advice has been printed and reprinted elsewhere—though it is generally spiced with a new twist or a new justification purportedly based on a scientific breakthrough. In January, 1986, alone, nine women's magazines featured eighteen different diets. These figures don't include all the diet tips that slip into the regular health and beauty columns of journals, nor do they include the pieces in newspapers, Sunday supplements, and other publications. And in addition to these established staples, a whole new genre of magazines, with titles such as *Body Beautiful* and *Today's Health,* has emerged to satisfy the seemingly insatiable demand for information about fitness and diet.

What are these diets that inundate us? Their number and variety are bewildering, especially today when concerns about salt, cholesterol, fat, and additives complicate the picture. Many physicians and nutritionists, the AMA, and various branches of the federal government have tried to publicize which are the healthy and sensible diets and which are quack ones, but with little success—and they certainly never denied the merits of diet consciousness. When Theodore Berland tried to rate the diets for *Consumer Guide* in 1983, he had to wrestle with eighty different plans. Among them were fasts and semifasts, high-protein, low-calorie diets, high-fat and low-fat diets, both low- and high-carbohydrate diets, balanced diets that simply cut calories by reducing portions and eliminating frills, and unbalanced diets that promoted one food or, if you were lucky, one food group to the exclusion of all others.[3]

Then there are the diets that vary more by their techniques than by their menus. There are those that let you indulge your weaknesses, like the Carbohydrate Craver's Diet or those that promise you brief vacations from the grueling regimen such as Fats Goldberg's Cheater's Diet, or the Rotation Diet. Others let you make limited choices from prescribed lists while still others rigidly plot out your meal plan and warn that even the slightest deviation spells failure. Some advise you to eat several small meals a day, while others insist on only one large meal. There are psychologically oriented diets that range from "thinning from within" to self-hypnosis to behavior modification. The latter presume that adults need to re-educate themselves about where, when, and how to eat and even how to chew—behaviors usually learned in childhood. Each period seems to produce its own characteristic style of diet books. While many diets are merely revised versions of older ones, these revisions and the newer diets do not emerge in a vacuum: They are linked to shifts in social rhythms and living patterns. The latter half of the eighties has produced "life-style" diets like the Fast Track Diet and sports-related diets that promise to make us more successful athletes at the same time that they help us shed fat. Now, we are told, we can literally "eat to win."

These diets reflect important changes in diet philosophy and presumptions. In the recent past, dieting usually meant an interruption in normal eating habits, a period of unpleasant deprivation after which the successful dieter would begin eating as he or she used to (or almost) and like everyone else. Although experts constantly explained that permanent weight loss involved a permanent change in eating habits, this was not something successful diet books stressed. Gradually, many of them began to include maintenance as well as weight-loss guidelines, and in recent years it has become axiomatic that a dietetic regimen should be everyone's daily regimen, not a brief, unpleasant interlude. While regularized eating patterns may be better than bouts of deprivation, this new, permanent dietary approach is perhaps even more insidious.

Low-fat, low-calorie, sugarless meals are being touted as the only healthy, sensible way to eat. Even more surprising, these diets are no longer described as, at best, painless. Now they are described as satisfying ways to eat. Through nouvelle cuisine, a decorative, diet-conscious translation of haute cuisine, small-portioned, low-calorie meals have become pre-eminently chic. Perpetual deprivation has become a fashionable way of life.

The growing prominence of "health-food" concerns contributed to this change. Health-food faddism has moved from the fringes to the mainstream of American life. Many experts caution that diets high in salt, fat, cholesterol, sugar, and artificial additives can be unhealthy if they are eaten to the total exclusion of other, more nutritious, foods. But today, many experts and a growing segment of the general public believes that these substances, even if they are part of a well-balanced diet, are unhealthy in and of themselves. We call foods containing them *junk foods,* and we've coined the term *junk-food junky* for people who are hooked on them. The worst indictment brought against them is that they are high in calories yet low in essential nutrients. Our passionate quest for healthy foods reflects, in part, our profound caloric anxiety.

We are increasingly concerned with eating "healthy," natural foods, yet to a large extent eating itself has ceased to seem natural at all. People used to eat in order to get energy—that is, calories. Today, industries that siphon off those calories, or make prepared meals limiting them, are cornering the food market. "Lite" versions of many foods abound. Sales of low-calorie frozen foods have risen 15 percent annually for the past several years. Between 1984 and 1985, sales of brand-name frozen diet dinners jumped from $500 million to $1 billion. Diet sodas now account for 20 percent of all soft-drink sales. Restaurants, too, defer to the calorie conscious and often include low-calorie meals on their menus. Entrepreneurs, gauging the intensity of the public's desire to eat out, eat well and *still* diet, have responded cleverly to these once-incompatible urges. Restaurants, fast-food chains, and take-out eateries specializing in low-calorie foods, such as Skinny Haven and Diet D'Lites of America, are suddenly appearing and succeeding. Today, even McDonalds has reponded to these new demands by expanding its menu to include salads.[4]

Dieting by oneself often proves ineffective, so millions of Americans flock to group organizations where they try to shed pounds communally, hoping that group support will provide that extra push to start and keep them losing pounds. Weight Watchers, the best-known of them, has attracted 13 million people over the past twenty years. Approximately 500,000 eager reducers attend the 16,000 classes held weekly across the country. Despite these large figures, Weight Watchers is far from the only organization appealing to the group-minded.[5]

Group efforts are only one of the support systems to which frustrated reducers have recourse. They also turn to the countless psychiatrists, psychologists, and group-therapy programs that specialize in weight reduction. They try to find out how and why they got fat in the first place and hope therapy will help them work through the emotional problems they believe are behind their weight problem. Still others appeal to the growing ranks of reputable and disreputable diet doctors and nutritionists, and often attend them in the growing number of spas. The wealthy spend $1,700 to $2,500 a week to diet and exercise at spas like the Golden Door, La Costa, and Palm Aire, but spas can be found in all price ranges. Recently, specialized health resorts have begun advertising themselves as ideal vacation spots for couples—much as dieting has been transformed into gourmet eating by nouvelle cuisine. Since the sixties we have even had spalike programs for children and teenagers.

Still other Americans turn to the plethora of diet aids sold in supermarkets, pharmacies, health-food stores, and through the mails. In 1985 we spent $200 million just for over-the-counter diet drugs made of caffeine and amphetamine-related substances, and millions more for concoctions like kelp, grapefruit extract, herbal concoctions and growth hormone pills. One company, Herbal Life, might serve as a symbol of the successful diet-related business. The company, founded by Mark Hughes in 1980, cleverly combines diet-reducing concoctions, health supplements, and an evangelical atmosphere, and it has grown spectacularly since its modest beginnings. In its first year it sold $2 million worth of its goods; by 1984 sales had reached $500 million.[6]

Food supplements are only one form of diet aid. Americans also spend millions more on mechanical aids, many of them elaborate contraptions that sound like vestiges from a prescientific age: slimming pajamas, plastic wraps that "melt off" fat, obesity creams, and cellulite removal creams. Conversely, high tech has also entered the field. In 1984 more than fifty different computer diet programs were available.[7]

Even these myriad possibilities don't exhaust the reducers' options. The most desperate, or richest, turn to acupuncture, jaw wiring, gastrointestinal bypass surgery, gastric stapling, or liposuction, a procedure in which small pockets of fat are literally suctioned or vacuumed out of the body.

Yet bald statistics do not accurately reflect how deeply "diet-mania" affects American culture. It is at the personal level that we see the effects most vividly, with family and friends made into partners, audiences, or enemies in relation to the dieter's crusade. Family meals become bizarre contests of strength and temptation, and many dieters avoid social engagements altogether, staying isolated until they feel thin enough and so able to participate in the primal social rite: breaking bread with friends.

The presumptions that fattening foods shouldn't be eaten, and that everyone needs to or at least wants to watch his or her weight, have crept into the language and imagery of our daily lives. When a friend phones and says, "God, I was bad this weekend," we don't expect to hear about sexual licentiousness or about cruel temper and behavior. Instead, we expect to hear about how much our friend ate. Restaurateurs, when not catering to their clientele's obsessions, assault their defenses with desserts described as "sinfully rich," or as the "all-out splurge." Journalists often introduce their January articles with an offhand remark about how we all have to diet now that the holidays, with all their fattening goodies, are over, and their spring articles frequently presume that we are all watching what we eat to get ready for the bathing-suit season. These issues have become givens in our culture, and even the most oblique reference to diet and weight loss is picked up immediately by most Americans.

This proliferation of fat-fighting aids reveals only part of our obsession. A new weight-control strategem has captivated us: exercise. Just ten years ago moderate exercise was recommended as an adjunct to diet. Today diet is seen as the natural adjunct to vigorous exercise; which supposedly produces not only healthier bodies but ideal and idealized ones. This belief has catapulted us into a public love affair with our Olympic athletes, whose victorious moments are replayed endlessly on television ads, along with exhortations to buy one product or another. The media overwhelm us with images of taut, sweaty, leotard-clad bodies and with exercise advice. They promise us that with exercise, we too will manage to mold an ideal form, one that is, above all, fat-free and flab-free.

No sentient American can escape the pressures of this fitness blitz. We exercise—or feel guilty because we don't. And the imperative is spreading. Ten years ago vigorous exercise was seen as the province primarily of young men. Today no one is considered too old—or too young—to work out, and women have smashed the sex barrier that once excluded them from this "male" domain. If the exercise bug, as a self-conscious rite, is most pervasive among the rich and the white-collar, college-educated, its milder strains are now infecting groups who have less money and less leisure time.

In 1961 only 21 percent of American adults exercised regularly. By 1982 the percentage had leapt to 60 percent. A mere fifteen years ago joggers and bodybuilders were part of an extremist fringe. Today it is estimated that 20 to 30 million of us jog or run, and bodybuilders like Arnold Schwarzenegger, Sylvester Stallone, Lisa Lyon, and Cher are among our most prominent physical ideals. If we don't jog, run, or work out with weights, we speed walk, swim, bike, or do aerobics. In the five years between 1977 and 1982, the total revenues of health clubs jumped 116.7 percent.[8]

In its earliest phase, when jogging was the most popular activity, the exercise fad required little more than a good pair of shoes and a nearby street or park. But the fad diversified, becoming more specialized and focusing on all those muscles jogging didn't affect and on the different forms the body could take when strictly disciplined. Suddenly, Americans had to—or wanted to—start spending money on their workouts. Sales soared for shoes and clothing designed specifically for exercise. Between 1981 and 1982 exercise-wear sales leapt by 60 percent and showed no signs of abating. In 1983 leotard sales hit a new record, with 30.2 million of them sold. In 1984 department-store trade journals excitedly reported that exercise-wear was the hottest-selling item of the year, and they rhapsodized about the more fashionable leotards to come. Women liked to sweat in style, and sweating itself became stylish.[9]

At first, Americans went outdoors to exercise, but then they began to bring their routines into the home. Between 1978 and 1983 sales of home exercise equipment leapt 150 percent, propelled by, among other factors, the phenomenal success of Jane Fonda's workout video. Other celebrities and fitness gurus quickly followed Fonda's lead, and today self-help and exercise videocassettes are commonplace.[10]

Moving beyond the impersonal option of exercise videos and the spate of television exercise programs, the wealthy began to hire their own private fitness experts who might charge up to $300 an hour. Many also built spacious, superbly equipped workout centers in their homes. These airy rooms, with their gleaming equipment, are oddly reminiscent of medieval torture chambers, which themselves contained ingenious contraptions for the human body. Such punitive instruments contrast sharply with the opulence of these homes—much as the wealthy's often spare diets invert their capacity for plenty.

While advocacy of exercise can be traced back to the ancient Greeks, to the Renaissance, and up through the Enlightenment, exercise crazes are a more modern phenomenon. America has had such crazes before—most notably in the post–Civil War period, at the turn of the century, and after World War I. Each had its own character, befitting the different perceptions prevalent at the time of the human body, the individual, and the body politic. The contemporary phenomenon is unique in its duration, comprehensiveness, and extremity. Whereas in previous eras exercise was viewed as invigorating and/or spiritually regenerating, to us it is exalting and an end in and of itself. Ordinary men and women strive for skill levels comparable to those of Olympic competitors or of professional athletes and for the attendant "highs" of supercompetition. That we strive to be superathletes rather than merely athletic is evidenced by the startling 34 percent of American adults who work out a minimum of five hours a week and by the large numbers who participate in contests like marathon and triathalon races. In 1983, 157,000 runners completed the grueling marathon. There is no more loneliness for the long-distance runner. The triathalon, with its biking, swimming, and running segments, also crescendoed in popularity. The first triathalon, held in 1975, had only thirty participants. After ABC's "Wide World of Sports" televised the Iron Man Triathalon in Hawaii and popularized the event, the number of contenders leapt: In 1983 it reached 250,000 nationwide.[11]

The fitness obsession has entered our lives in countless ways, affecting everything from our schedules to our sex lives. We don't just spend money on it, we also spend lots of time. Paradoxically, at the same time, it remains an isolated occupation. We haven't integrated it with our ordinary activities. We haven't eschewed labor-saving devices so we can perform physical labor when we do our daily chores. Most of us still drive instead of walk. We still use gas-powered lawn mowers instead of the old manual ones. We keep buying remote-control devices for our televisions so we don't even have to get up to change channels. Instead, we search for extra chunks of time to fit exercise into our daily schedules. Singles have moved from the bars to the gyms, where they flirt over barbells instead of drinks and get high on endorphins instead of alcohol. For many, leisure now means work: getting up at the crack of dawn— or earlier—to fit workouts into overcrowded schedules or passing up drinks for the gym. The press tells us how star-level corporate executives religiously squeeze workouts into their day and imply that this vigor and discipline are part of their success. We read, for example, that Pepsi Cola president, Wayne Calloway, exercises hard for an hour before appearing at his desk at 5:45 A.M. and that Thomas Monaghan, president of the world's largest privately held fast-food pizza chain, Domino's Pizza, does forty-five minutes of floor exercises and runs 5½ miles six days a week..[12]

Lesser luminaries do the same. Predawn residential streets across the nation are filled with bicyclers, joggers, and speed walkers. In Santa Monica, California, an upper-middle-class community, a three-mile grassy strip is used by twenty to forty exercisers at 5:30 A.M. on any weekday morning. They pound the pavement in small groups or with only the company of their ubiquitous walkmen.

Our standards of acceptable public appearance and private habits also reflect the change. The craze has revolutionized fashion. Garb once appropriate only for the locker room, gym, or dance studio has become the height of chic. The "Age of Sweats" has replaced the "Age of Denim." As *Stores,* the trade journal for department stores, explained, "This is a clothing line that reflects a complete new life-style, evokes a stay-fit ethic that has captured the imagination of the entire country." Not only do we want to show off the fat-free bodies we believe exercise will give us, we also want to wear the fashion badge of the exerciser. And while twenty-five years ago a "lady" never "sweated," but merely perspired, today women sweat—and discuss the reasons why—with pride.[13]

Why has all this happened? Why are we so preoccupied with our weight and with diets? Why are we exercising so feverishly? Why do we spend billions of dollars a year and so much time and energy fighting bodily signs of our prosperity—and of our humanity? Sadly, the obsession has so much power over us that we rarely even stop to ask these questions. The reasons for what often amounts to compulsive behavior are so deeply imbedded in our structure of beliefs that we rarely see them objectively.

Simply put, we pursue thinness and fitness in response to a now-invisible aesthetic and moral structure. We believe them to be healthier, more beautiful, and *good.* The unusual alliance between our beauty and health standards gives the imperative to be fat-free a special potence and has bred the ancillary convictions that thinner is also happier and more virtuous.

This is a complex cultural phenomenon, and there are broad historical reasons for its development. A matrix of influences—medical, social, political, demographic, aesthetic, psychological, and ideological—converged to create it, and the elements of this matrix support and perpetuate each other.

Idealogically, health concerns are the bottom line of our obsession. We believe in the concept of an "ideal" or "desirable" weight, one that correlates with less disease and with longer life expectancy. Many experts even capitalize the term *Ideal* or *Desirable Weight* to stress its sanctity. Health authorities incessantly warn that any excess fat, any increase above this desirable weight, is dangerous. "[Being] 20 percent above desirable weight constitutes an established health hazard," concluded a conference of experts at the National Institute of Health in February, 1985. This was hardly news. We have heard the same pronouncement for more than three decades. The list of diseases associated with overweight would make any rational human being choke on his or her next forkful: stroke; diabetes; high blood pressure; cardiovascular and pulmonary disease; diseases of the liver, kidneys, and gall bladder; certain cancers, especially those of the colon, breast, and uterus; increased risk of surgical complications; aggravation of conditions like arthritis and osteoporosis; and even appendicitis. The list seems to grow longer and more menacing every year, and though experts periodically add or even subtract from it, all these possibilities are jumbled in the popular—and often, professional—imagination. The only morbidity/mortality categories in which the overweight come out better than their thinner counterparts are tuberculosis and suicide. Today, many authorities claim that obesity itself is a disease, not just a cause of disease.[14]

These warnings would not be very alarming if most of us felt we were safely in the desirable weight zone, but we have been told otherwise. The standard of healthy weight has become progressively lower over the century, and experts have stated emphatically that an *average* weight is not the same as a *healthy* weight. Exactly how many of us are too heavy is anyone's guess: Different studies accept different "ideal" weights and use different methods for measuring fatness. Regardless of which criteria are used, experts insist that a good portion of us are overproportioned—anywhere from 20 to 50 percent of adult Americans. *Time* reported in January, 1986, that the *average* American male is 18 pounds over his desirable weight, the *average* female 21 pounds over. "Ideal weights" have become harder to reach not only because they have gotten lower but also because average American weights seem to be moving in the opposite direction. We are regularly told that a century-long trend continues: Americans keep getting heavier. *Time* ushered in 1986 with the old but still unsettling news that "[the] U.S. population ranks as the world's fattest" and that the problem is steadily worsening.[15]

We have good reason to be frantic about eating right and exercising. The demand that we get down to our ideal weights is based on the presumption that we can control our body size, that there is no reason for anyone to be fat. The incontrovertibility of mathematics is used to justify this demand. Scientists explain that one pound is equivalent to 3,500 calories. If we take in 3,500 calories more than we burn off through activity, then we gain a pound of fat, and if we reduce our intake by 3,500 calories, or burn them off through exercise, then we lose a pound. We have developed a mechanical model of body weight that makes reducing seem as simple as doing first-grade arithmetic.

We have still another reason to be frantic about our weight. Various influences, bolstered by a bewildering and shifting array of statistics, have caused a fundamental distortion in our perception of normal body size. Instead of the obese being the extreme end of a relatively normal-weight population, the whole population has been convicted of near-obesity and is prey to the fits, fads, and fashions—in medicine and other fields—that make up the obsession with slenderness.

Fueling our obsession with weight loss, authorities warn that weight gain can be insidious, caused by trivial lapses that add up fast. Harvard nutritionist Dr. Jean Mayer, for example, explained that "you can become very fat by eating just 1 percent more than you need every day." An extra slice of bread and butter at every breakfast, without compensatory exercise, "is all it takes to add up to a whopping 10 pounds or so in a year." Dr. Philip White, former director of the AMA's Council on Food and Nutrition, pronounced, "The catch is that gaining weight tends to be an ever-upward cycle—in this field, an ounce of prevention is worth 30 pounds of misery."[16]

None of us—even the genuinely slim—can escape the advancing paranoia because no limit has been set on desirable slenderness. When is thin thin enough? Many authorities insist that every increment above ideal weight brings disease and mortality closer while every ounce below it pushes them further away. Professor Jules Hirsch explains that "there's no one point at which obesity occurs. What we're telling people is that obesity is any excess fat and the danger increases on a sliding scale." No one warns that being too thin may have its hazards, save in the extreme case of anorexics. The inescapable conclusion is that the leaner you are, the better your health and your chances of escaping disease. So even the lean have reasons to be leaner.[17]

Further complicating the issue of weight is the fact that concern has expanded from the simple issue of body mass to the composition of that mass: the ratio of fat to lean tissue. As a result, today even the lightweight are told they must beware of invisible but lethal fat deposits.

Our new nutritional concerns can be seen as a parallel development. What we eat is as pressing an issue as how much we eat and requires the same compulsive attention to detail as does our calorie count. We are constantly reminded that prosperity and technology have revolutionized our food supply—for the worse. This "revolution" has not just caused obesity; it has also contaminated our food supply and ruined any healthy balance in our diets. The Senate Select Committee on Nutrition and Human Needs, headed by Senator George McGovern, introduced its 1977 committee report with the news that "the eating patterns of this century represent as critical a public-health concern as any before us." This conviction has moved from the fringes to the mainstream of American thinking. The committee report was both symptomatic of this shift and helped to accelerate it. Although the facts remain controversial in scientific circles, the popular press has taken the advice for moderation to extremes and assures us we get too much fat, cholesterol, salt, sugar, and additives, and too little fiber, natural grains, vegetables, fruit, and calcium. We are warned that this diet contributes to the same diseases associated with obesity. It seems more than coincidental that the most condemned substances—fat and cholesterol, salt and sugar—are the very ones we consider the most fattening. Their onus of being weight-producing may have led researchers and the public to embrace, unquestioningly, preliminary research that suggested they might be pathogenic in and of themselves. These new convictions have powerfully reinforced our dietary obsessions.[18]

Disease prevention is not the only reason we eat right, watch our weight, and exercise with such fervor. We are now also in search of "wellness," a kind of superstate of mental and physical well-being. We believe that slenderness and its perpetual pursuit can produce profound psychological and emotional transformations, revealing another self beneath the layers of fat and flab. This other self is a more successful, effective, happy human being, magically able to overcome both professional and personal problems. Jane Fonda even argues, in a blend of romantic and almost religious rapture, that exercise and eating right might rejuvenate us spiritually and help us recapture the innocence and purity of our childhoods. "Best of all," she writes, "you may rediscover the child in you who was lost along the way."[19]

At the heart of the wellness concept is the most romantic notion of all: the suggestion that we might postpone, halt, and even reverse the aging process itself. While some scientists are doing research on aging and on human mortality, many wellness buffs—and even some reasonably accredited scientists—are promising that we may soon penetrate the secret of the aging process and with this knowledge, actually extend Homo sapiens' normal life span. In short, we might break the death barrier. While many search for a magic elixir, others stress diet and exercise as the keys.

Those who remain impervious to these romantic hopes have other incentives, or more aptly, coercions, for obeying the wellness creed. The health industry, national and state governments, and private corporations have been influenced by it and have helped spread it. In its 1982 publication, *Wellness at Work,* Blue Cross/Blue Shield provided guidelines for private corporations to set up fitness programs. And ever since the White House Conference on Food, Nutrition, and Health was held in 1970, the federal government has been increasing its outlays for public programs and for education and scientific research about nutrition and exercise. The Surgeon General's 1979 report, *Healthy People,* explicitly outlined the new government health goal—"to encourage a second public-health revolution in the history of the United States," by which it meant ending Americans' careless health habits, such as poor diet, underexercising, and overweight. Since McGovern's subcommittee report was released, federal departments have been reorganized to act on this new priority. Nutritional education and policy setting is now part of more than thirty programs administered by five different departments, among them the Department of Health Education and Welfare and the Department of Agriculture. HEW set up a central Nutrition Coordinating Committee, and in 1979 the Secretary of Agriculture announced new priorities for his own department, shifting from "a policy of sole concern with production of food to a larger concern that includes the diet and nutrition needs of consumers." The National Center for Health Education and the Office of Health Information, Health Promotion, Physical Fitness, and Sports are only two of the many agencies that have sprung up to respond to this new priority. As a result of the McGovern hearings, the government began considering budgets for advertising campaigns that would promote healthy food rather than the processed food so heavily advertised by private industry. And it began pressuring private industry to improve the quality of foods available to consumers. While one must applaud the government's efforts to address the quality of life and not focus solely on production and profit, these programs and attitudes also have endorsed and bolstered our obsession with diet and weight loss.[20]

Such federal policies trickled down into society. State governments began following suit. Arizona expanded its Nutrition Services Staff from 3 to 140 in nine years; Connecticut set up an amply funded Lifestyle Council; Michigan increased the budget of its Office of Nutrition from $94,000 in 1975 to $250,000 in 1979; and in 1987 the state of New Mexico went on a diet with the collective goal of losing 35,000 pounds. Even more directly influential, many school districts have recently expanded and revised the nutrition curriculum for the primary grades. Others have banned vending machines selling "junk foods" from school campuses.

Those of us immune to the pressures of the schools and government cannot stay immune to pressures from the workplace. Corporations, among them Xerox, IBM, and General Motors, have begun instituting voluntary or mandatory wellness programs. Some hire professional groups like Executive Health Examiners to examine the weight and health of company executives—and to urge those who don't measure up to do something about it. Others, responding to ads like those for Weight Watcher's At Work program—"There's more to a lean operation than office systems. We work where you work. We trim corporate fat."—provide meeting space at their facilities so employees can easily participate. By 1982, nearly twenty New England companies supported the At Work program. Other companies have more elaborate and thorough wellness plans. They include everything from nutrition counseling to full gym services replete with trainers, classes, showers, and even laundry facilities. When Thomas Monaghan of Domino's Pizza opened his new corporate headquarters, it included a $750,000 fitness center; PepsiCo has exercise facilities in eleven of its plants and a $2 million exercise center at its corporate headquarters. The pressures on overweight and/or unfit employees, both direct and indirect, are enormous. Monaghan offered to pay one of his staff members $50,000 if he lost weight and ran a marathon within a year, but few corporate employees have such attractive incentives, or need them. Employees are acutely aware that leaner junior executives earn more money and move more quickly up the corporate ladder than their heftier counterparts, and articles in the trade journals frequently describe the fate of the overweight executive. "Fatter Execs Get Slimmer Paychecks" was the title of Robert Half's 1974 article in *Industry Week,* and Sylvia Auerbach discussed a related problem in a 1982 article entitled, "Obesity: An Obstacle to Managerial Success."[21]

Many recent critics of the diet craze have blamed the mass media and the fashion industries for idealizing impossibly slender models of beauty and for thereby creating Americans' obsession with weight. They are ignoring the pervasiveness of the weight-loss imperative, how deeply it invades the daily lives of all Americans. Every authority, every institution in our society urges us to fight our fat. We cannot help but see those fatty layers as abnormal, almost as purulent growths that threaten our health and our success in life. We essentially have transferred our fear of the diseases we believe fat will cause to the fat itself. Overweight and obesity now seem to us to be illnesses in and of themselves—illnesses we have been told we can cure if we just diet and exercise enough.

Aside from our pursuit of health and its psychic corollary, wellness, another even more powerful lure drives us—particularly women—toward the creed of slenderness: beauty. The concept of beauty has a long, complex and variegated history but today the fashion industry and advertisers have decreed that slim and fit are beautiful and that fat and flabby are worse than ugly: They are hideous. And mere slenderness is not enough. Our ideal women, from dancers and Olympic athletes, to professional beauties like fashion models and Miss Americas, to the socially celebrated like the Princess of Wales, are women whose thin bodies appear to have not an ounce of subcutaneous flab. And these celebrities of beauty keep getting thinner. One recent study showed that twenty-five years ago, the average model weighed 8 percent less than the average American woman. Today, the average model is 23 percent below average weight, and American women everywhere want to look just like her.[22]

We have virtually redefined beauty. Today it means only the perfect body. The face has lost its priority as the measure of loveliness. The most exquisite, flawless visage does not win praise if it has the misfortune of being attached to an overweight torso. Fashion magazines no longer focus primarily on clothes and cosmetics; their emphasis is on bodies and how to perfect them. The media inundate us with news about how celebrities got their perfect forms, and we greedily read about the dress sizes, weights, and weight histories of the rich and famous. The sad ups and downs of Elizabeth Taylor's weight have been fodder for the press for years, but she is only one of many luminaries whose battles with weight we eagerly review.

The rich and famous are our paradigms, and we expect them to realize the preposterous body ideals we fall short of. Those who fail to do so are ruthlessly pilloried. Christine Onassis, at 200-odd pounds, was called "poor little rich girl" by the popular press. Readers were titillated by pictures and stories about this woman whose high weight made her seem a misfit in her glamorous world. Nor does fat fit comfortably into the elite world of politics, particularly for the wives of politicians. Mrs. Richard J. Hughes, wife of the former governor of New Jersey, and once 80 pounds overweight, was compelled to report that "New Jersey voters have elected my husband . . . governor twice, knowing he had a fat wife." Fatness, even in the wife of a candidate, can be a political liability, as if, in a bizarre equation, it somehow reflects on his probity or competence.[23]

Our impression that the slim are always rich, beautiful, and glamorous is borne out by recent studies that showed women's weights varied inversely with their husband's income level: the higher the husband's income, the lower the wife's weight. The studies did not speculate about why this was true. Perhaps slender women are more upwardly mobile simply because they attract the hearts and hands of ambitious men who seek stylish mates. But weight consciousness has become part of everyone's campaign for upward mobility. How much we have come to identify status and slenderness is underlined by the now-familiar quip, "A woman can never be too rich or too thin." In essence, in our increasingly visual, competitive, industrial society, appearance—especially the shape of the body—has become as heraldic in its way as any standards set by Renaissance princes.

Celebrities and the rich are not the only ones who have to be slender. So do the rest of us. We cannot resist these heraldic standards, but the overweight have trouble meeting them. Any woman who wants to buy clothes to look presentable, let alone chic, must bow to the standard. The fashion industry designs with the perfect body in mind. Unsightly bulges and a surplus of adipose tissue make even the most exquisite, costly dress look frumpy. Even worse, the clothes advertised in magazines and catalogs, and those that hang on department store and boutique racks, invariably come only in smaller sizes, usually 4 to 14. Until quite recently, when "big women" rebelled, the bigger woman was banished to a lonely no-man's-land with few options for beautifying herself.

Fashion leaders compel us to be slender in another way as well. They have not only deemed fat hideous; they also have deemed it inexcusable. Scientists laid out the simple equation—eat less and exercise and you will lose weight and reshape your body. They placed the fate of our health in our own hands. Beauty experts do the same with beauty by popularizing these medical pronouncements. Whereas once adornment was a fundamental part of beauty culture, and mystery and transformation were at its heart, today, beauty is a matter of absolute exposure and absolute will. If we diet and exercise, we are assured, we will achieve it. The press lures us with bold headlines such as "Shape Up! Diet Dos and Don'ts from Dozens of Celebs" or "America's 10 Sexiest Beauties Show You How to Have Your Best Body at Any Age." Barbi Benton, a former *Playboy* Playmate who achieved fame through her long liaison with Hugh Hefner, claimed she had an altruistic motive for reappearing as a *Playboy* centerfold at the age of thirty-five. She wanted to show other thirty-five-year-olds that they could stay beautiful, too. An interview with her was capped by her comment, "If you're thirty-five and don't look good, it's your own fault." The assumption is clear: Age is an enemy of beauty, but it need not be. If we discipline ourselves enough to do what she does—exercise three hours a day and eat an ascetic diet of chicken, fish, and vegetables—we, too, will preserve the source of our beauty, a youthful body.[24]

The pursuit of beauty—to the extent that it can be separated from fashion—has seemed a far more worthy goal than fashionable chic, since ideals of beauty are part of the aesthetic and moral structure of human life. Health has always seemed a virtuous goal. But today, stylishness, beauty, and health have become inextricable, mutually dependent goals, proclaimed and enforced by experts and the popular media alike. This intermeshing has given the injunction to lose weight special power and worthiness. Even *Ms.* magazine, which rarely concerns itself with fashion, exuberantly emblazoned "The Beauty of Health" on a recent cover.[25]

Beneath this endless catechism about beauty and health lies a more powerful message. In the nineteenth century, cleanliness came to be regarded as essential to decency and even as "next to godliness." Today thinness, too, seems a prerequisite for decency and godliness. Certainly we believe the converse, that overweights have undesirable qualities. We presume them to be lazier, slower, less athletic, and more immature than their normal weight cohorts. We also presume they lack self-discipline and self-respect. Otherwise, they wouldn't be fat. We believe thinner is healthier and more beautiful, but even more, we believe it is a reflection of character, moral strength, and goodness. When we get angry with ourselves for gaining weight, or when we prod our loved ones to drop a few pounds, we are only trying to help ourselves and them meet this moral standard.

Behind beauty is truth, and behind truth, especially in our hopeful American society, is happiness. Indeed, we seem to believe that the pursuit of thinness will bring the ecstasy and fulfillment that religious devotion used to promise. Cetainly we are convinced that thinner plus fitter equals happier. Who would deny that the fitter have better health, more energy, more drive, and more success? Who doubts that the fitter have more sexual enjoyment, more sex appeal, and more fun? We have come to believe these things so thoroughly that we cannot accept that a fat person—regardless of his or her financial and social successes—is truly successful or happy.

Lest we doubt it, every social interaction reconfirms it. Who has not found that the first words uttered by someone one has not seen for a long time are: "Oh! You've kept your weight off," or "Oh! You've lost weight. You look wonderful." To say the opposite—"Oh you've put on weight!"—would be the height of social impropriety even though you and that someone know these are the thoughts that remain unspoken. How many of us dread reunions when we will be sized up by old, close relations or friends because we are fatter than before or eagerly anticipate them because we are thinner and more muscular?

Americans are obsessed with watching their weight, eating right, and exercising for understandable reasons. From without, monoliths are urging us to do so, and from within we are compelled by assumptions about beauty, self-worth, success, and happiness that have been tortured into a religion of slenderness. Never before have so many institutions in our culture intermeshed to legitimize and support an extreme. Except for the recent spate of "big is beautiful" advocates, no authority—whether doctor, teacher, coach, clergyman, feminist, political leader, or parent—has stood up to moderate, let alone question, this extreme. All these authorities believe in the creed. And never before have so many people believed that the shape of their lives depended on the shape of their bodies.

It is understandable why we do. The creed is persuasive. It meshes with American thought and values. We trust science and demand happiness. We believe all diseases and infirmities can eventually be cured and that well-being is a constitutional right. In the creed, science seems to have given us the prescription for a longer, healthier life, not by erecting some strange, new scientific theory, but by building on two familiar ideas. One is our faith in the effectiveness of rational, scientific control. Just as it allowed us to tame the wilderness, explore outer space, and invent our technology, so we believe it will allow us to succeed on this new frontier: perfecting our health and prolonging our lives. If we carefully measure the input and output of this machine, our body, we can tune it until it is functioning perfectly. The mechanical imperative meshes with a biological one. Our Darwinian age now believes literally in the "survival of the fittest," and we have come to believe that fitness—like the defeat of aging—is within our control.

The creed also meshes with traditional American values, particularly our democratic self-help ideology. We believe there is equal opportunity for all; that is, that anyone, whatever his or her race, religion, or circumstance of birth, can belong to the aristocracy of the beautiful people if he or she has the industriousness and discipline to diet and exercise rigorously.

We pursue thinness and fitness with a fervor that borders on the religious. If sloth and gluttony have always been condemned as sins, we have taken those sins as the cornerstone of a new faith. We believe in physical perfectibility and see its pursuit as a moral obligation. The wayward are punished with ugliness, illness, and early death. The good get their just rewards: beauty and a blessedly long, happy, and fulfilling life. The virtue that presumably will put us on this road is our ability to control one of our most fundamental instincts—eating.

We have, in effect, an Eleventh Commandment. We have come to believe thinner is healthier, happier, and more beautiful as though it were handed down on Mount Sinai. But these are not divine truths. They are prejudices with a complex history. They have led to a false religion that does not deliver what it promises.

2

The New American Creed Re-examined: Too Close to the Bone

Amy just celebrated her forty-first birthday. She is a successful lawyer with three kids and a devoted if slightly workaholic husband whose expanding business went public last year. Amy has the energy, organizational skills, and judgment—an understanding of what's important and what isn't—to administer her tripartite empire. She's managed to "have it all." Yet Amy awakens each morning hating herself and resolving she will try to be "better" that day. Her problem: She never has been able to lose the 20 pounds she gained with her second pregnancy. Her husband can't understand why she now prefers sex under the covers or why she hates the beach. Amy is 5'5" and weighs 135 pounds. Even though she is within the Metropolitan Life Insurance Company's "desirable weight" for her height, she *knows* she is "fat." She swears to "starve" herself, like she did when she was younger, and to squeeze some extra exercise in between her rushed after-work grocery stop, late car-pool pickup, and the after-dinner homework sessions, scout and Little League meetings, and business/social engagements. Some days she manages, but the few vanished pounds return after even minor lapses in her regimen. And she starts to hate herself again, knowing that behind the façade of her success, she is still a failure.

Amy is not alone. She is one of the millions of women and men affected—even obsessed—by the new American creed of slenderness and fitness. But the creed, like a one-eyed Jack, has a treacherous, hidden side. Its vaunted rewards never quite arrive. It has not brought Americans more health and happiness. Rather, like all extremes, it has had terrible consequences, especially for women. It has thrust us into obsessive rituals and distorted our perceptions and priorities. And it has spawned a dogged sense of failure, self-hate, and behavioral disorders. Many, like Amy, have glimpsed this other, hidden side, but they still don't question whether the pursuit really makes them feel better, look better, or handle their lives better. It's time to do so. Our new religion cannot deliver what it promises, for its very premises are flawed.

What Kim Chernin called our "tyranny of slenderness" and our consequent compulsiveness about the food we eat and the bodies we put it into have turned eating disorders into a national epidemic. We can no longer regard them merely as cases of individual pathology. Experts estimate that 5 to 10 percent of adolescent girls and young women suffer from *anorexia nervosa,* the self-starving disease. Six times this number may suffer from a more recently discovered disorder, the binge-purge syndrome, known as *bulimia.* It is not surprising that bulimics initially were called "failed anorexics" or that anorexia nervosa has been called the "good-girl syndrome." Anorexics fulfill, to a grotesque extent, the standards of our new religion. They fight fat, watch their weight, diet, and exercise with frantic virtue and virtuosity. They have mastered their bodies. They have in excess that self-control the rest of us try so desperately to achieve. In earlier centuries, people who exhibited such mastery over hunger were categorized either as saints or as possessed by the devil, or, like the sixteenth-century Fasting Girl of Couflens, they were regarded as marvels whom travelers flocked to see. Today, that awe has become a horrified fascination, not because of the rarity of the phenomenon, but because of its increasing commonplaceness.[1]

These eating disorders were once rare and occurred primarily among upper-middle-class girls in early adolescence. Now they are filtering down the social ladder to classes once thought to be immune, and they are infecting a broader range of age groups. We are finding that ten- and twelve-year-old girls have the syndromes and that middle-aged women have engaged in this destructive behavior for years, a fact which underlines that the roots of the obsession were laid some time ago. These syndromes are even beginning to appear in other nations, as if they were exported along with other facets of American culture. Although it is not as life-threatening, obesity is the flip side of anorexia nervosa. It, too, is marked by a disturbance in the pattern of self-control over appetite. It, too, is widespread, though it is far more prevalent among the poor than among the prosperous classes in America—despite the fact that obesity has historically been associated with overabundance.

Eating disorders are the ugliest underside of the new creed. Lives are ruined—in some cases, ended—by them: as many as 19 percent of hospitalized anorexics may die from the disease. We must witness the grotesque spectacle of people starving to death amidst plenty or of people trapped helplessly in obsessive cycles of gorging and vomiting, slaves to impulses they cannot control. These behaviors are extreme, but they are extremes on a long continuum. What is most disturbing today is that an ever-increasing number of Americans, especially women, share the symptoms even though they do not reach the pathologic category. Anorexia nervosa has become the paradigm of our age, and we as individuals, and as a nation, suffer because of it.[2]

Our national abhorrence of fat and flab is a difference in degree, not in kind, from the anorexic's abhorrence of it. We, too, view with horror every ounce gained, every bit of subcutaneous fat. We, too, have come to see fat as an unnatural growth, akin to a cancerous tumor. We have come to see it as a disease and as a disgusting disfigurement. And we now consider it dangerous, an actively invading enemy that can engulf both body and soul. Describing the biochemistry of fat cells in highly colorful terms, a recent *Newsweek* article underscored how treacherous this enemy tissue is: "Far from being sluggish, [fat cells] are among the most chemically active cells in the body, sniffing the blood for traces of dessert, ever ready to send a squall of protest brainward if they sense deprivation . . . . Time and again they emerge phoenix-like from the ashes of last month's diet; even on the threshold of starvation, shriveled fat cells hang in limp clusters, clamoring for lipids . . . fat cells may shrink, but they never die."[3]

Our national abhorrence of fat is matched by our abhorrence of fat people. Prejudice against them keeps mounting. We stigmatize their "condition" because it has come to seem a form of plague, of evil. The root of this prejudice is our belief that the fat are responsible for their fatness. We believe people have absolute control over their body size. Even the most liberal, compassionate people will cluck their tongues about overweight friends and ask why they "let themselves" get fat. Our belief leaves no room for the sympathy we extend to other abnormalities or illnesses delivered by an unkind fate, such as blindness, deafness, or deformed limbs. Fatness strikes us as an avoidable "crime," an attitude underlined in 1965 when a new "reform party" proposed a tax on fat people. As social psychologist Erving Goffman explained, such attitudes exacerbate prejudice: "Whenever the stigmatized are believed to be the cause of their own condition, the irrational, prejudiced attitudes are exaggerated."[4]

The overweight in this country feel, only too keenly, the brunt of this prejudice. Studies spanning the last twenty-five years document how it infiltrates every aspect of a "fat" person's life. In any competitive situation, whether it be applying for college, a job, a promotion, or a sports team, the overweight are passed over in favor of their slimmer competitors. Catherine McDermott, a 5'6", 249-pound woman, sued Xerox Corporation for withdrawing a job offer because of her weight. She finally won the case—but only after an eleven-year battle in the New York courts. Most overweight people do not attempt legal battles because it is not clear that legislation will protect them (in 1979 a federal judge ruled that employers had a right to set appearance standards), because health is often used to justify such discrimination, because the discrimination can be subtle, and because overweight people themselves often feel their condition is indefensible. The prejudice operates in less official ways as well. Teachers tend to favor and expect more of their normal-weight students than of their overweight ones. Doctors treat their overweight patients in patronizing and often cruel ways, regarding them as recalcitrant patients who won't follow orders.[5]

The overweight suffer bitterly from these prejudices. Recently, "fat" women have tried to fight back by organizing groups that provide them with emotional support and that expose the depth and illegitimacy of these attitudes. *Big Beautiful Woman* and *Radiance* magazines proclaim "big is beautiful," just as blacks once coined the slogan "black is beautiful"—and for similar reasons. If these magazines are upbeat, earlier writings by fat women are painful to read. They are tragic testimony to the fact that fat is a license for abuse. A member of the National Association to Aid Fat Americans (NAAFA) recounted her experience when she went to a new doctor because of a cold: "I walked into his office and he looked at me and said, 'I'm not going to treat you unless you lose weight.' I said, 'I just want some cough medicine so I won't cough myself to death.' He said, 'OK, I'll give you some . . . but if you don't lose twenty pounds in two weeks, don't come back.' "[6]

Such abuse comes as much from strangers as from family and friends. Women recount how their childhood and adolescent fatness elicited contemptuous outbursts from mothers who called them "fat slobs" and "repulsive" and who had them try every weight-reducing scheme and monitored every morsel of food they put in their mouths. Adulthood did not bring a reprieve. At family gatherings, distant cousins would pull them aside and unceremoniously ask, "When are you going to do something about your weight? I hate to see you this way."[7]

In the popular media, the overweight are treated with similar contempt. Heroes and heroines are never fat. It would be unthinkable to cast a plump person in a romantic role: It would violate the very canons of the medium. On television or in the cinema, the fat are usually comic characters, buffoons or servants, and often their weight is one of the main comedic subjects.

The popular media seem unable to depict the heavy leading normal, complex lives, and the real social lives of the obese reflect these restrictions. They often are regarded as unworthy as objects of love, let alone of sexual desire. For them, the courting game is often fraught with heartache. Many don't even try to play. This prejudice is visited even upon men who find overweight women attractive. The NAAFA found that men who dated their members often were ridiculed or accused of being perverse, or of suffering from neurotic fetishes or from low self-esteem. The women in the NAAFA are generally at the extreme end of the normal weight-distribution curve, but similar, if less exaggerated, negative judgments are brought even on those who are only moderately heavy. When men walk out on wives who have fattened over the years, one hears little condemnation. Instead, friends are apt to say, "She shouldn't have let herself go."

Such attitudes are buttressed by the whole repertoire of negative traits we associate with the overweight. Because lack of self-control is perceived as the cause of fatness, the fat are seen as weak-willed, morally flabby, and immature. Psychoanalytic explanations for overweight have encouraged us to view them as emotionally disturbed and sexually maladjusted. And we believe they are slow and lethargic, mentally and physically. Such biases are held so widely in our culture that even grade-school children absorb them. Studies reveal that youngsters point to photos of fat children when asked whom they would not choose as a playmate. When asked to describe these children from their photos, they use pejorative terms like "ugly" and "stupid." Fat has become synonymous with these terms.[8]

Societies have never been particularly kind to deviants—those who are outside the norms in physical appearance or behavior—but the most tragic aspect of our prejudice against fat is that it affects people who are not remotely deviant. Our standard of normal body size has become so thin that average-weight people—the norm—are considered abnormal. Our culture has elevated casual physical variations into mental and moral grotesqueries. This is especially true for women, who are expected to meet the ultralean fashion standard. Sociologist Marcia Millman reported that for them, their 20 to 30 pounds above the fashion norms can be a social and possibly occupational liability, and we are all acutely aware of this. When we get angry with ourselves for gaining weight, or when we start prodding our daughters or sons to drop a few pounds, we are only trying, in part, to protect ourselves or them from becoming victims of this terrible prejudice. We are also responding to a fundamental cultural conviction: We believe that fatness is indeed a major obstacle to happiness and to our ability to realize our potential.[9]

In effect, our creed has created another oppressed group in America. Studies dating from the 1960s reveal that "obese" adolescent girls have personality traits similar to those of other oppressed minorities. They exhibit "low self-esteem and depression," "passivity, obsessive concern with self-image, expectation of rejection and progressive withdrawal." They feel isolated and hopeless. Already in the fifties, some psychiatrists such as Hilde Bruch and Albert Stunkard, began to argue that the negative traits believed to cause overweight—laziness, immaturity, lack of drive, depression—were often *responses* to this punitive cultural attitude, not causes or results of fatness. They were also among the first to notice that compulsive overeating was sometimes triggered by despair caused by this prejudice, which contributed to a vicious circle of denial and abandon.[10]

Bruch's most successful treatment of childhood obesity was with children whose parents did not share this punitive cultural attitude, who did not devalue them because of their fatness, and who did not see their body weight as their primary characteristic. Much of Bruch's work with these children was done in the thirties and forties, before our standards of "normalcy" had become so distorted. Today, it is unlikely that overweight children would find such a generous attitude in their homes. The obsession has become too powerful and too unforgiving.[11]

Our creed has not only created a new oppressed minority; it has also created and sustained a network of neuroses. Food is not a problem just for those with eating disorders: Millions are hooked into a perpetual dieting syndrome. Statistics indicate that 95 to 98 percent of those enrolled in reducing programs regain their weight, and then some, within two to seven years, and then they begin another round of dieting. Careening between compulsive, deprivatory periods and periods of plenty, they are not unlike the bulimic who alternately starves and gorges.

Even for many of those not on such a yo-yo, food is a problem. What we can and cannot eat, how much we should and should not eat, where, when, and how we ought to eat have become overriding concerns, even matters of national policy. Our new "health-food" anxieties have piled on top of our caloric anxieties. Their combination engraves in stone our belief that "good" foods—the unfattening, natural ones—promote health while "bad" foods—the fattening, fat-laden, salty, sugary, refined ones that too often taste good—can be death-wielding. It is as if every time we put something in our mouths, we must re-evaluate our life-expectancy hopes. We feel compelled to be as obsessive about food as any bulimic or anorexic.

In a sense, the eating pattern of much of the nation is disordered. All societies set up complex food rules, but in most of them, food is considered a necessity. In contemporary America, we have come to the odd conclusion that it is not a necessity. Eating has become a moral issue. We must ask ourselves if we are "entitled" to nourishment. We have to be "good" enough— work out enough, diet enough, and above all, be slim enough—to deserve it. We have distorted the exhortation not to overeat into the conviction that eating itself is a suspect process, that our bodies need only the barest minimum of food, and that eating more is "bad." We are encouraged to feel guilty if we eat the bad and enjoy it. The Blue Cross book, *Wellness at Work,* enthusiastically cited the success of one health program because participants reported an important attitude change. As one participant expressed it, "I still eat my pizza, but [now] I feel guilty about it."[12]

The very pleasures of the palate have come to be regarded as sinful. *Esquire* magazine recently ran an updated version of the Seven Deadly Sins which made it clear that the concept of gluttony has changed. We did not read about an avaricious appetite worthy of a Dantean hell. Instead, the writer, a woman, described a "gluttonous" evening as one when she crawled under her bedcovers and ate, with voluptuous delight, *one* chocolate-covered Klondike bar. There was no hint of excessive quantity, of moral judgments compromised by the lust for food. Today, gluttony refers to getting secret and sensual pleasure from a "bad" food. Eating for survival is a war of vigilance; eating for pleasure is a sin.

Many now blame the foods themselves for their failures at self-control, and argue that these foods are addictive—hence the popular terms, *sugar junky* and *junk-food junky.* In an era when addiction and substance abuse are paramount concerns, these terms put many foods into a sinister category even though they are applied to the nourishment we need to live. Some people may indeed suffer from addictive problems with food, but today even people with normal eating patterns view themselves as bordering on the pathological. Jay's Potato Chips' old advertising jingle, "Can't stop eating 'em, can't stop eating 'em . . . " has become a nightmarish possibility for all too many of us. We no longer regard such eating habits as a rather normal and forgivable self-indulgence.

If the eternal vigilance of anorexics is extreme and obsessive, it is again a difference in degree, rather than in kind, of how we all believe we should behave. Even those of us who manage to get svelter forms stay locked in rituals of diet and exercise. The battle against appetite and fat never ends. Pizza entrepreneur Larry "Fats" Goldberg, author of the best-selling *Controlled Cheating*, went from 320 to 160 pounds by using the diet he invented and subsequently published. But his dieting days, he knows, will never end. "Food is an obsession," he admits. "I'm hungry all the time. I try to help other people who are dieting. I know . . . the pain, the honest-to-God physical and mental pain of deprivation, the pain of being hungry." Even medical authorities who endorse and disseminate the creed are aware of these unfortunate effects. Dr. Jules Hirsch, one of the nation's leading obesity experts, warns that successfully keeping weight down "requires not only constant vigilance . . . but often persistent discomfort." Today, Americans are urged to put themselves on programs that parallel anorexics' pathological regimes.[13]

Even growing children are infected with these attitudes. Many conscientious parents put infants and toddlers on low-fat, nonsugar diets and ask for advice from doctors about how to get rid of their baby's baby fat. Recently, researchers have found that many nine- and ten-year-old girls and boys are trying to "undereat" and to stay away from "bad" foods that might make them "fat." And, not surprisingly, the medical literature is beginning to report that many of these babies and children suffer from stunted growth, delayed puberty, and failure to thrive.[14]

These have been the creed's effects on the nation as a whole. Its effects on women have been much more pernicious. Eating disorders occur primarily among women. Nine in ten diagnosed anorexics are female, and those who do not go to such punishing extremes make up the vast bulk—more than 80 percent—of people who join weight-reduction programs and get hooked on the dieting yo-yo. Normal women, far more than men, exhibit the behaviors and attitudes associated with anorexia and bulimia.[15]

This obsession has produced widespread distortion of body image and consequent feelings of self-loathing among women, not unlike those found in anorexics and bulimics. It has intensified women's traditional self-consciousness and socially enforced tendencies to equate worth with appearance. Now thin is never thin enough for them to feel they are not fat, and every detail of their anatomies is scrutinized endlessly and found wanting. The ancillary effect is that many women believe they are not *good* enough: good enough for their marriages, their jobs, their children, and their lives.

The depth and breadth of this epidemic of distorted body image, with its resulting self-hate, surprised researchers who first explored it. During her research on middle-aged women in the late seventies, sociologist Lillian Rubin found that "well over half of them" complained about being fat and wanted to lose weight—even though few "were anywhere near fat and most [were] not even discernibly overweight." Drs. Wayne and Susan Wooley, of the University of Cincinnati College of Medicine, were stunned by the results of a national survey of 33,000 women that they did in conjunction with *Glamour* in 1984. Seventy-five percent of the respondents thought they were too fat, even though only 25 percent of them were over the standards of the Metropolitan Life Insurance Company's weight tables, which themselves are below average American weights. Even those who were *underweight* were not satisfied: 45 percent of them felt they were "too fat"; 66 percent of them often wanted to diet because they felt "too fat." A 1988 University of Michigan study of normal-weight freshmen men and women found that only 15 percent of both sexes were satisfied with their weight—evidence that this body distortion is spreading among men—but that only women were disturbed enough to try to reduce.[16]

Two feminists, linguist Robin Lakoff and Raquel Scherr, conducted a somewhat different investigation among college women, also in 1984, but the results they got were similar. Lakoff and Scherr wanted to expose the extent to which cultural standards of beauty have oppressed women. They had assumed that the co-eds would want to have beautiful faces and blonde hair—a presumption that seems terribly dated. All of these young women, even those who rated themselves as "attractive" and used a "liberated" definition of beauty—that it consisted of health, energy, feeling good and self-confident—had one and only one overriding concern: the shape and weight of their bodies. These were never good enough. They all wanted to lose 5 to 25 pounds, even though most of them did not appear remotely overweight. They went into great detail about every flaw in their anatomies and told of the great disgust they felt every time they looked in the mirror.[17]

Most disturbing was the intensity of the women's desire to be slimmer, which did not correspond at all with the degree to which they were—or perceived themselves to be—overweight. A typical response in the *Glamour* survey was the plaintive comment, "There isn't a day I don't wish I were thinner." Perhaps nothing underlines this distorted body image more than the complaints of women who struggle with 100, not 5 or 10 pounds. In a recent letter to *Ms.,* a woman wrote that if she lost 100 pounds, she might get herself down to a "fashionable" size 16 or 18. Yet, she found that her slender friends who tortured themselves about 5, 10, or 15 pounds frequently turned to her "with straight faces" and said, "I know how you feel; I have the same problem." The writer astutely concluded, "They do *not* have the same problem.

And that *is* the problem." She was right. Many women who feel they are 5 to 10 pounds overweight believe their overweight is as debilitating as it is for those who need to lose 100 pounds to get within a normal weight range.[18]

In 1982 *McCall's* ran a story entitled, "Why We're Never Satisfied with Our Bodies," which recounted similar distortions. Women, whom the author assured us had "fine, well-developed bodies," described their figures in terms usually reserved for the extraordinary. One had "huge" hips, another a "grotesque" stomach, a third had "repulsive" thighs, and three had "misshapen" breasts. Even allowing for the hyperbole that has crept into our daily language, the invective was extreme. When these women's weights crept up a few pounds, the invective delivered against their bodies became even more extreme. The problem has become so pervasive that in 1984–85, the popular press ran eight articles on women's distorted body images. *Glamour* tried to find some solutions in pieces such as, "How to Make Peace with The Body You've Got."[19]

We have come to dread weight gain so much that many women fear it even during pregnancy—though it is a normal and necessary aspect of procreation. The pregnant woman, with her fecund belly, has virtually been banished from our repertoire of beautiful female images. At least in visual terms, many now view pregnancy as a distortion of the body, not as one of its natural functions. (This attitude may have had its original impetus between the thirties and fifties when obstetrical theory held that such weight gains could lead to the complication of toxemia. But subsequent research revealed that weight gain does not cause toxemia and that the healthiest mothers and babies were produced in pregnancies in which the mother gained 25 to 35 pounds.[20])

For many women, however, the medical issues are irrelevant. Their fear of weight gain during pregnancy makes them impose limitations on themselves. A number of women I spoke with reported that they exercised and "didn't feel like eating" throughout their pregnancies. When their doctors admonished them, they felt a secret pride. When alarm at the small size of their bellies prompted doctors to order sonograms to check fetal growth, they explained that their powerful stomach muscles kept them from "showing." Two days after delivery of their small but healthy infants, they were back at the gym, soaking up the "oohs" and "ahs" of other women who could not believe how quickly they were returning to prepregnancy shape. Today, women rarely feel there is a time when weight gain is acceptable or even normal. A woman with child is as likely to call herself fat as pregnant.

The ascetic diet and exercise regimens women are adopting today can also cause physical abnormalities. Sexy as they may look, large numbers of women who sustain these regimens suffer from infertility and amenorrhea, or cessation of menstruation. Once seen primarily among ballet dancers and anorexics, it is becoming increasingly prevalent. Researchers are finding that weight loss, low fat-to-lean ratios, diets, and exercise can independently or, more often, in combination, cause this abnormality. It has been documented among obese women who lost 10 percent of their body weight but who still remained obese and among women whose fat-to-lean ratios fall below 22 percent. Exercisers are especially vulnerable. Recent studies suggest that 20 percent of women who exercise to stay in shape and 50 percent of endurance athletes have menstrual irregularities including amenorrhea. Among competitive athletes, the incidence is increasing: Only 10 percent of the women competitors at the 1964 Tokyo Olympics had these symptoms compared with 59 percent of those who participated in the 1976 Montreal Olympics.[21]

Even if a woman is not particularly interested in having children, more than fertility is at stake. These studies suggest that such hormonal imbalances may promote ovarian and endometrial cancer and increase the risk of osteoporosis. Physically active women who cease menstruating for a year or more often develop progesterone and estrogen deficiencies, much like those that accompany menopause. The effect is similar: diminishing quantities of bone mass. After just one year, there can be a diminution of 10 to 15 percent. Ironically, the very exercise these conscientious women think is keeping them young may be aging them. The lean bodies they are trying to mold may be more akin to those of old women than to those of prepubescent girls.[22]

The kinds of diets promoted by exercise gurus and adhered to by their disciples may aggravate the problem. One key as to whether or not an athlete becomes amenorrheic is her diet. In one study, those who consumed 25 percent fewer calories than their regularly menstruating coathletes exhibited symptoms of amenorrhea. More than 80 percent of these women were eating less than the Recommended Daily Allowance for protein, which may have been a contributing factor. In short, those perfect, healthy-looking bodies of our beauty celebrities who conscientiously stick to semivegetarian fare, may be anything but healthy. Somehow, we have devised an image of—and a program for—female beauty that threatens a vital function of the female body: procreation.[23]

Our creed has not just distorted our body images and our relationship to our bodies; it has also distorted our priorities in life. Fear of fat has made many women hesitate to have children, and slenderness has come to be such an independent value that the benefits it is supposed to bring often become subordinate to it. This, too, is more true for women than for men, in part because prescriptions and proscriptions relating to diet and exercise are reinforced by the world of fashion, where standards of slenderness are most extreme and most insistent. Many women regard their weight as the central issue of their lives, the primary obstacle to self-realization, the matter that must be resolved before other issues, such as careers or romance, can be addressed. A variety of research studies and the voluminous literature by women cured of their eating problems uncover the same warped attitude.

This distortion of values even extends to issues of health—clear evidence that for women, health is not the main objective of slenderness. Kim Chernin, in her path-breaking book, *The Obsession: The Tyranny of Slenderness,* dared to record the daily behavior and attitudes that rarely enter scientific studies but that reveal the depths of this distortion. A friend with an undiagnosed disease—cancer of the stomach was one possibility—rejoices because its acute attack made her lose 5 pounds. She admits to Chernin, "I'd like to tell you . . . that I'd willingly gain back the 5 pounds rather than go through that horrible pain again. But I honestly don't know whether that's true." Her friends had also seen this weight loss as the "bright side" of her illness. Their attitude is not unique. This distortion is also reflected in the envy that tinges our fascination with anorexia nervosa. Psychiatrist Hilde Bruch sensibly observed that the "fear of hunger is so universal that undergoing it voluntarily arouses admiration, awe and curiosity." But today, women have more than curiosity. They want to emulate this behavior. Popular jokes abound about women who wish they could "catch" the disease—but they are only half-joking. Certainly such women are not striving for health but rather for a way to rid themselves of their stigmata—their extra pounds.[24]

Even if its logic could be divorced from the behavioral havoc it wreaks, our new religion would still have this ugly underside of pathological behavior and moral and emotional confusion because it is based on flawed logic and flawed scientific premises.

A relatively moderate caution to watch our weights, eat right, and exercise boomeranged into an imoderate, even hysterical injunction to get underweight, to undereat, and to exercise strenuously. One of the classic formulations of what produces better health and longevity demonstrates the extent to which we have gone to extremes. Dr. Lester Breslow, former consultant for the Presidential Commission on Health Needs of the Nation and Dean of the School of Public Health at UCLA, published his Breslow Prescription in 1972. He and his research team, after a long-term study of 7,000 men, found that those who lived the longest and were the healthiest had seven characteristics:

1. Three meals a day, no snacks
2. Breakfast every day
3. Moderate exercise two to three times a week
4. Seven or eight hours of sleep a night
5. No smoking
6. Moderate weight
7. Alcohol in moderation only

If we accept these habits as behavioral prescriptions, it is easy to see that moderation is the key, yet our standards for thinness and fitness have become extreme, and so have the methods we use to achieve them. They cannot produce a sense of well-being.[25]

We believe "eating right" is tantamount to not eating. Yet, undereating, or its variant, dieting, does not make people happier, more energetic, or more effective, nor do they find themselves bursting with renewed sexual vitality. More often, they find they are hungry, and they suffer from the ill-effects of undernourishment. Yet only a few authorities have dared to go against the tide and point out the price we pay for chronic dieting.

Food is a complicated issue. Biological, cultural, and psychological factors all affect our eating habits. Hunger and appetite are two distinct, if related, entities. Appetite can remain unsated even when hunger has been satisfied. The degree to which we have distorted our attitudes toward food and eating is underlined by the scientific literature about caloric deprivation. It falls into two distinct categories. One is concerned with the overweight person's apparent inability to control appetite and lose weight. The other chronicles the terrible effects of hunger, starvation, and semistarvation. The former presumes people eat because of desire, the latter that they eat because of desperate biological need. But ironically, the number of calories consumed by the dieter and the victim of semistarvation is often the same. Only some experts have noticed this parallel and used it to explain why so many Americans do not lose weight easily and why dieters end up locked in wars with themselves. Quite simply, they are reacting the way victims of semistarvation react. No matter how well-fed they look, they are hungry. And semistarvation, even if caused by self-imposed diets, produces startlingly similar effects on all human beings, whether they live in the midst of plenty or dearth, whether they are fat or thin.

Chronic undernutrition creates biological as well as emotional distress, but physicians and experts have tended to shrug off dieters' complaints as signs of weakness or poor motivation. Only recently have they begun to see these complaints as bona fide signals of biological distress. And only recently have we become aware of the fact that chronic dieters also suffer *emotionally* from undernutrition. They become irritable, tense, inefficient, and often depressed. Anne, a former model whom I met during a lecture on weight obsessions, described her own growing realization of these effects: "I'm a mother now and my kids come first. But I noticed that at around 5:00 in the afternoon, I started to snarl at them. I knew I was hungry and that if I ate something, like a bowl of ice cream, I'd be fine. Except, I'd get fat. And I wanted to be *thin.* So now, at 5:00, I have a bowl of ice cream. I'm not model-thin anymore [she is still very slim], but everyone, especially me, is sure happier around the house." Undernourishment has unpleasant effects on all people, regardless of their starting weights. It certainly does not give them that radiant health and energy described in our popular media.[26]

Our dietary beliefs threaten our psychological balance as well. The former model, Anne, also illuminated this complicated issue when she turned on a woman in the audience who, in the litany of health authorities, had suggested she eat an apple instead of ice cream. Anne leapt to her feet and angrily retorted, "I spent five years in analysis to give myself permission to eat ice cream when I wanted ice cream. No, an apple wouldn't do!" Which is not to say anything against apples, but which is to underline the point that our diet fetish frequently leads to a dour, ascetic life-style, to a fear of the pleasures of the palate, one so deeply ingrained that some of us need psychoanalysis to be freed from it. Instead of rejoicing over the blessing of our culinary plenty, we fear it, and we are teaching the same fear to our children. The joyless, regimented diets we are encouraged to follow seem rather like the proscriptions the nineteenth century attached to sex, when it was to be only for procreation. We have wholeheartedly rejected this sexual austerity, but we have replaced it with dietary rules that are equally austere.

Our environment makes the struggle still more difficult. In an age of plenty, with restaurants crowding our landscape, with gourmet fare and snack foods affordable and at hand, with advertisers tantalizing us with their goods, and with a great deal of disposable income in our pockets, how are we to resist? Many argue that this historically unprecedented plenty necessitated our creed. This is an overly simplistic explanation, but certainly, our ample food supply intensifies our struggle. Our life-styles and our body ideal have diverged.

In dieting we are not even exchanging one sensual pleasure for another, although we often think we are. We may believe that dieting men and women are the sexiest, that those who read the *Joy of Sex* instead of *The Joy of Cooking* have more robust sexual appetites, but evidence suggests that just the reverse is true. They may look sexier, but dietary deprivation seems to inhibit, not enhance sexual appetite. We have somehow come to believe that chronic undernutrition—and the slenderness it brings—can be an aphrodisiac.

Ironically, dieting, the very method we use to control our now-suspect appetites and to vanquish our unruly bodies, itself may provoke obsessive behavior and binge-eating. It may indeed *cause* both eating disorders and obesity itself through what is now termed *diet-induced obesity*. Sadly, in trying to control our eating, we court the very problem we think we are solving.

The relentless exercise regimes to which we subscribe are subject to the same flaws and fallacies as dieting. Evidence indicates that excessive exercise does *not* produce better health; that more fiction than fact supports the notion that it will protect us from heart disease. Indeed, much evidence suggests that the punishment inflicted on the overexercised body harms it, not helps it. Nor does strenuous exercise give us greater well-being, energy, or sexual vitality, or help us get other aspects of our lives under control. More often, it does just the opposite.

We have confused fitness, the ability of the body to do work, with health, the absence of disease and in a semireligious search for the grail of health have strained ourselves beyond our own capacities. Sports injuries abound and they have turned sports medicine into a thriving subspecialty. The injuries that once were the accepted liability of dancers and professional athletes are beginning to afflict the general population—those who have no professional or monetary reason for subjecting themselves to such ills. We have come to ignore the messages of our own bodies in our belief that we are perfecting them, just as we have come to ignore the natural and pleasurable promptings of appetite.[27]

Although there is considerable evidence to the contrary, we have come to believe that a half-hungry, compulsively exercising nation will be a more productive, successful nation. We have come to endorse a way of life worthy of the strictest Calvinist. We do so because we absolutely believe that thinner is healthier. But this, our most fundamental "scientific" premise, is the most flawed. An enormous amount of national and international evidence is accumulating that indicates that thinner is *not* healthier, that those who enjoy the longest lives and the best health are either of average weight or heavier— and that those with the poorest health and life expectancy are almost consistently the thinnest in the population. The "desirable weight" to which we are all encouraged to reduce is *not* the healthiest weight. Our very conviction that fat is dangerous is wrong.[28]

Indeed, it also appears that, contrary to current scientific orthodoxy, not all people were intended to have the same weight and fat-to-lean ratios just because they are the same height. There is considerable variability in human tendencies for fatness and weight gain, just as there is in other species. People cannot totally control these tendencies: They do not have absolute control of their body weight. And often, weight reduction puts them into a physiological state of semistarvation even though they still look "fat" by our current standards.

Our creed has spawned a series of paradoxes. We discriminate against the overweight, yet 25 to 30 percent of us presumably fit this category. Are we a nation of self-haters? We live in a presumably liberal culture in which differences are not only accepted, but even celebrated, yet we have developed a narrow, rigid standard of body size. We live at a time when feminism has liberated women, yet women are trapped into hating the natural curves of the female body. We live in an age of unprecedented plenty, but food has become an enemy, not a blessing, and we have been urged to stay half-hungry. We live in an age of sexual liberation, yet we must control one of our most compelling drives—the one for nourishment.

The purpose of this book is to discover how we developed these beliefs, for the battle against appetite and ample flesh is a modern phenomenon. In the past thirty years, we have redefined overweight and obesity, revised our concept of normal body size, and set up new norms about what constitutes overeating. We have also redefined beauty and goodness. Social, moral, and aesthetic values, and political and economic developments all interacted to produce these changes and to produce our new creed. In the following pages we will trace how these different developments converged and turned a preference for slenderness into a new religion. We will trace how a moderate caution was converted into an extreme, hysterical injunction, and we will investigate why the creed has so much power over us. Most importantly, we will discover how distorted our values and our beliefs about the body and food have become.

THE DEVELOPMENT OF
THE MYTH

3

When Thin Wasn't In: A Selective Overview of Fashion and Beauty, Antiquity to 1830

"Since time immemorial, youth has set the universal standard of physical beauty and the reason is simply that a shapely, firm young face and body are more attractive sexually and aesthetically than bulges, sags, and wrinkles," Hugh Hefner proclaimed in the twentieth-anniversary issue of *Playboy*. But Hugh Hefner was wrong. Consider this: "A small foot, a round, plump thigh and a fat backside speak to the prick straight," the Victorian Frank Harris wrote in *My Secret Life*. And he added, "Few men will keep long to a bony lady whose skinny buttock can be held in one hand." Over the centuries, the standards for a beautiful body have changed considerably.[1]

I know I often curse the ill-timing of my birth. If I had lived before thin and fit were in, when the women painted by Rubens or Renoir were the ideals of female beauty, I would never have had to diet, never have to hate flesh swelling on hips and thighs. I always linger over these paintings and art historians' descriptions of them. Art historian, Anne Hollander wrote that the abundant flesh of Rubens's nudes was "alive with eddies and whirlpools . . . . Nameless anatomical bubbles and unidentified waves agitated the . . . adipose tissue of these nymphs and goddesses." Hollander's choice of words is instructive. It cuts through our modern prejudices and allows us a vision of excess flesh as richly erotic and sensuous. The art historian, Sir Kenneth Clark, captured these qualities even more poetically. He wrote that "Rubens' nudes seem at first sight to have tumbled out of a cornucopia of abundance . . . . They have the sweetness of flowing water."[2]

Such descriptions are persuasive, but if we were to view these "nymphs" as contemporaries, rather than as expressions of a safely distant aesthetic, we would undoubtedly call them fat women whose flesh probably jiggles with every movement and whose "bubbles" can only be identified as that modern blight, cellulite. They do little to relieve a modern woman of her feeling that fatness is ugliness, that *any* excessive flesh, let alone a wallowing abundance of it, is unpleasant. She knows very well that if she looked like a Rubens nymph and paraded in a bikini at the beach, the other beach-goers would shatter her illusions quickly. They would evaluate her according to contemporary tastes. In matters of fashion and beauty, it's hard to be a majority of one. Others invariably become the mirror in which we see ourselves.

In short, we are very much victims of our own times, and this alone should tell us, though it doesn't, that our standards are transitory and external. The ideal of "thin" beauty that we have today is really a complex of social and psychological behaviors and attitudes toward beauty and health, toward the body, and toward food. By briefly examining how these behaviors and attitudes differed in the past, we can gain a perspective from which to assess the foundations and validity of our current beliefs.

Even though the female body has not altered significantly for thousands of years, in Western culture its ideal shape has been transformed periodically, not merely shifting from thin to plump, but also emphasizing different parts of the body. Until recently, only Western culture evidenced these wild shifts of taste. Two factors seem to be principally responsible for this phenomenon, though they also reflect broader changes in attitudes and beliefs: our artistic heritage and the nature of our tradition of dress, which has evolved as the phenomenon of fashion.

The beliefs that inform many of our aesthetic views derive from the ancient Greeks, who developed the notion of the nude as an art form. As Kenneth Clark pointed out in his analysis of the form and its history, *The Nude*, *nakedness* is a flawed, human state, while the *nude* is the naked form transformed and idealized into Beauty. The Greeks conceived of human beings as potentially godlike, while the Christian mind, carrying Platonic dualism to its extreme, tends to see divinity only in the human spirit. The flesh and its animal instincts are burdens, sinful obstacles to perfection. The Greeks recognized no such dichotomy. As Clark put it when describing Aphrodite, "Perhaps no religion ever again incorporated physical passion so calmly, so sweetly, and so naturally that all who saw her felt that the instincts they shared with the beasts they also shared with the gods." This belief was the core of their humanism— the reason they idealized the body in their art and why it became an aesthetic subject in its own right. Although our own beliefs and traditions have been altered by myriad influences, we have retained the sense that there is a profound link between the human body and aesthetic ideals and symbols—and that the body is perfectible.[3]

This viewpoint is unique to the West. Clark reminds us that other cultures did not develop a similar attitude about human flesh as an aesthetic subject. He noted that "the idea of offering the body for its own sake, as a serious subject of contemplation, simply did not occur to the Chinese or Japanese mind, and to this day raises a slight barrier of misunderstanding."[4]

These artistic canons fell into abeyance after the fall of Rome, but during the Renaissance, artists rediscovered and revived them. The idea of the nude as an expression of perfection re-entered Western culture, but what constituted that perfection had altered. The combined Hellenic and Christian heritage left Europe with conflicting standards about the body and its potential for good- ness and beauty, and historical and artistic developments themselves changed perceptions of the body. Consequently, successive European artists kept modi- fying the physical characteristics of the nude, especially when they portrayed women.

One effect of the preceding traditions, particularly the influence of Church teachings, was to make women the nexus of many of the concepts about man's divided nature, his divinity, and his fallibility. Consequently, while men were portrayed primarily as either Herculean—muscular and massive—or Apol- lonian—blonde and lissome—women were subject to a variety of changes. This tendency became even more pronounced toward the eighteenth century as the female came to be considered a more suitable subject for the nude than the male. Woman's body, not man's, was identified with Ideal Beauty, and that beauty became eroticized and secularized—a turning point of considerable significance and one that came in tandem with other profound historical changes, especially in concepts about woman's nature and biology. While ideas about the male nude were neglected or left almost undisturbed, those about women continued to evolve as artists tried to reconcile contemporary tastes with artistic traditions and with their own private visions. If she was lucky, a woman found herself born in an era that idealized the shape nature had given her.

An influence parallel to that of art in the creation and perpetuation of ideal types was fashion. The nude describes the ideal unclothed body, while fashion directs what the clothed shape should be, and in life, this outer self has proven to be as important to the conception of women, and their conception of themselves, as the hidden form. Art and fashion, of course, have long in- fluenced each other, and in turn reflected a variety of social and cultural standards. The very principles behind fashion, a dress system peculiar to the West, caused the proliferation of ideal body types. Fashion, as we define it now, was essentially developed by the Europeans sometime between the twelfth and fourteenth centuries. The term referred to two radically new principles in dress—tailoring and stylistic variation. Until this period, Europeans wore a tuniclike garment inherited from the Romans, which was draped around the body. But between the twelfth and fourteenth centuries, creative tailoring—cutting and sewing—replaced draping. Material began to be fitted and molded to the body, which also meant that the body could appear to be remodeled. Clothing items became progressively more elaborate, more decorative, and less functional, and they began to redefine the bodies beneath them.

In tandem with the art of tailoring came the new principle of originality. It became a goal of fashion, and styles altered at an ever-quickening tempo as the centuries progressed. To understand how unique this concept was, we need to compare it with the other predominant dress system, customary dress. Customary dress is, as the name implies, based on custom. While it seeks to resemble, as closely as possible, the model of the past, fashion seeks with equal fervor to differentiate itself. While customary dress seeks individual anonymity through its requirement that everyone wear prescribed and traditional clothing, fashion emphasizes individual identity—within limits—through its emphasis on originality. Other cultures were well aware of these differences and were often puzzled by and critical of them. The Shogun's Secretary at Yedo in 1609 criticized the Spanish style of dress, observing that the Spaniards "are so inconstant that they are dressed in a different way every two years." He attributed this instability to the "nation's levity and the levity of the governments" and boasted that his own country's costume had not changed for "over 1,000 years." In essence, clothes in Europe became simultaneously declarations of personal style—and of individual humans—as well as expressions of a person's place in the social order.[5]

This heritage may explain why there has been a succession of "ideal" body types, framed by clothing, but it doesn't explain why one particular style replaces another, nor even why certain preferred body types emerge. Scholars have tried to find some coherent pattern in the cycles of the various styles that have seized the Western imagination. They have also tried to understand the main impulse behind fashion and dress in general. And they have tried to penetrate the even bigger mystery of why people follow fashion at all, subjecting themselves to remarkable discomforts and expending a great deal of time, energy, and money to do so.

Despite the interest in it, the subject of fashion has generally been considered trivial, at least until recently. Fashion has its shallow, frivolous, and competitive aspects, but it also functions on a much more profound and compelling level. Only by understanding how fashion functions can we understand why and how the present imperative to be thin is both so powerful and so unusual in the annals of fashion history.

Apart from the need for protection against the elements, modesty—the "fig leaf" or "decency" theory—has been the West's oldest and most durable explanation for dress. The teachings of the Church stressed that after eating from the forbidden tree, Adam and Eve knew the sin of lust, and so rushed to hide their nakedness. Humanity followed suit. For centuries, clothing was condoned for serving the demands of modesty, although excesses in luxury of dress and adornment were often severely condemned. They were attributed to that ubiquitous human weakness, vanity. These attitudes remained dominant in the West long after fashion was introduced, even while clothing's heraldic functions were universally accepted. Church leaders, humanists like Erasmus, and other moralists commended clothing's usefulness for modesty but condemned fashionable excess as a frivolous, worldly distraction from worthier concerns—an indictment that surrounds the pursuit of fashion and physical beauty in our own day as well and one that once worked to keep the excesses of fashion in check. In general, the reasons for stylistic change were seen as incomprehensible, and Dame Fashion was often described as a deity who capriciously and irrationally decreed new forms. It was generally believed that people adopted these new forms because they were "actuated by the delight in novelty and the passion for display."[6]

In the nineteenth century the development of the social sciences inspired more systematic theories about fashion. Anthropologists and later, psychoanalytic theorists argued that sexual display and eroticism—not modesty—propelled the dress of all societies. Fashion itself, with its stylistic variations, could be understood as a response to "shifting erogenous zones." As one body zone lost its erotic charge, interest shifted to a different spot. In essence, they inverted the notion of clothing as a handmaiden to modesty. It was not designed to conceal but rather to call attention to erogenous zones. Other late nineteenth-century theorists focused on Marxist concepts and on the tense competition between classes. Thorstein Veblen, in his *Theory of the Leisure Class* (1899), argued that all conspicuous consumption was designed to vaunt social status. He suggested that the more impractical a clothing style, the more it symbolized someone who didn't have to work; the more costly the clothing, the more it symbolized one's wealth; the less functional the adornments, the more they symbolized the great privilege of the wealthy—conspicuous waste. The less advantaged classes had the unfortunate habit of quickly imitating their betters' innovations. A store clerk, for example, adopted the gloves or the cane of his better. When the crinoline came into fashion in the late 1850s, even plantation slave women tried to imitate this fashion by putting stiff vines into their petticoats. In this scenario, stylistic changes were explained by the elite's efforts to stay ahead of those beneath them on the status ladder. Still other late-nineteenth-century theorists, such as the Frenchman, Octave Uzanne, and the German, Max Von Boehm, came up with a more encompassing theory. They argued that fashion reflected the *zeitgeist* or spirit of an age. They emphasized the remarkable unity between the politics, social dynamics, aesthetics, and even interior decoration and eating habits of an epoch and its dominant clothing styles.

In the twentieth century some psychoanalytic thinkers followed the nineteenth-century anthropological view and described dress as a form of sublimated sexuality while others, struck by the fact that men's clothing no longer changed much from year to year while women's changed more than ever, and by the emergence of Paris dress designers and of a modernized clothing industry, contended that designers and industrialists were motivated by economic self-interest. They forced women to keep buying new clothes no matter how extensive their wardrobes, by perpetually introducing new styles. Two other theories have gained popularity recently. One derives from semiotics and suggests that clothing is a form of communication that operates on the same principles as language and changes in the same way language does. The other derives from art historians such as Anne Hollander, who suggest that fashion is an art of image- or picture-making and that it evolves along principles of its own, much as art does.[7]

Variants and combinations of these theories have dominated thinking about fashion until quite recently. But in the past few years, feminists opened up a new debate about the meaning and function of dress and, more precisely, of fashion. Lois Banner, Susan Brownmiller, Robin Lakoff, and Raquel Scherr, among others, contend that fashion and the very existence of ideal female beauty have oppressed women and have even been the root of their oppression. Only women, they argue, are valued according to their beauty or sexual desirability. In effect, they combine the erotic and status theories of fashion and put them into a political context, charging that patriarchal societies often impose painful, debilitating styles on women to enforce and symbolize their oppression and to deflect them from more serious pursuits. They consequently also attack fashion polemically, as moralists have for centuries, as vain and frivolous, and lament that women have been enslaved by such superficial structures. They suggest that the only solution is to do away with fashion standards altogether and replace them with "natural" dress or beauty.[8]

What sense can we make of these theories, and what insights can they give us about our own obsession with slenderness? The theories developed in the nineteenth and twentieth centuries deepen our understanding of how dress and fashion function. All of them have validity, for clothing is multifunctional, and the characteristics they outline have all operated to one degree or another; only the relative importance of each changes from culture to culture and from epoch to epoch. In fact, these theories are themselves documents for a study of the history of fashion, and they reveal the way we are influenced by expressions of physical ideals. In a sense, in our own time, filled with figurative popular media but dominated by de-mythologized, nonfigurative art, fashion has become one of the primary areas where our physical ideals reside.

Fashion is propelled by deep impulses, which it shares with all dress systems. Dress and adornment are basic to all human cultures. Even the most primitive tribes find ways to decorate the body. The overwhelming importance of dress and adornment is underscored by the fact that from the moment we slip out of the womb to the moment of our deaths, we alter our natural appearance. For every situation, we seek appropriate ways to present ourselves. How we choose to dress is a complex cultural phenomenon. Clothing is simultaneously a material object, a social signal, a ritual, and a form of art. It is different from all other cultural objects because it is worn on the body and thus becomes part of our image of what human beings are. Every facet of a society, from its economic base to its social structure, from its values about human beings and their bodies to its loftiest spiritual and aesthetic ideals, influences the forms and rules of dress. Each culture sets up its own rules, and in following them, people defer to and perpetuate fundamental social values and norms.[9]

Clothing, in both its functional and decorative aspects, serves social psychological, and symbolic functions. On the social plane, clothing is a crucial signal in every human interaction. Like language, it is a form of communication with its own syntax, vocabulary, and varied connotative meanings. And like language, it differs in different cultures, with each culture determining which groups should be identified and differentiated whether because of age, sex, geographic origin, group affiliation, status, occupation, or wealth. The more complex the society, the more complex these signals. Each culture also determines which situations, and even which emotional states, require special clothing. In Europe, for instance, even as late as the nineteenth century, mourning attire was mandatory for bereaved families, and its details altered according to both the individual's relationship to the deceased and to the length of time since the death. Even in less dramatic and less codified situations, clothing can convey our moods and even our attitudes toward a situation, event, or person. In many primitive and modern cultures, attending a wedding in workday clothes would be construed as an insult to the families involved or as evidence that something was grossly wrong in the offender's life. In pre-industrial societies, inappropriate dress can upset the social, psychic, and ritual balance of the community.

In this sense, clothing functions not just like language but also like a theatrical prop, establishing a setting and a mood and informing an audience of expected behavior. It also works as a psychological prop for the wearer, setting up his or her sense of self in relation to the situation and events. For example, appearing in a bikini on a modern American beach is fine, but appearing there in a bra and panties is not. A girl is decidedly undressed in the latter, even though an uninformed observer would think the outfits identical because the same parts of the body are covered—or uncovered. But the girl is wearing private attire in public, showing a gross misunderstanding of the social situation and sending confusing signals about her expected behavior. She seems to be in the midst of dressing or of undressing, not yet ready to present herself.

In some societies, such as Islam and pre-Meiji Japan, dress rules are enforced by law. But in modern Western culture, though specific aspects are sometimes regulated (for example, the restriction on public nudity, or the tie requirement in restaurants), the general rules are not legally enforceable. People obey them because they are rooted as deeply in society as language and because society exacts obedience to them in the same way it exacts obedience to other social norms. As the social critic Quentin Bell observed, "there is a whole system of morality attached to clothes," and violating it "excites censure that is almost exactly comparable to dishonorable conduct."[10]

Clothing is more than a manifestation of obedience to social norms. It also acts on an intimate psychological level, becoming a symbol of deeply held beliefs about the individual's relationship to the external world. Anthropologists have found that in societies where it is believed that dangers to the self come from the outside world, self-boundaries are protected through elaborate masks and clothing, while in societies where safety is believed to be derived from continuous and conscious self-control, clothing is correspondingly less important and may even be regarded as an impediment to developing inner strength. In our dress habits, we reflect and perpetuate whole systems of beliefs about the self and the world.

Clothing acts on a psychological plane also because it affects our very sense of ourselves and—most important for the issues we are considering here—our bodies. Its weight, sounds, and motion, its feel against the skin, and its constraints mold our physical reality. It affects how we move and experience our bodies.

Dressing is also a virtual process of self-creation, of self-portraiture. It reveals the way we see ourselves and the way we want others to see us. We select from all the choices our culture gives us and use them to define ourselves. We reveal our estimation of our attractiveness, of our qualities and personality traits, and of our social position, which is why social psychologist Erving Goffman argued that clothing is crucial to an individual's "identity kit."[11]

Clothing is a physical object, dressing a ritual filled with all the meanings we have just outlined. Fashion is our type of dress system, the dominant aspect of our ritual of dressing, and it operates on these same principles. In obeying fashion, we are bowing to powerful constraints about self-presentation and about how others should interpret our attitudes, behavior, and identity. The enormous time and energy women and men devote to being attractive is simply another of civilization's many demands and, possibly, pleasures. For in dressing, we are engaging in a game, a plastic art, and in a process whereby we partially create ourselves. We are involved in social and private play, play of the profoundest type. We are, in essence, trying to transcend our uncivilized, animal state, to make ourselves human. Nietzsche, in *The Birth of Tragedy,* even argued that "We derive such dignity as we possess from our status as art works." Fun, fantasy, humor, artistic creativity, and our deepest human aspirations exist in the dress constraints of everyday life.[12]

Fashion is a dress system that very much reflects the concerns and rhythms of the West. Declarations of status, modesty, erotic intent, drama, and opulence have all, at one time or another, been the most important function of fashion. For the functions, norms, priorities, and rules of fashion have changed over the centuries almost as much as styles have. They need to be analyzed in the same way as other cultural norms and values. They, too, are a product of transformations in society, from those in the social and economic structure to those in attitudes about the body and its functions, about food, about the roles of men and women, and about aesthetics, health, and medicine. If fashion evolves according to its own internal rules, it also evolves in response to these other cultural transformations.

We seem to have moved a long way from questions about twentieth-century American women and their obsession with dieting and slenderness. But in fact, we have only provided a perspective from which to understand and evaluate it. The degree of slenderness we cherish today has never before been an aesthetic or sexual ideal, though it was, at times, a religious ideal. Before we take too much comfort from this fact, we must remember that obesity has never been an ideal either. And gluttony, by very definition, has always been a negative characteristic in Western culture, categorized as one of the deadly sins—but gluttony, as we shall see, has not always been associated with fatness. We do know of cultures that prize fatness. Some African tribes seclude brides-to-be to fatten them before marriage, and certain Polynesian groups have had great reverence for women who reach 200 or 300 pounds. They keep their Queen and her ladies sedentary, feeding them until they attain these proportions. Nevertheless, the fight against fat is not a modern invention. There is evidence that the surgical removal of fat—a not uncommon phenomenon today—was also practiced in Roman and Byzantine times. The Greeks reputedly envied the wasp-waisted Etruscans who, it was believed, had found a magic potion that kept them slim. And the reports we have about obese people's efforts to lose weight—reports that begin, somewhat obliquely, in the sixteenth century and that become more numerous in the nineteenth century—testify to the difficulties and frustrations reducers encountered, which is evidence not of how widespread the phenomenon was, but rather of how difficult reducing has always been. But to find evidence of individuals concerned about excessive fat is not to find an entire culture orienting itself around ideals of slenderness.

It is fair to say that the range of body types in the past was no different than the range we know today. What has changed is the body type—or types—that have been set up as ideal, the extent to which people have tried to change their appearance to meet this ideal, and the methods they have used to do so. We can tell much by looking at artists' idealized and realistic depictions of the nude and at contemporary fashions and attitudes about those fashions—two different phenomena which, however, especially in past centuries, were closely interconnected. In addition, we can look at important differences in the values and images associated with fatness and thinness, the body, health, and in attitudes about food. It is far beyond the scope of this book to analyze all these issues in detail. Instead, we will briefly survey the successive changes so that we have a framework in which to evaluate our current obsession with thinness. At the risk of oversimplification, we can delineate five major periods in body-size ideals, although certain themes persisted through many periods, and variations existed within any one period.

The Greeks are an appropriate starting point, as they are, in a sense, the originators of our standards of female physical beauty, most perfectly expressed through their Aphrodite images. These became the classical standard for European artists, and they continue to be powerful images in our own day. And the Greeks of both sexes were much concerned with slimness. Hippocrates considered fat a disease, and Socrates is supposed to have danced every morning to keep his figure. But their definition of slimness was quite different than our own. The Aphrodites are beautiful, and one cannot help feeling inspired by the statues that have come down to us. But for all their beauty, would a modern American woman want Aphrodite's figure? Probably not. By our standards, harmoniously proportioned though she is, Aphrodite seems fat. There is a very decided layer of soft adipose tissue under her skin—not a bone nor a muscle shows through. She is too ample, too stolid, too rooted to the ground to approximate the steamlined look we cherish. Her arms look too fleshy, her thighs much too heavy, her belly too full. She is short-waisted, and short-legged. Admittedly, her breasts are exquisite, and she betrays no irregular, ugly bulges. But her flesh looks a little too soft, a little too far from the underlying bone and muscle, and it threatens to jiggle if she walks—with a graceful, stately flow, to be sure—but jiggle nonetheless. We like our bodies smoother, sleeker, tauter. If she were elongated, her curves straightened, she would approximate more closely our own ideal.

The Greeks abhorred both gluttony and obesity, on the one hand, and excessive slenderness on the other. Both extremes violated the Greek veneration for moderation and decorum. Fat people were the actors in comedy or the objects of contempt. In an ancient misogynistic poem by Seminodes of Amorogs, the catalog of horrors a man can expect from different types of wives are vividly detailed. The woman like the "long-haired sow doesn't take baths but sits about/ In the shit of dirty clothes and gets fatter and fatter." The skinny woman doesn't earn Seminodes's praise either. He warns us that the wife who is like a monkey "hardly has an ass and her legs are skinny. What a poor wretch is the husband/ Who has to put his arms around such a mess!" A Hellenic vase dating from the fifth century B.C. underscores how the Athenians felt about figures that were either too fat or too thin. It depicts a fat youth and a thin one in the gymnasium. They are so embarrassed about their respective sizes that they hang back while two better-formed fellows throw the javeline and discus.[13]

In the transition from Aphrodite to Venus, that is, from Greece to Rome, Aphrodite's body size remained the same. Evidence suggests that Roman women dieted to preserve their figures, and the vomitorium was an adjunct to banquets during the Roman Empire, though presumably its purpose was to let guests relieve their overfull stomachs so they could continue banqueting rather than to control their figures. But despite this preference for a moderate-sized form, the Romans did not regard the body and its shape as the medium of religious and aesthetic ideals, as the Greeks had. Beauty was expressed through ornamentation, not pure form. For them, certainly, the body was never tied so intimately to a sense of the spiritual and to religion. To satisfy their craving for beauty and elaborate self-presentation, Roman women concentrated much more on jewelry, cosmetics, and other adornments, than on the shape of their figures. In any case, like their Greek counterparts, their bodies were draped and rarely seen; modesty forbade their direct display.

A new recognizable ideal did not emerge until the late Middle Ages. In the years between the Fall of Rome and the late Middle Ages, attitudes about the body and its representation had changed considerably. Early Christianity rejected representations of the naked form for their pagan associations and as violations of the second Commandment. Early Christianity also rejected the notion that the naked body could be a thing of beauty, or rather, that physical beauty itself was an abstract good unfettered by man's mortality. The body itself was seen as a vulnerable, fragile, vulgar vessel of the soul, its appetites dangerous temptations that led to sin and damnation. Nakedness was associated with Adam and Eve's Original Sin and their expulsion from the Garden of Eden. If, for the Greeks, the body could be a source of pride, a reminder of the divinity in man, for the early Church it was a source of shame and humiliation. In the rare instances when artists did depict it, they did so for religious themes that showed the body in torments—in scenes of martyrs, of the Apocalypse, and of the Expulsion itself—or of abstract beatitude.

Clothing reflected this attitude. Men and women concealed their bodies in flowing, thick garments that were similar for both sexes. This clothing served two functions: One was modesty or piety. Even the head and neck were covered; only the hands and face could be seen. But dress was also a badge of rank, and nobles and Church leaders were *obliged* to dress grandly for the pomp and pageantry of medieval ceremonies, to show God's grandeur—and their own—on earth. This rank was revealed through colors, fabrics, and ornamentation, not through any alterations in style or body shape.

Ascetic Christianity and its negative attitude toward the body slowly changed between 1200 and 1500. During the late Middle Ages and the Renaissance, the human body once again came to be seen as an object of beauty, and clothing became a prominent aspect of its celebration. Many developments caused this change, from the influence of the Crusades, to the new flourishing of trade and the emergence of towns and a middle class, to the rediscovery of the classical world, the revival of learning, and the emergence of humanism.

In thirteenth-century Italy and France especially, the concept of ideal beauty was revived and developed in the visual arts and in literature. Influenced by these and other changes, the Church revised its prescriptions for art, ruling that depictions of human history should no longer end with the Apocalypse, as had been the case for centuries, but rather with the Final Judgment and Resurrection. The bodies rising from their graves were to be naked and beautiful, befitting Matthew's description of the event. Spiritual perfection could now be embodied physically, as it was before sin. With this new emphasis on Resurrection and with the triumphant humanism of the Renaissance, the nude was reborn—and modern fashion was born. As the pre-eminent costume historian, François Boucher, put it, with these developments, "greater importance was attached to the perfection of the female body, and indeed, to outward appearance in general." Men and women "translated this search after formal beauty into costume."[14]

The physical ideal conveyed to us by the paintings of clothed women between 1350 and 1500 was in fact quite slender. By this time, distinct fashions had come into their own, and men and women's clothing diverged in distinctive ways. Men abandoned the long, flowing robes formerly common for both sexes and adopted short costumes. Women wore robes that formed a long, slim A-line, a continuation of the elongated styles of the preceding period, but now the bodice was fitted closely to the body, revealing the outline of the bust, and the waist was often accentuated by a band under the breasts or around the waist itself. The look, in essence, was the attenuated Gothic ideal in human form, a look that had come to be equated with elegance. In the illustrations of the period (such as the miniatures in the Duc de Berry's *Book of Hours* and those on tapestries) and in the paintings, we see similarly sinuous, elongated forms with slender arms and slender waists dressed in gowns with long, flowing trains. Yet to assume from this that slenderness was the accepted ideal would be to discount the evidence of the nudes, which reflected more than one ideal.

Three rather dissimilar traditions of the nude emerged during this period, reflecting different standards and bringing with them different associations: the Gothic nude exemplified by Jan van Eyck's work, the nude of the Italian Renaissance, exemplified by the work of Sandro Botticelli, and what Sir Kenneth Clark calls "Venus naturalis," that is, nudes designed to show secular human beauty and vanity, exemplified by the *Vanitas* of the School of Memling and that by Giovanni Bellini.

The Gothic nude is startlingly slim. As portrayed by the De Limbourg brothers in the "The Fall" (from the *Très Riches Heures* of the Duc de Berry), and by van Eyck in his Ghent Altarpiece, the nude Eve has arms and legs that border on modern thinness, though it does not in the least resemble our own. If these Eves have limbs that are slim and smooth, they show no hint of a well-toned muscle, and their bellies are huge, gracefully swelling ovals that, to our eyes, makes them appear to be almost five months pregnant. They are short-waisted—necessarily because of their stomach—short-legged, and narrow-shouldered. Most of us would not want to look like them. Clark has observed that few young women of the period were likely to have had these contours, just as few young women today have them. They were an ideal of beauty. He conjectured that Eve's shape, and especially her belly, could be explained by her Judeo-Christian background. The humbleness and weakness of this vessel—the body—were transformed into an image of beauty, but a beauty full of humility and modesty, one that underscored both the primordial function of the female body and the vulnerability of human flesh. Humility, however, does not entirely account for this protuberant stomach. As styles evolved in the fifteenth century, fashionable and erotic attention also focused on and accentuated this protuberance. The long, flowing, heavy robes were gathered in a great, graceful bunch at the waist, and bags of padding were strategically placed there to reinforce the effect.

Botticelli's Venus is quite different. He was influenced by Neoplatonic ideals, and the Greek Aphrodite is at the heart of his feminine aesthetic. His Venus is remarkably like the Greek Aphrodites, only she is etherealized, with none of the weight and earthiness of the original. But she certainly is not thin. Her body is sweetly full, round and sensuous.

Juxtaposed against the slender Eve and the sensuous Venus, we must put the *Vanitas* of the same period and heroic portrayals like that of Konrad Meit's *Judith*. All these women have the large Gothic stomach and proportions, but they are far fleshier than Eve and even than Aphrodite. To us, they seem fat, like the "before" photos in ads for weight-loss aids. Yet the *Vanitas* in particular represented worldly beauty, and such luscious fullness, with its dimpled flesh, apparently was considered highly erotic.

Ironically enough, the age that brought us Botticelli's Venus and these other intense strivings for human beauty, was also an age of ever-present physical deformity. Well into the eighteenth century, the life of most Europeans was filled with insecurity, fear, and what can only be called, from a modern perspective, brutality. Death, disease, and physical grotesquerie abounded, and primitive medical science could do little about them. During the fourteenth century the plague killed off close to one-third of Europe's population. The Black Death took the highest toll, but other epidemics were still terrifyingly virulent and rampant. If the rich tended to suffer somewhat less than the poor, they still were rarely spared. Accidents, crime, and disasters were as common as disease. They were not, as they are today, failures in a well-ordered system but rather omnipresent dangers. Fires could destroy whole towns, lack of sanitation contaminated food and water supplies. Wild animals and rabid dogs lurked everywhere, even near towns, and brigands and robbers threatened constantly.

These conditions affected the way people looked and felt. Deformities were commonplace—something that is hard for us to understand in modern America, where even teeth are straightened and prettified. Crude obstetrical techniques left their marks on women as well as on offspring. Crippled legs and arms, bad teeth, and skin diseases were physical constants. Nutritional-deficiency diseases took their toll and left their deformities. Smallpox left hideous disfigurements. Fleas, lice, and other vermin were so accepted a part of everyday life that removing them was an integral part of normal social life. In fourteenth-century Montaillou, a French village, delousing provided a time for intimacy, for gossip, for planning trysts, and for spreading heresy. In 1773 a French government official described some villagers as they walked out of church: Many were "atrophied, hunchbacked, deaf, blind, one-eyed, bandy-legged, bloodshot of eye, lame and twisted, harelipped . . . . " Few people could easily meet the standards of beauty presented on canvases and pedestals.[15]

Despite these overall conditions, people did strive for beauty. Sumptuary laws, designed to regulate the number of clothes and quality of materials appropriate to each rank in society or to protect favored industries, were enacted with increasing frequency as the frenzy for opulence and adornment led to violations of the hierarchy. The lower classes and the great mass of peasants participated in fashion in only a very distant way, in part because of poverty, in part because a customary dress system was also emerging which required that individuals wear the special costume associated with their occupation as well as their rank.

We also have ample evidence that the elite attempted to change certain natural attributes to match the fashionable ideal. In Renaissance Italy, men and women bleached their hair to make it blond, and women removed all the hair from their eyebrows, foreheads, and temples. But we have no evidence that they tried to remodel their shapes to approximate the nudes. Instead, they worked from the outside in, using fabrics, padding, and corsets to make their public appearance resemble the ideal.[16]

Only among some religious ascetics of this time do we see thinness valued, but, it was not actually thinness that was sought, rather mortification of the flesh, subordination of the corporeal to the soul, holiness. Although by the sixth century the Church had adopted a moderate stance on fasting, one that certainly did not condone self-starvation, an increasing number of what one historian calls "holy anorexics" appeared between the twelfth and fifteenth centuries. Historian Rudolph Bell has drawn parallels between modern anorexics and these early Church female saints who exhibited similar symptoms—hyperactivity, denial of hunger, and dangerously low body weight. There are many convincing similarities, but the parallel is not entirely justified. While food abstinence was more characteristic of women who sought holiness, many male saints and religious ascetics also tried to deny and control their appetite for food. More important, the motives of the female saints were completely different from those of today's anorexics. They did not want to be thin, and they certainly did not want to be beautiful, nor did they associate thinness and beauty. They did not suffer from distorted body images: rather, they saw bodies themselves as distortions of the soul. Their impulse grew out of medieval Christianity, which described the body as a polluted vessel that trapped the soul and prevented otherworldly purity. Mortification of the flesh through self-flagellation, fasting, and other self-inflicted torments was seen as a way to pay penance for sins, to release the soul, and to achieve salvation for oneself and for others. The thirteenth-century "holy anorexic," Margaret of Cortona, did not just starve herself. She also tried desperately to destroy her natural beauty and at one point bought a razor to cut her nose and lip because, she explained to her confessor, "with the beauty of my face I did harm to many souls. Therefore, wishing to do justice upon myself, by myself, for this offense to God and to transform the beauty of my body into ugliness, I pray you to permit me . . . to offer to Christ the King the sacrifice which I propose." The fourteenth-century saint, Catherine of Siena, who became a model other holy females tried to emulate for the next two centuries, also did more than just not eat. At times, she forced herself to eat the repulsive—spiders and, once, the puss from a woman's putrefying wound. These features of ascetic Christianity did not survive the sixteenth century. The Church, suspicious of even these early anorexic saints, came to regard the self-starving woman as possessed by the devil, not by the divine. By the eighteenth and nineteenth centuries, though "miraculous fasting maidens" still occasionally appeared and were popularly deemed saints, female religiosity was expressed primarily through good deeds, not through heroic submission of the flesh.[17]

At the end of the fifteenth century, during the High Renaissance, two new ideal nudes evolved which continued and accentuated the differences between the nudes of the previous period. In Italy, Leonardo da Vinci and Raphael were painting more ample women, and shortly thereafter, Titian and Giorgione were celebrating fully fleshed forms with wide pelvises, ample expanses of stomach, and, to our eyes, remarkably stout arms, exemplified by Titian's *Venus* and *Venus with the Organ Player,* and Giorgione's *Concert champêtre.* Struck by the new Italian taste for bodies "full in flesh," Montaigne remarked that Italian artists "fashion them large and stout."

But these richly fleshed nudes contrasted sharply with another ideal that emerged simultaneously and that has generally been categorized under the heading of *Mannerism.* These nudes, exemplified by Bronzino's *Allegory of Passion,* Cellini's *Nymph of Fontainbleu,* and, especially, by Cranach the Elder's *Judgment of Paris,* are much more in keeping with our own preferences—though not a muscle nor a bony angle is visible. The Gothic nude had become elongated and more slender and graceful, with narrow, tapering limbs and a narrow torso on which the great Gothic ogival belly had been reduced to a delicate, though still noticeable, curve. Kenneth Clark aptly observed that these narrow, delicate bodies appear ill-designed for childbearing and the tapering hands and feet ill-designed for physical labor. They seem, rather, an embodiment of French chic, which tends toward these unclassical proportions and elongation.

Such nudes were widely disseminated as decorations and in popular prints— one even appeared on the title page of Erasmus' New Testament—but it is not clear whether women sought to look like them. Certainly, high art created ideals by which real-life women were measured. For three centuries, the phrase "belle comme une Madone de Raphael" was a standard expression of praise. But it is unlikely that women struggled to match the body ideal, in part because such varying body standards existed, and in part because of the clothing fashions of the period. The fashions that evolved seemed designed to make people look twice as large as nature made them, and they concealed the body totally, from their impossibly large, stiff ruffs around the neck down to the feet. The soft, flowing robes of the previous century gave way to stiff, straight formality and form, befitting the difficult century of Reformation and Counter-Reformation. The female torso was encased in a rigid bodice lined with stiff canvas and edged with heavy wire, which ended in a point below the waist and which compressed the breasts and, in essence, bound the upper half of the body into a cylindrical shape. Sleeves were puffed and full, particularly at the shoulder. Below the bodice, skirts of heavy, rich fabrics spread out in a great expanse. They were held out by the farthingale, a bell-shaped underskirt on which hoops made of cane, whalebone, wire, or switches of wood were sewn. The female body looked like two cones inverted on top of one another. Toward the middle of the century, the French modified the farthingale into a peculiar circular roll fitted around the hips, from which the skirt fell precipitously. These fashions did not conform to nor show off the natural human form but rather seemed designed to display the sumptuous materials the wearer could afford to buy, and to create an image of regal grandeur and artistry. The body virtually served as a scaffolding on which to mount this display, and women resembled ambulatory sculptures or canvases. While gross differences in body size could not be concealed by all this material, certainly a wide range of differences was camouflaged by them. And even in France, which was most receptive to the Mannerist ideal, women did not want to be thin. In 1595 a Dutch caricature of the new styles read, "Come, fine young maidens with your skimpy thighs/ Soon we shall make them round as Paris' prize."[18]

In the early seventeenth century a new bodily ideal evolved, one that was far more compatible with the overblown fashions of the day. The nude fleshed out—and at its most extreme—blossomed into the proportions of Rubens's nudes. To our own tastes, nothing could be more unfortunate than this effulgence of flesh. And yet, these figures compel us to acknowledge their beauty. They teem with the fullness, vitality, and richness that marked the baroque era, a period in which the emerging faith in a beneficent natural order still seemed reconcilable with the Triumph of the Sacrament. Even more, there was an exhilarating sense that much in the world might be subject to human understanding and possibly control—a faith that would culminate in the Enlightenment. If Rubens's women would look less than lovely in bikinis, they nonetheless were perfectly suited to convey this new sense, and the Rubenesque ideal eventually supplanted the slender Mannerist nudes. Fulsome, dimpled flesh was cause for celebration, not for disgust.

We have little evidence as to whether seventeenth-century women dieted or indeed ate to match the contours of the Rubenesque nude. Again, fashion so concealed the body that only extreme deviations would be noticeable. The first wife of Henry IV, Marguerite de Valois, earned considerable public contempt when in her later years, long after her divorce from Henry, she alternated between addiction to piety, learning, and lechery, and even dressed herself as she had in her youth. Contempt for her stemmed as much from her lewd behavior as from her enormous bulk which, reputedly, could block a palace doorway. This was also the century in which France, under the Sun King, Louis XIV, created elaborate court fashions and established its hegemony over European fashion. Beauty of appearance was crucial in this environment, but beauty was more closely tied to the elaborate styles that covered the body than to the natural form underneath.[19]

In any case, this aesthetic celebration of the flesh had its corollary in more fundamental attitudes toward the body and its primal urges. At least until the sixteenth or seventeenth centuries, Europeans had a matter-of-fact and unembarrassed attitude toward the body and all its functions—including spitting, belching, urinating, defecating, farting, copulating, nose blowing, eating, and even nudity itself. All these functions were considered a normal part of public life. They were taken for granted and were even a main subject for humor in palace and peasant hut alike. The "civilizing process," as historian Norbert Elias calls it, entailed the pacification of nation states, of individuals, and of bodily appetites and functions. Christianity did not automatically "civilize" people and give them the refined standards we know today. Early etiquette books point to these changes. The learned humanist Erasmus revealed in 1530 that a new modesty was developing about farting in company. He debated quite seriously whether it was healthier to retain wind or expel it and quoted experts on the subject before concluding that the ideal solution was to cough when farting to cover the sound.[20]

Attitudes toward food and eating were similar. "Binge-eating" was common, but it was not prompted by neurotic needs. All classes alternated between periods of plenty and scarcity. The fear of hunger and starvation dogged everyone. Even the nobility could expect to eat only what they got from their manors, and poor harvests plagued them just as they plagued the peasants. Technical and practical limitations made storing and preserving food difficult, and primitive transportation prevented regions with good harvests from coming to the aid of those with poor harvests.

Table manners as we know them emerged only slowly did not yet put brakes on appetite. Silverware came into fashion slowly, as did individual plates, glasses, and napkins. Food was eaten out of a common plate with the fingers; greasy faces were wiped clean with the sleeve or the hand. The idea of carrying on polite conversation during meals would emerge only in the sixteenth and seventeenth centuries. Louis XIV's enormous appetite was commented upon by his diarists, and the Princess Palatine described the gorging that went on among the French nobility. The Duchesse de Berri presumably ate herself to death; Montaigne, at the end of the sixteenth century, remarked on his own greed at the table: "So hurried am I that I often bite my tongue and sometimes my fingers . . . my greed leaves me no time to talk."[21]

There was, however, an external constraint on excessive appetite. Gluttony *was* deemed a sin, but fatness was not considered evil by association. The two were not clearly related. Gluttony was considered the sign of a disordered appetite, when one ate more than one's measure. By the Renaissance, medical warnings were added to moral warnings for the glutton. Falstaff knew that "the grave doth gape/ For thee thrice wider than for other men." Luigi Cornaro, a Venetian nobleman whose gluttonous habits had brought him to the brink of death at the untimely age of forty, reformed his diet in 1497, and lived to be ninety-eight. Near the end of his life, he published *Discourses on a Sober and Temperate Life* in which he shared the secrets of his regimen. The book was so popular that after its initial publication in 1557, it was translated into several languages and reprinted until the nineteenth century. But even Cornaro was not primarily interested in body weight. His concern was with the way a temperate diet could produce miraculous transformations, restoring youthful health, vigor, and appearance. It reflected the emerging Renaissance belief—one that would be important in later diet history—that human beings could control their health and fate if they controlled their food intake.[22]

As noted earlier, with the exception of extreme ascetics in the early Middle Ages, hearty appetite, up through the eighteenth century, was generally regarded as normal and unthreatening, and food as a necessity and a pleasure. The famous Fasting Girl of Couflens in 1660 was viewed as a marvel, a worthy object of pilgrimage because she had defied one of the most basic of human needs. The Church, interestingly, condemned the "arrogance" of fasting more harshly than it condemned gluttony. Fast days, of course, were a common feature of early modern life, but official fasting did not always mean going totally without food either in pre-Reformation Europe or in Puritan New England. It meant abstaining from meat, or skipping a meal, or eating only plain foods, or not getting sensual pleasure from food. As late as the nineteenth century, fasting popularly meant that one did not eat meat, bread, cereals, or starchy vegetables. But people could still claim to be fasting even if they ate fruits, greens, juices, teas, whey, mineral water, tobacco, and opium. It was generally believed that people needed hearty, solid victuals to survive, and not until the late nineteenth century do we find the fasting person who eats nothing at all held up as more moral and virtuous.

Many historians have observed that the personality traits typical of pre-modern Europe were very different than those typical of our own. Elias, among others, argues that medieval and Renaissance people were emotional, impulsive, and temperamental. While these were traits ideally suited for life in medieval and early modern Europe, they would not remain so as social, economic, and political structures changed, as kings monopolized violence and centralized power, and as economies became increasingly rationalized and centralized. By the time of the Enlightenment, man was idealized as a creature of reason and refinement, his animal-like qualities and impulsiveness disdained. In the same period and perhaps for similar reasons, the evolution of manners radically changed people's behavior. In the seventeenth century particularly, a great cultural divide began to separate the courtly aristocratic classes and the popular classes, who proved slow to adopt these refinements.

Emotional and physical self-control, restraint, and an aversion to anything animal-like became the hallmarks of the civilized person. As a result of the civilizing process, the body slowly came to be seen as an object that had to be controlled, its natural functions either hidden from public view or modified by "niceties."

Indeed, as we move into the eighteenth century, we find attitudes and a body type more familiar to us. The full-bodied forms of Rubens and Rembrandt were refined and became petite and compact. The last hints of the Gothic belly disappeared, and the waist became tiny, edging toward the hourglass form. With the brief exception of the Revolutionary years in France, when the Empire style prevailed, this tiny waist remained the central feature of woman's shape for the next hundred years. Skirts might billow in peculiar ways, the bustle come and go, but the tiny waist remained. Despite this tiny waist, however, the ideal form was not slender by any means. The bodies depicted by Watteau, Fragonard, and Boucher were juicely plump and shapely, the hands and feet small and delicate. And the nude herself had become more explicitly erotic, stripped of her mythic settings, caught unaware while she lay on her sofa (as in Boucher's *Miss O'Murphy*) or as she bathed (as in Fragonard's *Women Bathing*).

These eighteenth-century artists were in fact reflecting profound changes in attitudes toward the body—woman's body in particular. Fairly consistently, from antiquity to the eighteenth century, women had been regarded as having less control over their sexual and sensual appetites than men. Women suffered from excessive lust, not men; women were more inclined to libertinism; Eve, not Adam, had eaten from the forbidden tree. Medical treatises and popular and learned opinion attributed this difference to the peculiar physiology nature had given to women. Describing common views of women in the early modern period, historian Natalie Davis wrote, "Her womb is like a hungry animal. When not amply fed by sexual intercourse or reproduction, it was likely to wander about her body, overpowering her speech and senses." But gradually, men came to be seen as the creatures of lust and women as the creatures who had little of it. Base—or recreational—sexual appetites were unknown to them—at least in theory. The female orgasm, which for centuries had been viewed as normal and even essential for reproduction, ceased to be associated with conception, and its very existence was questioned. Paradoxically, this revision of woman's nature may have contributed to the eroticization of the female nude and fashion. The new privacy and shame now attached to the undressed, exposed body converted it into a forbidden delight, one rich with covert sexual promise. Simultaneously, women's clothing could more directly convey this eroticism in a civilized way precisely because females were presumed not to have sexual appetites. There was an innocence, and a new seductiveness in their sexuality.[23]

Oddly enough, the fashions of the day did not seem to describe a plump form. Instead, they described a remarkably slender, erect torso with great billowing skirts shaped by *panniers* or hoops that assumed various forms. Portraits from the era can leave us breathless in disbelief at the studied narrowness of the bodice, which nonetheless had a square, often low, décolletage that revealed a pearly, plump bosom. In part, this was achieved by the boned bodice and the stays that had become popular at the time, and in part by the contrast afforded by a straight bodice and a voluminous skirt. Although we have little direct evidence about actual body weights in this period, we do know that the fashionable body was not slender by our standards. Madame de Pompadour, the mistress of Louis XV, who was renowned for her beauty and fashionable taste, purportedly once complained that courtly life was undoing her health. She was becoming skeletally thin: She weighed 111 pounds. Madame de Pompadour probably was between 5'1" and 5'4". Today we would hardly consider 111 pounds a dangerously low weight for a woman of this height. In fact, we probably would consider her close to ideal.[24]

Yet now, for the first time, we hear about English girls of marriageable age dieting to attain the tiny waist, the willowiness, and the pallor prized by fashion. Women and girls were attempting to alter their natural bodies not through clothes and cosmetics, but from within. The eminent historian, Lawrence Stone, gives many examples of the deprivations mothers and expensive boarding schools imposed on young girls to meet the standards of the day. At the time, however, women usually relied on stays and corsets, rather than on alterations in diet, to mold their shapes. In 1675 the staymakers had become powerful enough to form their own guild in France. Their purpose and justification for doing so was to "educate the bodies of the young into the newly fashionable slenderness." The reducing diets and slenderness we value today had not yet come into vogue—women still relied on what they put *on* their bodies to mold the shape fashion desired.[25]

Even more profound change was brewing in this period. Fashion was being transformed by political and social developments. In essence, the centuries-old aristocratic dress code was dying out, along with the aristocratic political system. Splendid, colorful dress had once been a serious obligation for aristocratic men and women. It had been vital for the pomp and ceremony of royal society and for symbolically reinforcing the hierarchy of aristocratic society. These functions were becoming anachronistic in an age that argued for the equality of man, for rationalism and moderation, and in which the middle classes were claiming their right to political power. We needn't speculate about this connection. During the French Revolution, several manifestos for dress reform were promulgated, and laws outlawing certain kinds of dress were even enacted briefly. Throughout European society, the complex symbolic meanings of elaborate self-display were being diluted.[26]

The rising influence of the middle classes also brought with it the work ethic and utilitarianism, which regarded work as a moral imperative and which preached restraint. Attention to appearance, beyond what was necessary for propriety, was often deemed frivolous and vain. Self-ornamentation began to seem rather superficial, wasteful, and senseless. Interestingly, for the first time since the fourteenth century, men's fashions stabilized. Although male vanity was still a considerable force in the eighteenth century, and the Regency period was the heyday of the fop and the dandy, men's clothing became increasingly sober and restrained, much as in art, between the seventeenth and eighteenth centuries, the male body gradually ceased to be a subject for the nude. Only women continued to play the fashion game in the old way. Fashion and beauty thus became woman's domain.

The feminization of fashion and the eroticization of female dress coincided with significant eighteenth-century changes in courtship and marriage patterns. In earlier centuries, marriages for all social groups were arranged by parents, whose motives were largely economic and social. Kingdoms, noble estates, middle-class businesses and fortunes, and even peasant holdings were enlarged through marital unions, and noble pedigrees were passed on to new families. The betrotheds' sentiments played little if any role in the decision making. Often the young bridal pair remained strangers until their wedding night. Romantic and sexual love, at least for men, was reserved for the mistresses who were an accepted part of social life.

By the eighteenth century, particularly among the rising middle classes, arranged marriages were becoming passé. A central theme of late eighteenth- and nineteenth-century novels is the good daughter who heroically defies her parents' choice for a husband and runs off with a man who has inspired her passions and sentiments. These novels accurately reflected a new social reality: Young girls had to attract their own mates. Erotic beauty (suggesting sexual happiness), combined, of course, with modesty (suggesting sweetness and fidelity) could be a crucial advantage in the marriage market. As Lawrence Stone put it, girls now had to compete "with one another in an open market for success in which physical and personal attributes had to a considerable degree taken over the role previously played by the size of the dowry." It is little wonder that physical beauty became so important to women. Nor is it surprising that women often became trapped between erotic display and modest concealment. A woman had to combine, somehow, the allures of a courtesan with the demureness of a domestic paragon. The main purpose of female dress thus became the artificial display of erotic beauty, with status and modesty secondary, but still powerful, themes.[27]

But along with the feminization of dress came a new attack on the artificiality of fashion, a reflection of the division between "art" and "nature" that troubled the Romantic Age. Historian Valerie Steele observed that it was rather odd that France, the nation that led in the artifice of beauty, was also the nation in which "the idealization of the natural reached its most philosophic elaboration: nature, simplicity, and virtue were united, while the artificial, exaggerated and luxurious were denigrated as the product of 'corrupt' civilizations." Indeed, the new faith in Man, Reason, and Nature that came with the Enlightenment slowly set up a new standard: natural human beauty.

Rousseau, among others, argued that in a state of nature, humans were noble and pure. Society corrupted that purity. The same held true for fashion. In a state of nature, the body was innocent, beautiful, and healthy. Fashion, with its artificiality and constraints, corrupted all these virtues. Fashion did not make the human animal civilized and human; rather, it did just the reverse. The natural was more civilized and human, more noble.

Philosophical writings, even those as popular as Rousseau's, might not have had the enormous impact they had, had it not been for the fact that in England, a dress style was developing that seemed to give them sartorial reality. The English gentry, who had not experienced the lavish court system developed in France, were already adopting simpler, "rustic" modes that captivated the French. All these developments had two critical consequences. First, they set up an ideal of female beauty that was in direct competition with the one set up by fashion: Beauty should come from natural, not artificial means. For the next century and a half, the "natural, Republican maiden" would stand as a counterpoint, a foil, and a check for her artificial and fashion-conscious sister. Second, a corollary principle emerged: The natural body could and should be beautiful.[28]

It was not just attitudes toward the body and fashion that changed in the eighteenth century. The civilizing process was also changing attitudes toward eating. Indulgent gluttony was shifting to more regularized, controlled eating. With increasing security about the food supply, cooks for noble families suddenly had a new task: whetting the diner's appetite so that taste, not hunger, would keep him or her eating. The delights of "gourmet" food appeared as quality and subtlety of taste became the insignia of the noble table. At the same time, aversion to anything "animal-like" changed the way food was served. If England, with its country traditions, still served the hefty joint of meat at the table, the French had begun to serve delicate ragouts in which the animal origins of the dish were completely camouflaged. The gluttonous appetite, so common in the past, was now considered rude and coarse. By the mid-eighteenth century, extreme gluttony became an exception. Louis XVI shocked his court because he seemed to be a throwback to an older eating tradition. He lacked the new refinements in taste, manners, and quantity. As historian Louis Gottschalk explained, "By his appetite and by his appetite alone did the unfortunate Louis XVI revive memories of Louis XIV. Like him, he did not bother himself with cookery, nor with any refinements; . . . always afraid of not having enough to eat, he stuffed himself, going so far as to incapacitate himself at his wedding dinner, scandalizing his grandfather, Louis XV."[29]

The delicacy of the food now required manners and, above all, delicacy of appetite. If in the past, the natural oscillation of the food supply—and the sin of gluttony—had put external constraints on how much people ate over a year's time, now self-restraint was supposed to control quantity. A well-bred person should not make the crude mistake of overeating. Eating had become dining and it was an art. Writing in the first third of the nineteenth century,

J.-A. Brillat-Savarin, the first modern gourmand, contrasted true gourmands with "those pseudo-gourmands whose bellies are abysses and who eat up all of everything everywhere." True gourmands were "fit and pleasant guests who, while they savored each dish with right philosophical attention and gave to the fork all the time it demands, yet never forgot that a moment comes when reason says to appetite: 'Non procedes amplus' (Thou Shalt Go No Further)."[30]

Delicacy of appetite had become another hallmark of the civilized person. It was not the same as the moderation urged by doctors and philosophers, for it was based on voluptuous taste and refinement, not health. For Brillat-Savarin, this brought with it a battle between appetite and self-control and concerns about body weight. "I have ever looked upon my paunch as a redoubtable foe; I have conquered him and drawn the line at majesty; but before surrendering he fought well; and whatever good is contained in this chapter [On Obesity] I owe to a struggle of thirty-years duration." But Brillat-Savarin makes it quite clear that attractiveness and gentility, not health, are the reasons for his concern. A big paunch might suggest that one lacks breeding and refinement. For eighteenth-century women in particular, this imperative was strong. Slenderness may have come into fashion partially as a result of this change—certainly, the two arrived in tandem.[31]

During the eighteenth century we see changes in attitudes toward the body, toward beauty, and toward food that presage, in many ways, our modern attitudes. It is not surprising, then, that by 1830 we begin to see the first glimmerings of diet-mania in France and the United States.

4

Thin and Fat: America 1830–1900

The hourglass shape fell briefly out of favor in France between 1792 and 1820–25. Women started wearing latter-day versions of Roman dress, with the waistline up under the breast and the gown falling in graceful lines from there to the ankles. This simple dress, a startling contrast to the ornate and courtly costumes worn previously, was an expression of the Republican ideals that dominated France during the years of the French Revolution though its antecedents could be seen in the simple country gowns of the British upper classes. The Revolutionary government outlawed excessive finery that smacked of privilege and tried to find a national style more appropriate for a new society dedicated to Liberty, Equality, and Fraternity. Inspired by Rousseauean ideas about the impact of dress on both morals and health, the government sought a costume that would be ideologically correct and that would "work for universal regeneration." The revolutionary Committee of the Arts and artist J. J. David were commissioned with this formidable task. Their creations were never adopted—except by the students in David's studio—but women, without official guidance, established the Antique Empire style which, with various modifications, was imitated in Europe, England, and the United States.[1]

Ironically, given its origins, the style came to be associated not with moral purity and the enthronement of Reason, but with the decadence and lasciviousness of the Directory and the Napoleonic years. It became startlingly immodest in reputation if not always in fact. Revealing décolletage, sheer, light fabrics, and scanty underwear, when carried to extremes as they were by the *merveilleuses* of Paris, gave passers-by generous glimpses of the female form underneath. And this form was not particularly slender. Portraits reveal lushly fleshed, rounded bodies similar to the neoclassical nudes being painted by artists. But if slenderness was not desirable, the style's tendency to expose the body did require an acceptable shape, one with reasonable contours. Frederica of Prussia, the Princess of Orange, wrote in 1793 that "[this gown] is horrible on ugly, ill-made on old people, and excessively indecent on the young . . . . " Though widely accepted within a short time, the Empire style rapidly disappeared once the political and social chaos anu wild enthusiasm of the Revolutionary years ended. With the return of the Monarchy, order and restraint once again prevailed, but this chaotic period bequeathed two important themes to future discourse on dress. It reinforced and intensified both the idea of a "healthy" form of dress as desirable and the thrust toward the democratization of dress.[2]

Between 1815 and 1825 the Romantic Age succeeded neoclassicism. The waist returned to its natural place, skirts slowly became voluminous, and the hourglass figure, with its primary feature a tiny waist, began to be a celebration of woman's fragility and delicacy. Slenderness became an explicit fashion goal. To examine this phenomenon, which lasted roughly from 1830 to 1850, we shift to our principle arena, America, which now was developing its own fashion culture and where, prophetically perhaps, the fad was most pronounced.

The first identifiable trend toward slenderness can be traced in the United States because America now had its own domestic fashion authority, which interpreted and presented European modes for the American market—the fashion magazine. Sara Joseph Hale's *Godey's Lady's Book* first appeared in 1828 and soon became the arbiter of American ladies' taste. The fashion pictures were steel-engraved, and the popular image of the era has aptly been called the "Steel Engraving Lady." This lady was young and pretty, with tiny features and a rosebud mouth, and she exuded a demure delicacy and gentility. Above all, she was gracefully slender and willowy and so ethereal that it seemed even gravity could not affect her. She became the dominant ideal and, in 1850, demurrer Harriet Beecher Stowe angrily observed that "we in America have got so far out of the way of a womanhood that has any vigor of outline or opulence of physical proportions that, when we see a woman as a woman ought to be, she strikes us as a monster." Stowe's standard of what "a woman ought to be" was closer to the aesthetic of a Titian or Giorgione female than to that of the willowy Steel Engraving Lady.[3]

As we have observed, there were European roots to this American "craving" for slenderness. J.-A. Brillat-Savarin wrote in 1828 that had he been a doctor, he would have specialized in obesity because then he would have been "daily besieged by the prettier half of mankind, for to acquire or maintain the perfect mean between fat and thin is the life-study of every woman in the world." In support of this, he reported the case of his friend Louise, a beautiful young girl whose friends teased her about getting fat. She put herself on a regimen of just a daily glass of vinegar, and within two months, she died—one of our earliest recorded sacrifices to thinness. But Europeans still idealized other physical types, and American girls seemed to strive for an even slenderer form than did their European sisters. Foreign visitors repeatedly commented on the frail, slender figures they encountered here. In the 1830s, one visitor reported that the women looked "as though a puff of wind would break them in half or a drop of water soak them through." Others described them as "sylphlike" and "ethereal," which was precisely the effect they sought, although another visitor, Isabella Bird, remarked that the sylphlike elegance of youth deteriorated into an unpleasant angularity by the time they were thirty, and others noted that it led to a "loss of skin tone, to sallowness and gauntness."[4]

A complicated aesthetic, not merely a physical standard, lay beneath the Romantic Movements' emphasis on delicacy, ethereality, and slenderness, though initially it applied more to men than to women. The movement, given voice by French and German intellectuals and artists and codified by the English Romantic poets Byron, Shelley, and Keats, exalted the isolated individual, particularly in the guise of the embattled artist. The artist, as portrayed by these spokesmen, was associated with spiritual passion and suffering, with contempt for social conventions and crass material ambitions like money and success, and with a decided aversion to animal-like activities such as eating. In a sense, they were creating a new kind of aristocracy for a democratic age—an aristocracy of those with exalted sensibilities.

The Romantic did not control his baser impulses through reason and self-restraint, which were abhorred as bourgeois conventions, but rather through the natural refinement of his soul. Part of this enoblement was a yearning after unattainable, and frequently otherworldly, ideals, and women came to be one of the principle embodiments of those ideals. Beginning in philosophy and the arts—literature, opera, ballet, and painting—Romantic standards pervaded society, where they were tamed and domesticated. The Romantic hero came to be a man of unearthly passions and the heroine a woman of unearthly beauty. Such a hero, alas, needs a body, and it had to be slight as though to underline this lack of corporeality. The French writer, Théophile Gautier, recalled that during this period, when he was young, he could not "have accepted as a lyric poet anyone weighing more than 99 pounds." Such ideas quickly spread among the general public in America as well. The *Newark Daily Advertiser* put it quite blatantly in 1838: "Obesity is a deadly foe to genius; in carneous and unwieldly bodies the spirit is like a gudgeon in a large frying pan of fat, which is either totally absorbed, or tastes of nothing but lard."[5]

The popular romances of the day were filled with slender damsels who fainted, their white bosoms heaving, at the slightest coarseness or intense emotion. In ballet, women first went on point around 1830, allowing them a range of gliding, fluttering, otherworldly movements, and the appearance of Marie Taglioni in *La Sylphide* in 1832 began the long reign of the ballerina as the crown princess of ethereality. When her successor, Fanny Essler, toured the United States later in the decade, she was wildly acclaimed, and some historians speculate that she was the real-life model for the Steel Engraving Lady. Cheap lithographs of Essler, which exaggerated her slenderness, and other souvenirs were widely reproduced and adorned the parlors of urban tradespeople. The magazines of the day showed this romantic young woman gliding on the arm of her escort, who himself was slender and elegant. Her arm rested on his as though it had no weight.[6]

While in men fragility and slenderness denoted higher passions, in women they declared purity. Even illness became fashionable, a sign of delicacy and refinement, and tuberculosis in particular—because of the translucent pallor and emaciation it caused—came to be seen as an ennobling disease. Women supposedly possessed, like the poets, a more refined sensibility, spirituality, and innocence than men. They fastidiously avoided any exercise except dancing and regarded all bodily appetites as coarse. These romantic notions grafted perfectly onto the emerging image of the Victorian woman and helped establish more firmly the idea that women were morally superior, made of finer clay, and lacking in animal urges, especially sexual ones. In the late eighteenth century the middle classes had already begun to set up sexual self-control as the highest virtue for women, and ,Evangelical Protestantism reinforced this development with its own revision of woman's nature. It argued that women were naturally virtuous and established the idea that women could be agents of moral reform. Slenderness became the concomitant to an approved passionlessness. As we have seen, medical opinion had even come to dismiss the centuries-old notion that for conception to occur, a woman had to have an orgasm. Those who argue that slenderness comes into vogue when women become free sexual agents are wrong.[7]

These qualities were incorporated into the notion of "gentility," that insignia of breeding used in democratic societies. Emerging American society pursued gentility, decorum, and respectability thoroughly. And the mark of gentility became increasingly important in the 1830s, when Andrew Jackson's rough-and-tumble democracy extended the vote to nonpropertied men and society itself seemed to be in a promiscuous scramble. Americans were caught in an intense struggle for upward mobility—in New York City, for example, 10 percent of the financial leaders had come from poor families—and these newly rich groups were the most eager pursuers of marks of gentility.

At the same time, women's social position was changing. The relative equality of women and the work opportunities afforded them in colonial America—largely because of the scarcity of labor—ended with the new wave of immigrants. Women's sphere narrowed to the home, the arts, and religion. Population changes also transformed courtship patterns. The favorable ratio of women to men that had prevailed during the colonial era had given women a good chance to find mates even if they didn't put undue effort into the process. By the Jacksonian era, this favorable ratio had changed, and American women had to compete on an open marriage market much as their British sisters had been doing for close to a century. Gentility, the mark of a perfect lady, became progressively more important as ammunition for this battle. The lady had certainly existed in colonial America. What was new, as historian

Gerda Lerner points out, was that there now existed a "cult of the lady, her elevation into a status symbol." Magazines like *Godey's* detailed how that lady was to look and behave.[8]

A lady's pursuit of fashionable beauty was also particularly intense during this period because women had become the "ornamental sex." Men were adopting the sober, restrained bourgeois uniform, and the beginnings of ready-made men's clothing and the imitability of these styles propelled a new democratization in male dress. In France and England as well, but especially in democratic America, it was becoming difficult to distinguish a gentleman from a clerk because they were dressed so similarly. The bourgeois husband instead displayed his success through his wife's apparel. Her taste and her gentility were crucial to a family's self-definition and public status. Thus, while male competition in dress became less overt, female sartorial competition intensified, spurred on by the new fluidity between classes.

It is, of course, no surprise that this era, shaped on one side by the emerging Romantic tradition and on the other by shifting social and demographic patterns, saw the emergence of slenderness's grim companion: dieting. Harriet Beecher Stowe remarked that "if a young lady begins to round into proportions like the women in Titian's or Giorgione's pictures . . . she is distressed above measure and begins to make secret inquiries into a reducing diet." That such inquiries were secret suggests that unlike today, dieting was not considered a virtue nor a topic for polite conversation. There were a number of sources for diets, including the backs of cookbooks and popular literature, but no widely popular diet appeared until 1864 when William Banting, a coffin maker for British upper classes, published his "Letter on Corpulence." In it, he recounted how he had reduced from 202 to 156 pounds by following the diet French physiologist Claude Bernard had recommended for diabetics. It was a low-carbohydrate diet, consisting of lean meat, dry toast, soft-boiled eggs, and green vegetables. His book went through five printings in just one year and was republished for almost fifty years. The word *banting*—meaning slimming—entered the language, and the low-carbohydrate diet would be resuscitated, with new names, innumerable times in the next century.[9]

By 1850, some twenty or more years after its appearance, this early vogue for slenderness fizzled out, though body size continued to be a matter of some concern for women. In many ways this was the first incarnation of our own diet-thinness mania, which allows us to speculate about what circumstances create a slender ideal. There are striking parallels between this period and the 1960s, the decade in which our own obsession about weight became most pronounced. Most noticeable were the emphasis on youth as both moral arbiter and stereotype, and on the recovery of the purity and innocence it symbolized. The Romantics romanticized youth itself. In addition, they lived in a period of considerable political and social turmoil not unlike that of the 1960s. It was the "Age of Revolution" in which the old order was constantly under attack. Political revolutions occurred, reform societies proliferated, and idealists envisioned and often experimented with utopian communities where marriage, property laws, and sexual conventions were repudiated. There was a powerful and exciting—or dangerous, depending on one's point of view— sense that society could be re-created. As we shall see, even a health and a health-food movement of sorts emerged.

Crucial to the creation of new bodily ideals for women are redefinitions of woman's nature and role—even though these redefinitions are quite different in different periods. The eighteenth century revisions of woman's nature were more carefully collaborated. A variety of fields, from biology to theology, increasingly stressed sexual differentiation. Woman had been redefined as a creature of sentiment and purity of soul instead of as a creature of irrepressible passions. The cultural and social spheres of the two sexes deviated sharply. Women were to be guardians of beauty, culture, the arts, and religion; men were to be masters of the harsh realities, of the marketplace and politics. The cult of the lady was born and beside it the cult of the mother. Woman, refined creature of sentiment, was to adorn society and refine it through her artful rearing of children.[10]

Despite these common circumstances, the slenderness vogue of the 1830s differed profoundly from that of today. The Steel Engraving Lady equated slenderness with delicacy and fragility. Health and energy were not part of her aesthetic self-definition, whereas the 1980s woman strives for slenderness because she equates it with both of these qualities. Furthermore, the slenderness the Romantic woman sought was radically different from our own. She wanted a willowy look and perhaps craved the 17-inch waist Scarlett O'Hara boasted, but it was *only* her waist she wanted slender. She, and men, wanted the rest of the female body to be soft and sweetly fleshed, full of an "amorous plenitude," especially in the shoulders, bust, and buttocks. Balzac underlined this dilemma when he observed that the ideal was "[to] manage to possess lovely contours and yet remain slender." Thinness was considered ugly, a misfortune for women. Brillat-Savarin defined thinness, as those of his epoch typically did, as "the condition of the individual whose muscular flesh, not being filled out with fat, reveals the forms and angles of the bony structure." He went on to observe that "for women it is a terrible misfortune; to them beauty is more than life itself and beauty chiefly consists in roundness of form and gracefully curving lines. The most painstaking toilette, the sublimest costume, cannot hide certain absences, or disguise certain angles . . . . " Even ballerinas—the most direct representatives of the Romantic ideal—were lush by modern standards. As Dr. L. M. Vincent remarks in his book *Competing with the Sylph,* 1840 engravings of the dancer Fanny Cerrito, make her "appear as solid as the Chrysler Building and possibly as tough to lift off the ground." In common American parlance, the thin woman was given short shrift and compared to a "whipping post."[11]

Another difference was that mechanical means of altering women's figures were considered legitimate, even though other artificial methods, such as cosmetics, had become taboo for the respectable lady—whereas our own generation despises any unnatural contrivance. And many of those tiny waists were more the result of contrivance than of dieting. Corsets of the day, if tightly laced, could reduce the waist by about four or five inches. Although contemporary reformers and modern feminists point to the corset as evidence of the oppressive and unhealthy nature of female fashion, recent historical research indicates that few women laced themselves tightly. Most let a comfortably laced corset, the volume of their skirts, and clever sewing and use of material create the appearance of a lovely figure. In these days before ready-made clothing, the tailor or seamstress designed clothes for *somebody,* not just for anybody, and the art of this highly skilled individual consisted, in part, in camouflaging a client's flaws. The tailor had to "bestow a good Shape where Nature has not designed it; the Hump back, the Wry shoulder must be buried in Flannel and Wadding; he must study not only the Shape but the common Gait of the Subject . . . . " Dressmakers for fashionable ladies did much the same.[12]

Unlike today, few women of the period were likely to *expect* their body dimensions to be a specific size. The tailor and seamstress presumed everyone's body was different, and the notion of and methods for standardized sizing proved to be one of the biggest hurdles faced by pioneers in the ready-made clothing industry. The presumption that one garment might fit an indefinite number of people would only slowly make inroads, first for men, and only toward the end of the century for women.

The number of women affected by the slender ideal also differed from our almost comprehensive obsession because, especially in the United States, the ideal applied principally to young, marriageable girls. When Harriet Beecher Stowe described the vogue, she referred merely to "our willowy girls," and other writers also referred to its prominence among courting girls. Older women subscribed to somewhat different beauty standards. In fact, one of the oldest fashion rules has been that styles vary with age: Young girls, girls of marriageable age, young married women, and even elderly women have historically had distinct dress codes. It is only the latter half of the twentieth century that has seen the erosion of this stratification.

Throughout the nineteenth century, the mature woman expected to have different body dimensions than a young girl. She was expected to fill out as she aged. When women's magazines began including dress patterns in the 1860s, they provided standard measurements that presumed a young woman would have a 20-inch waist (though few met this standard) but that a mature woman might have a 36-inch waist. A mature woman was, by our standards, young. If, in the early twentieth century, a woman was not considered old until she was fifty, in the 1830s she could be considered old by the time she hit her thirties.[13]

Another reason the slenderness vogue affected far fewer women in the nineteenth century than it does today was because far fewer were caught in the fashion nexus. Despite America's egalitarian ideology, and despite the comments of European visitors surprised by how well dressed America's working and middle classes were, fashion was generally limited to the better-off urban classes. *Godey's Lady Book* and other fashion magazines were harbingers of a growing democratization and standardization of fashion and beauty, but in mid- to late-nineteenth-century America, the vast preponderance of the population was rural. Most women had limited access to fashion messages, and they tended to be swayed more by local community standards than by those emanating from the cities.

Nor can the apparent concern with diet be compared to our contemporary preoccupation. Women ate little, less because they wanted to lose weight than because hearty appetite was considered unladylike and ungenteel. The "civilizing of appetite" prohibited such a public display. In deference to this standard, Scarlett O'Hara's mammy urged her to eat *before* going to dances so she wouldn't embarrass herself by eating in company. Eating was not condemned—only public display of appetite was.

Many doctors, lending medical credence to this notion, reinforced the strictures on women's eating habits by arguing that women had such delicate digestive systems, they "could not eat heavy meats but must subsist on small amounts of light nourishment: toast, tea and a bit of chicken or bullion." Sectors of the medical community and dietary reformers like Sylvester Graham endorsed these associations between women and food, which were based on the new interpretation of woman's nature and on new medical theories. Many believed in "vitalism," which argued that all of the body's functions required "vital energy" or "nerve force" and that the body had limited quantities of it. If the body's equilibrium were disturbed by any immoderation, all of this force would be diverted to one bodily function, overstimulating this area and debilitating all other areas. Excessive intake of food, especially of meat and spices, would irritate the stomach, create nervous disorders, and worst of all, inflame the sexual appetites—all of which would result in debility.[14]

Above all, the slenderness ideal did not assume the monolithic proportions it has today because many other standards and authorities supported different aesthetics. European artists and Europeans in general certainly had more than one ideal. A big, handsome woman was still an ideal in England. The term *pretty* was reserved for the diminutive Steel Engraving Lady; *beautiful* was applied to a more statuesque, mature woman. But in the United States, the most powerful competitor to the Steel Engraving Lady was the girl with the natural beauty praised by Rousseau, whom we might call the virtuous Republican maiden. She was an antifashion ideal who symbolized the popular ideas that inner character was more important than outward appearance, that preoccupation with fashion smacked of aristocratic frivolity and decadence. She was rosier, healthier, plumper, and stronger than her fashionable sisters.

Young women of the period constantly had her image thrust before them. Moralists, many doctors, and some women authors attacked fashion-greedy girls, idealizing instead this modest maiden whose beauty shone, despite a plain or even unattractive face, because of her moral purity and strength. Feminists and reformers like the energetic Catherine Beecher, who wrote numerous guidance manuals and "how-to" books before the Civil War, railed against the life and ills of the Steel Engraving Lady. She was too sedentary, moving from the piano to her embroidery to her art work without ever getting any exercise. Her corsets were destroying her health and threatening the health of future generations—a conviction that led many reformers, such as Antoinette Brown Blackwell, the first woman to graduate from a traditional medical school, Mary Neal, Paulina Wright Davis, and others to tramp through the East and Northeast on the lecture circuit, condemning the evils of the corset. Beecher thundered that artificial beauty was not beauty at all. She idealized the Greeks and set up an equation between health, beauty, and strength. As historian Harvey Green observed, "Beecher's assertion of a causal relationship between 'health' and 'beauty and strength' was a breakthrough for the nineteenth century . . . . Beecher was one of the first popular commentators to suggest that a subjective and culturally determined attribute—beauty—was a function of health." Unlike our own generation, where this link is paramount, "healthy" then denoted a certain amount of plumpness. Again in contrast to our own uniform standards, this antifashion ideal was even described in those women's magazines that promoted the Steel Engraving Lady's slenderer, more fragile look. Popular fashion had room for more than one ideal.[15]

But more important than differences in the diffusion and intensity of the ideal is the difference in self-perception between that era and our own. Mid-nineteenth-century Americans did not perceive themselves as fat or suffering from obesity. They saw themselves as generally lean, an impression that European travelers repeatedly confirmed. Today we believe unquestioningly that Americans *were* leaner in this premachine-age era, but after carefully analyzing height and weight data, historian Hillel Schwartz concluded that average weights for heights for both men and women did not increase appreciably between this time and World War II, though people did get taller. Nor were mid-nineteenth-century Americans leaner than their European counterparts. Schwartz concluded that Americans in fact had the same weights for heights as Europeans, except that Americans were, on the whole, two inches taller. In short, body size is, to a large extent, a question of perception, and most nineteenth-century Americans did not see themselves as fat.[16]

Paradoxically, even though obesity was not considered a general problem, gluttony was. "We may safely take for granted, after long observation," wrote a *Southern Review* contributor in 1829, "that almost every man, woman, and child in this country habitually eats and drinks twice as much everyday . . . as is necessary." Dietary reformer Sylvester Graham and Catherine Beecher made similar indictments. Americans ate too much meat and fat and too many spices. (In fact, between 1830 and 1839, Americans' per-capita meat consumption was 178 pounds a year, a level that would not be attained again until the 1970s. Meat was served at all four daily meals, and butter was its ubiquitous accompaniment. "Mon Dieu," exclaimed one French visitor with great disgust, "What a country! Fifty religions and only one sauce—melted butter!") But, curiously, these gluttonous habits were believed to cause excessive thinness more than fatness. The main illness of the era was *dyspepsia,* a vague term that covered all sorts of gastrointestinal ills, from constipation to diarrhea, as well as other ailments. Dietary reformers argued that gluttony caused thinness because it caused dyspepsia. Food that was eaten could not be distributed to the body tissues. Even the connection between overeating and overweight was not very direct. Dyspepsia, not gluttony, was often also considered the cause of obesity. The eminent Dr. Russell Trall warned that fatness was a disease, but argued that "fat men, fat women, fat children and fat pigs are not examples of excessive nutrition so much as of deficient excretion."[17]

Dietary reformers were not aiming for a thinner population. When critics viciously caricatured Graham and his followers by depicting them as wraithlike and yellow, seated before a meager table, Graham and his disciples defended the diet by arguing that it would "yield handsome, robust bodies." Rather, reformers were aiming for a population that felt a sensation of lightness. Scale weight and heaviness had not yet been inextricably tied together—and, in fact, weighing oneself was not yet a common activity. Heaviness was an undesirable and unhealthy sensation within the body; it was not related to an individual's scale weight. As Catherine Beecher explained, "To feel the body heavy, when it is in fact light on the balance, shows a worse state of health, than to feel it weighty when it is really so. On the other hand, to feel it light when it is heavy on the balance, shows an excellent state of health"—a distinction that has been lost to modern Americans who rely on scale weight to determine if they are heavy or light, and whose perceptions are so skewed that they don't trust bodily sensations.[18]

Although most Americans would have opted for this buoyant feeling, the dietary reformers did not win many adherents. For most Americans believed people needed to eat meat and hominy grits and other heavy foods that would stick to the ribs. The health-food faddism introduced by Graham would nevertheless remain an important, if periodically dormant, theme in American life. It expressed, in an extreme form, the emerging conviction that how one ate affected one's moral and physical condition, and the worry that Americans did not eat healthfully.

More fundamentally, dietary and health reformers underlined profoundly new expectations about the body. Enlightenment notions about natural science had slowly spread the heady idea that human beings could control their health, that they needn't just resign themselves to disease and early death. These beliefs merged with religious aspirations. Perfecting the body became part of the wave of religious Perfectionism of the period, which argued that if people bettered themselves morally and physically, they would either hasten the Second Coming or could ensure they were not one of the damned. Being saved had become more a matter of free will than of predestination. Diet and—to a more limited extent—exercise were seen as tools for salvation. Though we have stripped away their essentially religious bases, the food regimes and the healthiness advocated by people like Graham and Beecher were prototypes of our new dietary catechism.

The presumptions of dietary and health reformers and of certain scientists and physicians—that humans could control their health and the state of their bodies and that God intended both to be unblemished—reflected the rise of a profoundly new worldview, one that changed expectations about the body. It made the sight of human suffering and of physical abnormalities more a cause for reform and scientific research than for pious resignation. This view, which had slowly evolved from the Renaissance through to the Enlightenment and on into the nineteenth century, is the basis of the modern mentality. With its full flowering in the twentieth century, it proved a crucial underpinning of the war against fat.

The vogue for slenderness was relatively brief. Already by the 1850s, the willowy Steel Engraving Lady began to be seen as rather insipid and simpering, and a more mature woman with a fuller figure began appearing in the fashion pages. Dress historians have been impressed by the almost linear evolution of the female ideal in these years. She seemed to grow more mature, more self-assertive, more confident, more worldly, and more solid and substantial as the decades passed.[19]

Mechanical contrivances were still used to mold the ideal female form. The cage-crinoline was invented in the 1850s, and instead of using a quantity of heavy petticoats to hold out their bell-shaped skirts, women could now use this petticoat, which got its fullness from its graduated hoops of whalebone, steel, or watch spring. As is fashion's wont, this device proceeded to move to extremes. The cage-crinoline got fuller and fuller for the next ten years, earning the ridicule of many men who found they could not even get close enough to offer their arms to the lovely ladies who wore them. By 1865 the crinoline had already run its course, and now the hoops and fullness were confined to the back—in front, the dress fell in softened, uninflated folds. In the 1870s and 1880s, fashion took a new and rather revolutionary course. The hoop was abandoned for the sheathlike cuirass-bodice, and for perhaps the first time in the history of European female dress, clothing clung to and exposed the outline of the female stomach and hips. "Ladies . . . must be encased in a sheath," wrote one beauty authority at the time. "The curiasse-corsage now moulds not only the waist, but encloses the whole figure." The whole figure, that is, except for the elevated bustle. By 1875 the bustle had melted into a long, full train, which prevailed until a facsimile of the bustle was revived again briefly in 1885. From then on, skirts became progressively narrower and less ornate, and attention shifted instead to the bodice and to the shoulders and sleeves, which puffed out and were often extravagantly adorned. Women were still compressed into the peculiar postures of the day—the Grecian curve and then the S-curve, which thrust out the buttocks and bust. Erotic focus was expanding to include an opulent breast as well as an ample bottom, and clothing was beginning to expose more and more of the female form. Nonetheless, with the increasingly narrower skirts, fashion started inching toward the slim-hipped form that would prevail in the twentieth century.[20]

But beyond the changing clothing structures and exterior forms, how big did these women want to be? Tastes during this period moved toward ever-greater voluptuousness and stateliness—tall, commanding, well-developed women— with, of course, the small, tapering waist a constant. In 1847 Hiram Powers's sculpture, *The Greek Slave,* with her ample form, toured the country and became, according to one contemporary, "the century's model of beauty for women." In later decades Americans became more receptive to and familiar with European art and tastes—which had never so exclusively or wholeheart- edly idealized slenderness—and the images of artists like Ingres, Titian, and Raphael became American ideals. By the end of the century, lithographs of voluptuous nudes, like those of Bouguereau, adorned the walls of working- class saloons as well as respectable middle-class establishments.[21]

In the 1850s the *Water-Cure Journal* ran "personals" that bear a startling similarity to those we see today. Single men were advertising for mates, and they began to specify, among other ideals, the body dimensions they favored. These specifications afford us an unusual glimpse of popular standards of the day. In general, the men wanted what one would-be suitor, HLM, wanted: "A form medium-sized, well-developed, erect, and plump (not gross, but full and round—I do not admire skeletons)." Other men were more specific. One sought a woman 5'4" and 120 to 140 pounds; another wanted a shorter woman whose weight would range between 130 and 160 pounds. High as these weights sound to us, they seemed to reflect national averages. Hillel Schwartz noted they were close to the average weights of women who had stepped on scales at various state fairs—one of our few sources about female body size in the period.[22]

These dimensions, and the shapes they represented, were paralleled by those of various "disreputable" public beauties. Early photographs of dance-hall queens and actresses reveal similarly ample measurements. Lydia Thompson and Pauline Markham of the 1860s and 1870s touring dance-hall group, the British Blondes, look positively enormous by our standards, and actress and singer Lillian Russell, America's sweetheart from 1879 to 1914, tipped the scales at 200 pounds in her later years. In 1880 novelist and etiquette authority Marion Harland declared that "to be thin is no longer the acme of feminine desires," and the following year, Harriet Hubbard Ayer noticed that "plump- ness is fashionable." By the close of the century, in the Edwardian period, the fashionable ideal was Junoesque: an amply bosomed, tall, statuesque figure. The fine figure, the *Pictorial Review* explained, was "perfectly free from all scrawny and hollow places [with a] bust as full, plump and firm as you could desire." Women may have sought small waists, but they wanted opulent curves—40-inch busts, thighs that might measure 53 inches around, and weights of well over 150 pounds. Pornographic photographs and Victorian pornographic literature invariably focus on broad-beamed bottoms and plump, juicy thighs, arms, and shoulders, and even on "soft" bellies. The lust for flesh seemed to include every part of the body. Beauty authority Annie Wolf reported that she had known girls to "pit the dimensions of their calves, one against the other, as evidence of health and natural charm."[23]

If this era sounds prelapsarian to us who have had to fight so hard against every drop of flesh, it did have its casualties. The thin woman was an object of scorn and even ridicule. When Sarah Bernhardt toured the United States in the 1870s, Americans widely acclaimed her talent but fiercely caricatured her scrawniness. Bernhardt was 5'2" and weighed 112 pounds—today we would no doubt consider her perfect. By the 1890s historian Valerie Steele observed, the "thin woman was given short shrift and was rudely told to 'cover some of her angles.' " A wide variety of pills, creams, and potions started appearing, designed, or so the ads promised, to produce a bigger bust and a more ample form. In 1905 the *Pictorial Review* advertised a mysterious product that promised the user would "gain fifteen to thirty pounds more in weight and round out the entire form . . . until [she was] entirely developed."[24]

But unlike today, the woman with an unfashionable figure was not doomed. Fashion was still a plastic art and an art, in some sense, of deception. The public body did not look the same as the private, undressed body. Clever seamstresses, a variety of figure aids, and the styles themselves allowed women to transform their appearance. When the crinoline became stylish in the 1850s, commentators remarked that it made every woman look tiny-waisted and ideally shaped. In 1857 a *Harper's* cartoon observed that the crinolines "make us all appear the same size. Why a Girl might be thin as a Whipping-post, and yet be taken for a decent figure." Thin women could also fill out their figures with a variety of ingenious devices that the corset industry invented and eagerly marketed. False breasts, thighs, and calves were available in addition to rubber backs and hips that had "natural" dimples designed into them. And individually constructed corsets reformed a multitude of sins. The prevalence of these mechanisms may partially explain why, when the corsetless look came into fashion in the twentieth century, a slim, sleek body was a must. To let the human form flop and bulge and hang as it naturally tends to do would offend sensibilities accustomed to controlled curves.[25]

Figure standards were less unkind than they are today in other ways as well. The weight favored in the period seemed to be very much in line with the average weight of American women. If the ideal waist was excessively small, women at least could avail themselves of the corset to approximate the fashionable look. In addition, beauty experts described more than one type of beauty. Unlike today, when only a Jane Fonda figure seems acceptable, the beauty writers of the Edwardian period described a trinity of beauties: Juno, Venus, and Psyche. If poor Psyche was the least admired because of her slender, girlish figure, she nonetheless had a place, albeit a subordinate one, in the hierarchy of beauty. But the most important difference between this era and our own is that a woman who lacked the ideal figure did not have to blame herself or her character for the failing, nor did she have to do any violence to her body. Her failure was not perceived as her fault.[26]

Not only did fashion favor flesh; so did health authorities. Doctors regarded hefty body weight and hearty appetite as signs of good health for all age groups, even though they considered obesity a medical problem. The New York City Bureau of Hygiene, for example, stressed to poor and immigrant mothers that fat babies were healthy babies. The same standard applied to children and adolescents, largely because thinness was associated with diseases that killed the young, such as tuberculosis and pneumonia, and because doctors believed a good reservoir of fat helped children survive infectious diseases. Certainly it was evident that the puny children of the poor succumbed far more quickly to death than did the more robust. Even well into old age, people were considered healthier if they were heavy. Elizabeth Cady Stanton, when she was in her sixties, was quite plump by our standards, but she was described as having "that plumpness which indicates superb health"—a judgment we would never hear today. This bias was so deeply entrenched that the fledgling insurance companies screened thin applicants far more carefully than plump ones.[27]

Another boost for plumpness in this period came from growing concern about the number of Americans suffering from what was known as neurasthenia or nervous exhaustion, a disease category invented by Dr. George Beard in 1869. In his view, this nervous exhaustion was the result of advanced civilization. Professional people, bureaucrats, artists, and others had overused their brains and neglected their bodies. Consequently, they were weak, thin, nervous, and unable to withstand the frantic pace of modern civilization. As in Graham's day, medical opinion held that every person had a fixed amount of nervous energy endowed by heredity. Neurasthenia resulted when an individual used more nervous energy than had been endowed to him or her.

Beard wrote pages and pages describing the multiple symptoms of neurasthenia—everything from headaches and insomnia to deficient mental control and spinal irritation, uterine irritability, impotence, hopelessness, and irrational fears such as claustrophobia. Hillel Schwartz astutely noted that most of the ills once associated with dyspepsia now were categorized as neurasthenia, and the focus of medical concern consequently shifted from the stomach to the head—though not entirely. What caused neurasthenia was "immoderate toil or worry, lack of food or rest." These bodily abuses could "induce an attack or even a chronic condition." The antidote was to have fat in the blood, S. Weir Mitchell argued, elaborating on Beard's theory. He contended that a large number of fat cells was essential for a balanced personality. Mitchell invented his famous—or infamous—treatment for neurasthenia with these ideas in mind. He enforced complete bed rest, allowed absolutely no distractions for the patient, not even reading, and he fed them. Fattening them up, he believed, would restore their equanimity and their energy. Plumpness was not only aesthetically acceptable; it had become a cure.[28]

The concept became immensely popular when Mitchell's books, *Wear and Tear* and *Fat and Blood* were published in the 1870s. They went through several reprintings, and *neurasthenia* became a household word. It struck a responsive chord because it addressed anxieties prevalent among middle-class Americans. They had become overcivilized; the elite did brain work while farmers and the lower classes did manual labor that kept them healthy, hearty, and temperamentally well-balanced. This intensive mental work and over-refined sensibility of the upper-middle classes had to be balanced by greater physical and emotional robustness if they were to survive.

That their survival was at stake struck many observers as a very real problem. German and Irish immigrants threatened to outnumber "native" Americans, for these sturdy folk were robust and procreated in great numbers. Americans did not. The birth rate for native Americans was dropping; 11 percent of women remained unmarried in the 1890s; there seemed to be an epidemic of infertility and amenorrhea among them. When in the 1880s, immigrants began to come from eastern and southern Europe, native Americans became even more alarmed. If they admired the earlier immigrants who were of the hard-working, upright stock that had made America great, the later immigrants struck them as decidedly unsavory. Racial ideas were as popular in America as in Europe at this time, and Darwinian notions reinforced their fears about this new breed that threatened to outnumber them. In the introduction to his *Descent of Man,* Darwin had written that America's success was the result of natural selection because the "more energetic, restless and courageous men from all parts of Europe have emigrated during the last ten or twelve generations to that great country and there have succeeded best." Americans heartily agreed, as they agreed later with the judgment of economist Francis G. Walker, who argued in 1899 that the new immigrants were "beaten men from beaten races; representing the worst failures in the struggle for existence."[29]

The native middle classes also felt threatened by other aspects of modernization—industrialization, urbanization, and social mobility—and by their apparent loss of cultural, political, and financial leadership. Labor strikes became more frequent and more violent; "upstart" immigrants, among others, were becoming fabulously wealthy as robber barons who made fortunes, often through unscrupulous tactics; and the government seemed to be falling into the hands of corrupt bosses, especially in the teeming cities. Native Americans wanted to reverse these trends and believed they could do so in part by becoming sturdier and stronger themselves. The slender, fragile romantic, swept by spiritual passions, became a decidedly undesirable image.

As well as endorsing a fuller form, concern about neurasthenia contributed to the first concerted health/exercise movement in America. It had special implications for women. Teddy Roosevelt, endorsing the German-inspired progressive views of the new physical culturists, planned to combat debility by encouraging all Americans to follow his example and lead a "strenuous life." Women, as the keepers of moral integrity and the source of future generations, were under special obligations. As the popular periodical, *Ladies' Home Calisthenics* explained in 1890, "The health of coming generations and the future of the nation depend in great part upon the girls. They are to be the coming mothers; and as such, obligations for the formation of a new race are incumbent on them. These obligations they can by no means fulfill unless they are sound in body and in mind." The fragility of the Steel Engraving Lady, like her slenderness, had to be repudiated, and a new image of vigorous femininity replaced her. And perhaps in this tremendous concern for fertility, we find one reason why the fashionable ideal now emphasized female sexual characteristics so much more explicitly. Women might not have sexual natures, but they certainly could not be averse to sex if the fate of the race depended on their willingness to reproduce. Certainly, too, this development contributed to the "natural" beauty standard that would emerge in the next century, and it afforded new license for public concern about and display of the female body. Fat in the blood, fat on the body, and a new physicality had become the hallmarks of the American female ideal.[30]

The rise of feminism in the last quarter of the nineteenth century reinforced this image of vigorous femininity. Women were joining reform societies or were going into the overcrowded, dirty cities, to help spread education and middle-class values to the "teeming masses" who had landed on their shores. This was work for confident, energetic, and imposing women. The Junoesque ideal was a stylized, eroticized, and refined version of the imposing, capable woman.

On the other hand, she was also an oddly refined version of the voluptuous stage beauties who often were the courtesans of the unprudish and expanding demimonde. These women, the mistresses—and sometimes eventually the wives—of rich and middle-class men, enjoyed liberties not accorded their bourgeois sisters, and they seemed to be threatening the domestic sanctuary. They, too, influenced the new ideal, and the slow infusion of their subculture into mainstream culture would be an important dynamic in later standards of beauty. Many of their freedoms—smoking, drinking, and the use of cosmetics and contraceptives—would soon be claimed by a new generation of women.[31]

Throughout this period, body fat had profoundly positive associations which we in the twentieth century have either inverted or rejected. On the one hand, it resonated with the amorous, erotic plenitude of the theater world, which was becoming more gay and uninhibited in the post–Civil War years— much to the consternation of many middle-class reformers. For the middle classes, it had different associations. It symbolized a lofty, comforting maternalism, a placidity and sweetness also captured by Renoir's nudes. Americans still believed that the female sex was made of finer clay than the male, that women upheld all that was best in civilization. This belief in the differences between the sexes was the basis of the suffragettes' demand for the vote and is the fundamental difference between early and modern feminism. As one suffragette told a congressional committee in 1884, "Without the purity, the spirituality, and the love of women," political institutions were "apt to become coarse and brutal." Middle-class women mothered their children and their husbands, and with their many reform organizations, they also tried to mother society. Their fully fleshed bodies resonated with the sweetness of the ideal mother.[32]

More generally, abundant flesh symbolized all that was best in middle-class life, especially its comfortable prosperity. The dignified paunch of a successful businessman bespoke a similarly well-cushioned savings account. Throughout this period, fat was explicitly equated with money, and the body was described as the bank. An excess of body fat, one writer of the period explained, was a "snug balance in the body bank and a comfortable reserve in the case of emergencies." Expenditure of energy, which burned fat, was equated in popular and medical language with withdrawals from one's savings account. A well-cushioned body was evidence of thriftiness. It was also equated with great reserves of energy. In 1908 *Harper's Bazaar* explained to its readers that "fat is force and stored up fat is stored up force." For the wives of successful men, fat was a "silken layer," its prestige underlined by the French terms used to describe it, *avoirdupois* and *embonpoint.*[33]

Even more, plumpness symbolized a clean, temperate life. Thinness was now identified with the unsavory side of romantic excess, with degeneracy and lack of control of the animal passions. The femme fatale's slenderness reflected her evil, dangerous nature. Thinness was not ethereal. It was Satanic. In contrast, plumpness bespoke decency, calm, and dignity.[34]

But already, in the midst of this generous environment, lay the seeds of its demise. Contrary trends were also emerging. New attitudes toward food slowly developed. On the one hand, the "civilizing of appetite" accelerated as the standards of elite French cuisine became more accessible through the proliferation of cookbooks. They spread information not just about what the elite ate but also about how they ate. Cookbooks for the better-off classes included vital sections on etiquette, place settings, and manners. As Americans became more eager to take their cues from French chefs, the culinary rules began to change. They were moving toward smaller and shorter meals.

On the other hand, a competing concern about healthy food and proper eating also mounted in this period. Historian Stephen Mennell astutely observed that English and American cookbooks of the nineteenth century showed a relative lack of interest in the pleasurable aspects of eating, in contrast to their counterparts in France. They stressed plain, simple country fare and economy instead of the epicurean relish evident even in French cookbooks aimed at the middle classes. Republican America held an even stronger prejudice against such "French fanciness" than did the British, one that American Protestantism, with its distrust of bodily appetites, ingrained deeply in the American psyche, though this was more characteristic of the Yankee North than of the South. Food was for sustenance, not for pleasuring the senses. In addition, America still had its dietary reformers, the prophets of "dietetic righteousness," the heirs of antebellum reformers.

These strains in America's culinary traditions were powerfully reinforced in the late nineteenth century when the concept of "scientific eating" emerged along with early discoveries about nutrition. Wilbur Atwater of Yale University, who led the movement in this country, determined the exact amount of calories and nutrients needed for health and efficiency. Taste, texture, color, and other qualities were stripped from food, which became, simply, units of energy. Middle-class reformers recommended economical meals for the poor based on Atwater's discoveries, and they believed similar standards would ensure the health and well-being of their own offsping. Cooking schools began to appear in the northeastern cities where the new professionals, scientific nutritionists—Fanny Farmer among them—taught and began to publish their ideas in increasingly popular books that would transform Americans' culinary habits and attitudes. They bequeathed to us their rather puritanical, ascetic attitudes toward food under the guise of health. In succeeding years, the notion of "proper eating," like the definition of "thinness," would be endlessly refined and redefined.[35]

Perhaps the most dramatic change in food attitudes was caused by Henry Tanner. In 1880 he began a much-publicized forty-two day fast in New York City under the supervision of "irregular physicians." He was testing the limits of man's ability to go without food. His experiment was widely publicized and eagerly followed. The New York *Daily Tribune* called it a "Starvation Comedy," a "wrestling match with the invisible fiend of hunger." Physicians who generally believed human beings could survive only twelve to fifteen days without food, were shocked by Tanner's demonstration that they literally could go without anything but water for such a long time. This was a stunning revelation, one that would influence medical opinions about how much food people needed to function effectively. From the 1880s until World War I, "hunger artists" captivated American and European audiences. They entertained with their feats of self-discipline and were immortalized in Kafka's story, "The Hunger Artist." They bequeathed to the future the awareness that periods of scant meals—and sometimes, even, no meals—would not necessarily jeopardize health.[36]

In the same period, anorexia nervosa came to the attention of medical authorities and was attributed to neurotic pathology. The idea of obesity as a nervous disturbance was first discussed in the French literature of the late nineteenth century, most notably in G. Leven's, *L'Obesité et Son Traitment.* Almost simultaneously, anorexia nervosa was diagnosed and named for the first time. Dr. C. Lasègue in France (1873) and Dr. William Gull (1874) in

England published articles describing adolescents with the perplexing disorder. Fasting women, of course, were not a new phenomenon. We saw them as "holy anorexics" in an earlier era, and in subsequent eras there had been "Miraculous Maidens" such as the Fasting Girl of Couflens in the seventeenth century, and some seventeenth-, eighteenth- and early-nineteenth-century medical literature described vaguely similar cases.

In part, the new diagnosis reflected the emergence of psychology as a discipline and the recategorization of diseases. Indeed, Tanner's fast was inspired by the fierce controversy raging over Mollie Fancher, a young invalid who claimed she did not eat. While many believed her—particularly those associated with the evangelical Protestant churches, Spiritualism, and Catholicism—the medical community, particularly the emerging neurologists, derided her as an impostor. Tanner believed in the soul's independence from physical functions and intended to prove the medical men wrong. A profound issue was at stake: Was the fasting woman a religiously inspired saint or a medical patient? In a secularizing age, when the boundaries of popular religion were consistently being eroded by science, the outcome was inevitable. She was a patient, suffering from nervous disorders.[37]

The new diagnosis was also a response to an increasing incidence of fasting girls from the middle classes and it seems likely that the disease emerged because of newly evolved constraints about eating and new tensions within the bourgeois family. It did not emerge in a period when "thin was in."

What motivated these adolescents from the comfortable classes to starve themselves? Of course, unlike today, the disease was quite rare. In this period, the most common psychological disorder among women was hysteria, which several modern scholars have characterized as an exaggeration, almost a parody, of the period's ideal of femininity. As we have seen, the "civilizing of manners" that was occurring involved the refinement or privatization of animal functions. Eating was one of them. By the late nineteenth century dining had become an even more refined art and bourgeois family life revolved around long, sociable meals in which proprieties were carefully observed. Good breeding involved self-control and restraint of bodily urges. As Norbert Elias argued, the civilizing process can work so effectively on youngsters that their inhibitions actually manage to anesthetize the drives themselves. Or else, in a passionate youngster who is being taught such behavior codes, these natural drives can be so diverted that "their energies find only unwanted release through bypasses, in compulsive actions and other symptoms of disturbance." In short, the civilizing process, by setting up a standard of behavior that requires rigid control of instinctual life, creates behavioral disorders. Quite possibly, the special diets advocated for children—bland and rife with foods that might not taste good but were "good for you"—also helped turn eating into a more highly charged adolescent issue than it had been.[38]

Historian Joan Jacobs Brumberg persuasively argues that developments within the bourgeois family—prolonged adolescence which caused prolonged dependency on parents, fewer children which resulted in intensified emotional relations between parents and children, and increasing pressures on young women to "marry well"—could generate their own psychopathology. The importance of family meals and the growing equation between food and love encouraged a young woman to express her unhappiness through food refusal. It was an emotionally charged act that aroused intense parental concern but did not violate the canons of behavior appropriate for a Victorian girl. It was "discreet, quiet, and ladylike, in keeping with the Victorian notion that women were expected to 'carry reserve further than the male.' " Anorexia nervosa was not yet linked to an expressed desire for slender beauty.[39]

More general trends emerged in this period which heralded change, just as the opulent ideal was at its peak. Fashion began moving in a new direction. In 1894 the Gibson Girl, drawn by Charles Dana Gibson, made her appearance and rapidly became the new epitome of American beauty. She was taller, younger, and more slender than the ideal she replaced, in part because her skirt was narrowing and straightening into a line that had not been seen since the 1820s. She also gave the first hints of athleticism incorporated into fashion. The new taste had spread so much that when Sarah Bernhardt returned to the United States in 1900, no one ridiculed her. And it had spread enough for reducing diets to begin appearing as an adjunct to fashion. In 1897 Lillian Russell, who now reputedly tipped the scales at 200 pounds, began the first of a long series of well-publicized diets. Nasty reviews comparing her to a white elephant presumably prompted her efforts.

But the Gibson Girl did not approach our body standards. She was still bent in an exaggerated S-curve, and she still displayed the voluptuous bust and buttocks the century favored. Theater managers still preferred actresses whose hips were larger than their ample busts. The immensely popular Florodoras, the chorus girls in a smash musical hit of 1900, were chosen for their beauty and their perfect figures. They were all 5'4" and weighed 130 pounds—somewhat less than had been deemed desirable for the Junoesque woman but certainly more than we consider desirable today. Nor did this slenderizing trend undermine all the old comfortable associations with plumpness.[40]

There were other disturbing portents in the late Victorian period. Plumpness may have been in, but at the same time, there was a surprising emphasis on the exact shape and size of the female body. Even though that body was clothed, its unclothed dimensions had become remarkably important—much more so than in the early Victorian period, when only the waist was described so specifically. The human body was still a private affair, but it was becoming more public: Clothing hugged the natural form more tightly, and more detailed specifications were being made about its dimensions and its healthiness. At the same time, the sudden profusion of fancy underwear seemed to bring fashion concerns ever closer to the intimacy of the private self. Before the late Victorian period, women had worn only simple, unadorned linens close to their bodies. These developments, in a curious way, were heightened by the new concern about athleticism, about women developing healthy, robust, natural bodies. But these concerns about the body were no longer attached to religious motives as they had been in the first half of the century. They were slowly being unmoored from their religious foundations and attached to more secular goals. This combination of trends would have important repercussions in the next century.

5

The Thin Preference Begins:
1900–1947

Rather suddenly, in 1908, the voluptuous hourglass figure fell out of favor. It was replaced by a body type closer to the one we admire today: slender, long-limbed, and relatively straight. We don't often see such radical shifts in popular taste. Paul Poiret, an up-and-coming Paris designer, proudly took credit for this transformation, which he believed was liberating for women.

In 1908 he introduced his sleek, "natural" look, soon called neo-Empire, and by 1910 it had become the fashionable silhouette. Poiret banished the S-curve, the exaggerated hips, and the voluminous skirts and petticoats of the past, and with them the Junoesque breasts and shoulders cherished by the Edwardians. "From now on, the breasts will no longer be worn," Madame Poiret recalled her husband announcing. Most startling of all, he banished the tiny waist women and men had revered as the acme of erotic beauty. Erotic focus was shifting from the waist and the breast to the leg which, in the words of one surprised *Vogue* writer, had "suddenly become fashionable . . . . The long skirt reveals plainly every line and curve of the leg from the hip to the ankle." Her surprise was understandable. Never before in the history of European fashion had the leg been so exposed or been the explicit focus of interest.[1]

Like a caterpillar emerging from its cocoon, woman appeared metamorphosed. By 1908 *Vogue* was using adjectives that we would come to know all too well: "How slim, how graceful, how elegant women look," it proclaimed. Slimness was becoming synonymous with grace and elegance, and for the first time, the body underneath had to be slim without the aid of rigid body-shaping undergarments. Poiret had brought the female body closer to the surface of clothes. The lower body, once kept private and hidden beneath outer garments, petticoats, and stays, suddenly became more exposed and more public. These dual changes created women's first struggles with weight reduction. Dieting would become Beauty's most indispensable handmaiden.[2]

Though the neo-Empire style of clothing passed, the radical change in body aesthetics it had given form to did not. Indeed, after World War I the taste for slenderness became more firmly entrenched. Even when the hourglass shape reappeared, the preference for slenderness did not fade. It rooted itself more firmly in American culture.

Why did this happen? Where did Poiret get the idea of setting up a curveless, slim ideal? And why did the public accept it and abandon deeply ingrained ideas about propriety, modesty, and beauty?

Fashion rarely shifts without some warning or internal consistency, and in some ways the public was ready to accept the new style. The trend away from voluminous skirts had begun gradually in the 1880s and accelerated in the 1890s, when the bodice and sleeves became the focus of attention. By the early 1900s this elaboration, too, was spent, and several dress designers, not just Poiret, were moving toward a new visual image. Simultaneously, specialized sporting clothes for women and the increasing popularity of the "tailor-made suit"—a feminine version of the male uniform—were tending toward this same reduction in volume.[3]

These two radical innovations—the preference for slenderness and the new exposure of the female body—were also responses to much deeper cultural changes which were altering perceptions of the human body and social roles and influencing ideas about behavior and health as well as aesthetics. They set the framework for what would become, as one writer put it, "the century of svelte." Indeed, in the first half of the twentieth century, the culture of slimming was slowly constructed.[4]

Between 1880 and 1920 life in America and western Europe was revolutionized, propelling society into the modern age. Industrialization, mechanization, and mass production produced the systems, the perceptions, the mentality, and the artifacts of the present: the bicycle, the streetcar, the automobile, the airplane, and the phonograph, moving pictures, and the telephone. Domestic life—at least for the upper and middle classes—was transformed by indoor plumbing, flush toilets, central heating, and the electric light bulb. With them also came new personal freedoms. Progress appeared limitless. With the machine as its weapon, humanity seemed to be on its way to mastering nature, defying ancient limitations of time and space, and producing a new sense of freedom and mobility.[5]

These new images directly influenced aesthetic standards and body ideals. Artists became enchanted with the machine and with speed, motion, and pure energy, and the developing crafts of photography and motion pictures gave them new insights into movement. Eadweard Muybridge's slow-speed pictures of a galloping horse revealed for the first time the details of successive movement. To capture this line of action became an aesthetic ideal, one that favored economy of form and disdained the opulence and extravagance of the past.

Line, energy, and action also explicitly entered the language of fashion. By the 1920s one observer noted that the chic look had become a "kinetic silhouette" based on the "principle of movement." From mechanical engineering to art to fashion, the technological age was creating new standards for the human body.[6]

Growing industrialization reinforced aesthetic principles. A slenderer human body could not only be beautiful, but serviceable and healthful as well, and doctors and home economists such as Juliet Corson, Sarah Tyson Rorer, and Fanny Farmer began to advocate thinner—if by no means attenuated— figures. There were direct attacks on fat, though with nothing like the intensity that was to come. Dr. Emma E. Walker explained in her *Ladies' Home Journal* "Pretty Girl Papers" in 1905 that it was better to be too thin than too plump because "excess fat" "makes one heavy and awkward." Susanna Cocroft, an influential beauty and health writer, agreed. "A woman," she explained, "over-burdened with flesh, untidy in outline, suggesting physical overindulgence, in a neat, tidy, attractive, artistic home, is like a cheap chromo in an expensive handwrought frame."[7]

Concerns about the body reflected concerns about the country, which was seen as suffering from overproduction and inefficient consumption. It seems paradoxical that in this era when underconsumption troubled the economy, the ideal body became more slender. But the paradox is more superficial than real. For the new and apparently permanent productivity profoundly changed economic theories. Historically, scarcity had been the economic threat. Now, Americans had abundance, but they learned that abundance could pose its own set of serious economic problems. It had to be carefully regulated. This truth was underscored for manufacturers, who found the quantity of their goods on the market, combined with fierce competition, reduced prices so much that they faced financial losses. It was underscored for Americans in general, who saw the phenomenal growth of big-business monopolies and trusts as danger-ous. There *could* be too much of everything. It is perfectly consistent that in this period, experts also began to talk about the dangers of overnutrition, of the body being as glutted as the marketplace.

In short, technological innovations, economic changes, and the ideology of efficiency all conspired to reinforce the slenderized ideal. The human body— both male and female—was to be as efficient, as effective, as economical, and as beautiful as the sleek new machines, as the rationalized workplace. It was these turn-of-the-century developments that forged the society we know today and that established the framework for our prejudice against fat.

Side by side with society's new perception of itself came new images of women and new standards about their behavior. With the rise of feminism in the 1870s, women had started going to college; by the 1890s they were, in a small way, breaking into professions like medicine, law, and journalism, and were marching for the right to vote. As described in chapter 4, middle-class women organized into groups that crusaded for moral and social reform, and they went into the slums and schools of their mushrooming, urban jungles to educate immigrants and help them learn middle-class habits and virtues. At the same time, young women joined the labor force in unprecedented and ever-increasing numbers. In the last third of the nineteenth century, the number of women with jobs outside the home tripled. They worked as nurses and teachers, in offices and the new department stores. The expanding economy and expanding professional horizons for women combined with feminist sentiment to bring women out of the domestic arena. In 1911 the most popular woman's magazine of the day, *Woman's Home Companion,* underscored the change with its new editor, Gertrude Battles Lane, who announced a new editorial policy. Women, she wrote, were "sensitive, thinking beings with many interests outside the home," and she promised that the magazine would address these larger concerns.[8]

Simultaneously, women were enjoying a new physical freedom. Gone, or going, were the days when doctors feared exertion would harm the delicate body of the Steel Engraving Lady and when fashion decreed it ungenteel to move vigorously or enthusiastically. The physical-culture movement had taken hold among America's upper and middle-classes, and the women's colleges were among its strongest proponents. Dress reformers and feminists contributed to this trend. They encouraged the emergence of a new woman whose beauty would be characterized by health, naturalness, and athleticism. They organized into groups, such as the Rational Dress Society and vehemently criticized the unhealthiness of fashionable styles—especially the corset—that prevented women from being physically active.

Athleticism was not simply endorsed by doctors and reformers; it had become fashionable among the elite. Between the 1870s and the 1890s, women began playing tennis and golf, swimming, and horseback riding. By the 1890s, despite fears among many about the effect it might have on women's reproductive organs, bicycling became the rage. Even social dancing had changed. The patterns of glides and turns that had dominated the ballroom suddenly gave way to the maxxie, the cakewalk, the turkey trot, the tango and, in 1912, the fox-trot. They were first danced, not in the ballroom, but in the burgeoning urban dance halls by working-class women and men; from there, they slowly moved up the social ladder. A generation of young people were initiated into a dance style that called for a vigor and agility akin to what was demanded in fashionable sports.

In part, the banishment of corsets and petticoats was a response to the new need for more practical—or, since practicality has rarely been a high fashion priority, at least for less unwieldy—clothing. Voluminous petticoats could be cumbersome in small working spaces, and they projected an image of domestic femininity that didn't seem to fit in the workplace. The tailored suit or shirtwaist and skirt came to be preferred because it suggested the same sobriety as men's tailored suits. But couturier styles were designed for the elite, not for lower- or even middle-class women. The new style responded to their needs as well, particularly their new conceptions of the female body.

As always, the public images of women reflected private images. The Gibson Girl was celebrated not only as a symbol of vitality and practicality but also as a new standard of beauty and erotic allure neither delicate and ethereal, nor matronly, like her predecessors, but young, vigorous, and independent. As one beauty writer observed, the "fat" woman had symbolized the family; the new slender woman symbolized "youth" and projected a "disquieting and alert glamour." The Gibson Girl evoked the feeling that active participation in courtship and its consequences was a pleasure for women, not just a duty or a path to motherhood.[9]

Yet again, as was to happen increasingly, the medical community came by different paths to endorse the dictates of fashion and aesthetics. While throughout the nineteenth century slenderness had been associated with sickness and fragility, now many health authorities cautioned against overeating and excess weight. Middle-aged stoutness no longer earned unequivocal praise; it had become cause for concern. As early as 1897 Dr. Charles Purdy of Harvard had warned in the respectable and widely read *North American Review* that "well-to-do Americans" had a tendency to be "unduly stout as they arrive at middle age." He attributed the problem to a set of factors that have become a litany in our own day. They ate too much "meat, starch and sugar," and they had "sedentary habits"—that is, they didn't get enough exercise. Ten years later, the *Atlantic Monthly* ran an article "On Growing Fat," which underlined that *stoutness,* once a complimentary term for people of all ages, had become at best ambiguous, at worst an "obnoxious adjective, barely tolerable as a noun." It certainly no longer described someone who was healthy. It was no longer even necessary to say people were "unduly" stout. Stout itself now described a condition of excess.[10]

The growing medical bias against fat did not emerge because Americans suddenly were in fact getting fatter. Available statistics indicate they were not. What changed were perceptions about how much fat was too much. Nor was this emerging bias the result of new medical breakthroughs. And it was not universally shared by the medical profession—yet. The turn of the century was a transition period, and older, positive notions about fatness coexisted, albeit uncomfortably, with the new negative notions. But there was a developing industry that legitimized the new cultural undercurrents condemning fatness and that spearheaded the attack against it: the insurance companies.

Life insurance had been virtually unknown before 1840, and by 1874 there were still only about 850,000 policies in force. In the next two decades, the industry experienced a rapid, if unruly, growth. It also became the subject of frequent government investigations as scandals erupted because policyholders' premiums often were used for highly speculative investments. By 1907 considerable regulatory legislation had been enacted, and the companies had to reorganize themselves along more conservative and "rational" lines. Their profits were now more dependent on selling premiums to a wider market and making sure that they sold primarily to people who would not die prematurely. Yet, screening applicants for low-risk life-styles proved difficult: How often someone engaged in dangerous behavior could not be gauged easily. The insurance companies began looking instead for simple health measurements that would predict, at least statistically, good health, which for them was quite simply an indicator of good business. Dr. Oscar Rogers of the New York Life Insurance Company began these investigations in the late 1890s, and although he had found that underweight applicants also suffered premature mortality, and even that tall people seemed to as well, he focused instead on the mortality connected with overweight, and it was this finding that was widely disseminated and that shaped the direction of future research. As Dr. Brandeth Symonds, another physician affiliated with the insurance industry, explained in 1909, the relationship between body weight and health had "had no commercial significance until insurance companies came into existence."[11]

In 1909, just a year after the appearance of Poiret's revolutionary designs, Dr. Symonds ceremoniously announced to a conference of doctors that all the old notions about the beneficence of fat were wrong. The idea that stored fat was as good as savings in the bank was unequivocally false. Statistical studies of insured lives, Symonds explained, demonstrated that being overweight—whether from muscle or fat—was a liability, not an asset for people entering middle age. It was not a "storehouse of strength" or of stored up force but a burden that had to be nourished and one that increased the risks of early mortality and of a host of diseases. He warned that being overweight, even 10 percent above the average, "universally shortens life." Five years later the Actuarial Society of America and the Association of Life Insurance Medical Directors published their own investigations on the mortality experience of 700,000 policyholders insured between 1885 and 1908. The results confirmed these earlier studies. And so, the insurance companies codified and endorsed the new trend toward slenderness.[12]

These increasingly influential ideas about fat translated the disparate conclusions and quests of the health community into sets of absolute statistics that came to seem like the benchmarks by which society must measure itself.

Unfortunately, the statistical methods and models the insurance companies used had serious flaws, and these flaws were grafted onto the perceptions that resulted. Their sample was limited to the privileged few wealthy enough to buy life insurance, and they did not form a very representative group in the population, tending to be white, Protestant, middle-class, and from the Eastern-seaboard cities. And, since life insurance was not yet a familiar commodity nor part of a prudent man's portfolio, the typical policyholder most likely was not typical at all. Furthermore, as Dr. Symonds admitted, there was a built-in bias in their results since thin applicants had been more carefully screened and more thoroughly examined than fatter ones because of the equation between slenderness and the main killers of the nineteenth century, the "wasting diseases." There were few female policyholders so companies could only speculate, on the basis of their findings for males, on women's average weights and on the effects of excess weight. Policyholders were weighed only when they bought their policies, so if they died twenty years later, their weight would be recorded as what it had been two decades earlier, with no adjustment made for gains in the interim. Variables such as clothing were not taken into account, and only about half the applicants were actually weighed, while very unreliable estimated weights were recorded for all the others. Yet, weight had suddenly come to have a significance it had never had before. Gradually, the scale (introduced in standard forms during the 1890s but widely available only in later decades) became the symbol of the medical examination, an image immortalized on some of Norman Rockwell's *Saturday Evening Post* covers.[13]

The new body standards affected everyone. By 1914 a writer for *Living Age* magazine noted with puzzlement that a "cult of slimness" had taken hold. Men, such as former President Taft (who weighed 355 pounds at his inauguration) and Kaiser Wilhelm III, whose ample girth had once earned them the admiring title of "big men" now found themselves trying to slim down so they would not be called "fat men." But as usual, women, pressured by fashion as well as by aesthetics and medicine, responded more acutely to the trend. Between 1894, when Charles Dana introduced the Gibson Girl, and 1907, when Poiret heralded a more attenuated silhouette, dieting became an ever-deepening habit for American women. Diet was both what you didn't eat and what you did eat, and the burgeoning science of nutrition buttressed the new craze.[14]

It was not just body size that became smaller in this period. Experts, with efficiency and economy in mind, began trying to determine the minimum amounts and kinds of food necessary for optimal functioning. The calorie was still a new concept, but in the 1880s German researchers were discovering how many calories people burned when they were at rest and when they were engaged in various activities. Following their lead, the American scientist, Wilbur Atwater, conducted his own experiments and concluded that a moderately active person needed the equivalent of 3,000 to 3,600 calories, including 120 to 130 grams of protein, a day. (Atwater converted his findings into food weights since calories were still unknown to the general public.) He concluded that anything beyond this quantity was unnecessary, self-indulgent, and ultimately wasteful. Atwater was not interested in weight reduction. A product of the age of efficiency experts and progressive reformers, his goal was to determine what he called the "pecuniary economy of food"—that is, the precise amount of fuel a person needed to work effectively—and he wanted to determine the cheapest way people could supply themselves with the necessary fuel. Atwater charged that the poor went hungry out of profligacy and ignorance, not poverty, and claimed that if they bought the cheapest nutritional equivalent of tasty foods, they could feed themselves amply. By the turn of the century Atwater had managed to set new nutritional standards for the nation, standards that were endorsed and promulgated by the Department of Agriculture and the new "scientific" cooks.[15]

But Atwater's standards did not remain in force for long. By 1905 physiologist Russell H. Chittenden of Yale had published the results of his own investigations, and he argued that Atwater had grossly overestimated the amount of energy and protein needed by humans and grossly underestimated the amount of fruits and vegetables required. He reduced the recommended protein allotment by half and, anticipating many of the gurus of our own age, he also advised that vegetables, fruit, and milk replace the heavy breakfasts, meat, and bread ordinarily consumed by Americans. Experts did not accept Chittenden's recommendations as readily as they had accepted Atwater's, but by the 1920s Chittenden's standards had replaced Atwater's in medical textbooks.[16]

Atwater and Chittenden were not particularly concerned with overweight, but their findings nonetheless marked an important turning point in cultural attitudes toward food. Like the insurance companies, they were establishing scientific standards about what had once seemed to be personal and nonscientific matters—body weight and food habits. Through both, food became an instrument of science, stripped down to a quantity of energy and deprived of all its sensual and emotional aspects. Indeed, it was Chittenden who first listed nutritional recommendations in terms of calories instead of grams, ounces, and other weights. These attitudes, also promulgated by the increasingly influential home economists like Fanny Farmer, reinforced the Puritan strain in America's culinary tradition, and this heritage was bequeathed to us.

If Americans in the pre-War period were not yet familiar with calories, they nonetheless had begun their battle to lose weight, combining old and—increasingly—new methods. Among these were the Banting diet and various regimens, such as apple and barley, tea and toast, or rice and date diets, which had once passed as remedies for dyspepsia. They tried to avoid saturated fats because already at the turn of the century, it was believed that they were heavy and hard to digest and that they accumulated in the intestines and even in the appendix. If these efforts didn't work, the overweight tried fasting, a practice that was no longer looked upon as dangerous.

They didn't limit themselves to diet. Although exercise was not regarded as a particularly useful weight-reduction technique—it was said to stimulate appetite—they did try moderate exercises like "rolling," which literally involved rolling on the floor to work off, or at least redistribute, extra flesh. Women also tried an assortment of other techniques designed to attack not appetite, but the fat itself. They massaged themselves with "obesity-removing creams" (known since at least the sixteenth century), tried electrotherapy, applied mineral salts, drank sour milk, or took three hot baths a day to "melt" off their fat. They could even buy the "famous medicated rubber garments" advertised in *Vogue* in 1912, which promised to "reduce your flesh" through their special "scientific properties." And they used emetics and laxatives which did not cause alarm as it would in later decades, for they were venerable remedies for disease and had been staples of traditional medicine.[17]

Though most weight-reduction techniques were old forms turned to new ends, two innovations did appear. The most popular was "fletcherizing," a method of slow mastication named after its inventor, Horace Fletcher, who claimed he had reduced his own 205-pound, 5'5½" frame to 169 pounds by using this method. The ideal Fletcherite was exemplified by a kindergarten teacher who in 1909 reported that she devoted "twenty minutes daily to the serving and enjoyment of a single cracker." Fletcher himself was a flamboyant and unusually fit character, and his system became famous when his feats of physical strength were widely publicized. It captivated even such illustrious figures as William and Henry James. Its popularity, however, was due as much to its other purported benefits as to its weight-reducing effects. It could reputedly strengthen and fatten up the puny as well as cure constipation—a dreaded disability of the era—"indigestion, bleeding piles, catarrh, pimpled skin and a variety of other ailments."[18]

The other new technique for weight loss stemmed from medical developments and reflected the muddled alliance between medicine and diet-mania that would become such a pronounced feature of our own times. Endocrinology was just coming into its own at the turn of the century, and researchers discovered that thyroid extract, mixed with iodine, could cause weight loss. As a result, thyroid-fucus pills became widely touted as a cure for obesity after 1893.

New research in metabolism and endocrinology suggested that thyroid extract was an ideal solution because experts of the period differentiated between types of obesity. Metabolic studies had indicated that some people burned calories at a faster rate than others, so experts divided obesity into two types: exogenous and endogenous. The two were regarded as quite different, and the difference seemed to be gender related. Exogenous obesity, generally associated with men, was caused by overeating and underexercising. Such fat people, who were typically characterized as "cheerful and responsive," with firm muscles and vigorous hearts, were easy to treat: "Prescribe lean beef, laxatives and golf." Endogenous obesity presented a gloomier picture. It was generally associated with women who were characterized as "sad" or "sour" and burdened with flaccid muscles and feeble hearts. Their chances for slimming were poor. The theory held that they were fat because of glandular problems, and thyroid pills presumably corrected the malfunction, making the sluggish body burn calories more quickly and efficiently. The fat woman, then, was not entirely responsible for her overweight condition. She was a victim of glandular abnormality.[19]

In short, Americans had begun a quest that would prove to be more frustrating than they ever imagined—getting their bodies to fit a standard size.

After World War I, the diet impulse spread in part because all those modernizing trends that had begun at the turn of the century and that encouraged a slenderized body accelerated. Earlier, positive associations with plumpness were further undermined. The link between fat and potential energy was turned upside down, replaced by the conviction that fat was linked with lethargy, laziness, and slovenliness. By 1931 Dr. Alonzo Taylor, writing in the *Scientific Monthly,* took as a given that "stout persons usually feel, and look, less fit." The drive toward slenderness also spread because researchers were finding more connections between obesity and premature mortality. The insurance companies reconfirmed their earlier findings in 1919, 1923, 1929, 1932, and 1937, and other studies began to relate obesity specifically to diabetes, hypertension, arteriosclerosis, and heart disease, all of which were increasing at alarming rates. By 1920 neurasthenia had ceased to be a legitimate medical concept, and with its departure from standard diagnoses went the perception that extreme thinness was a neurotic condition that should be combatted by weight gain. These developments can be explained as much by the cultural prejudices now attached to weight—which influenced both medical judgments and the direction of scientific research—as by the fact that more people were surviving to an age when they became both fatter and more vulnerable to degenerative diseases.[20]

The standards instituted by the medical and insurance communities were becoming more accessible and widely disseminated. The reorganization of the medical profession, with physicians now needing state licenses and board certification, along with new discoveries in medicine, had elevated the esteem in which doctors were held. They also had shown that one's state of health could be measured accurately only with special tools that revealed the secret, inner workings of the body: the stethoscope, the blood-pressure cup, and the laboratory microscope. After the War, the idea spread that people should have annual checkups so that doctors could assess these mysterious inner workings. At the same time, the insurance industry was enjoying an explosive growth as more industries and businesses bought health insurance and more individuals bought life insurance. Getting insured usually meant getting examined, and getting examined included getting weighed. As the health industry took on its modern configuration, health precepts spread among the public.[21]

The public was touched by weight standards in other ways as well. Penny scales, introduced at the turn of the century, became enormously popular. In 1927 the *New York Times* reported that the penny scales made millions— 40,000 of them had registered 500,000,000 weights in just one year. By 1932 even small, out-of-the-way towns had them, and one scale company reported that in a town of 3,500, with only two penny scales, there were 1,000 weighings a month. Weighing onself was becoming a national habit.[22]

Still, it was the heavy hand of fashion that did the most to reinforce and exacerbate weight consciousness, and therefore women were again the primary audience. Following the War, Poiret's slender style evolved into the boyish look of the flapper. Skirts shortened to calf length, waists loosened and lowered to the hip, breasts were to be flat and were often bound to make them seem small, and women discarded one of the most cherished marks of their sex— their long hair. The body under these clothes, ideally, had a "serpentine slimness." For the first, but not the last time, fashion suppressed the female shape, exalting instead boyish or prepubescent forms.

In setting up this ideal, fashion was again responding to larger aesthetic trends that made curves and fleshiness hopelessly passé. After the War, that perplexing movement, modernism, gathered momentum, pursuing lines of development begun before the War. While most middle-class people found themselves hopelessly befuddled by abstractionism, dadaism, surrealism, and the other "isms" that emerged, they set the aesthetic tone for the twentieth century and in diluted form saturated popular culture. Painters were among the most prominent exponents of the new views, and they were engaged in a bold search for what they thought of as essential forms. In the hands of Picasso, Mondrian, and Modigliani, the female nude became a series of lines, angles, or curves. In architecture and design, the Bauhaus movement, begun officially in 1919 with Walter Gropius at its head, elevated the functional and the practical, the ultrarational and technological. Artistic fascination with speed and energy continued. In creating what seemed to be a practical, sinuous look, fashion was responding to these new tastes.

In setting up a slender ideal, fashion also seemed to be performing one of its more venerable functions: competitive display of social status. In a curious inversion of popular imagery, the poor and lower classes began to be seen as stocky and plump rather than as thin and undernourished—or rather, plumpness began to be associated more insistently with the lower classes, particularly with female Jewish and Italian immigrants. Although America restricted immigration in the twenties, the ensconcement of earlier immigrants into society adumbrated the need to distinguish the patrician "native" from foreign interlopers.

This new preference for slenderness and the cult of the flapper also mirrored other social developments which both echoed those of the 1830s and anticipated those of the 1960s. Among these were an idealization of youth, cultural and social upheaval, and transformations in the image of women. The young, particularly the newly booming collegiate generation, were becoming a distinct and self-conscious cultural group. They were also becoming the trendsetters. Contemporaries acknowledged that "youth rules the world today and in no phase of life is it more apparent than in fashion." The new breed of young woman was often either a free-spirited college girl or a cynical and freewheeling sophisticate. Either way, she was picking up her newly exposed knees and casting off the shackles of gentility. The swirling nightlife of the working classes, with their dance halls and speakeasies and abandoned behavior, seemed to be invading the citadels of middle-class respectability through the young generation, who now demanded personal freedom, personal happiness, and fulfillment. Young women, in part intentionally, shocked the staid and respectable by smoking, by drinking bootleg liquor, by their passion for provocative dances, by their immodest styles, and even by wearing makeup: Only women of easy virtue had done these things in the past. And they cultivated everything but innocence. The youthful look was not supposed to be naive and pure; rather it was supposed to convey worldliness and sophistication, a casual insolence, and above all (and most shocking of all), a titillating sexuality.[23]

The serpentine slimness that at the turn of the century had been associated with the femme fatale—the dangerous but exciting vamp with an insatiable appetite for money, power, and sex, the exotic outlaw who enticed men to their ruin—had suddenly become mainstream and fashionable. The young flappers tried to cultivate this flavor of exotic and mysterious sexuality portrayed so well on the silent screen by Theda Bara, Pola Negri, and later by Greta Garbo. The term *sex appeal* entered the vernacular, and sex appeal, not modesty, demureness, or regal elegance became the goal for many women in both fashion and behavior.

With the popularization of Freudianism by such psychologists as Havelock Ellis and John Watson, the traditional Ideal Mother was being attacked in ways that encouraged this new sexualization of women. Many claimed that doting, "oversolicitous" mothers had created emotional invalidism among children. Watson charged that they overkissed and overwhelmed their offspring because they were channeling their repressed sexual hunger into them. According to these standards, sexuality was not imcompatible with maternalism. On the contrary, women had to be sexually expressive in order to be good mothers.

To many, these developments seemed to threaten the sanctity and security of the family. With personal fulfilment and expressiveness becoming paramount; values, duty, economic necessity and tradition no longer promised to cement the marital bond. Cultural authorities, from sociologists to fashion writers, painstakingly revised concepts about marriage in response to these changes. Affectional ties and personal fulfilment were now seen as the primary cement for the marital bond.

The standard for a model wife changed accordingly. She was sexualized. Women were urged to channel their energy into their marital relationships, not just into their children. They were advised to keep alive the romance of their courtship days, to be lovers, not mothers, to their husbands. This meant maintaining an alluring, slender form, and set the stage for our own generation's assumption that a woman's sexual attractiveness is one of the linchpins of her marriage, an ever-more powerful presumption in modern times. Women's magazines and manuals also shifted their emphasis accordingly. They no longer included just recipes and child-care suggestions. Now they also gave helpful hints about this new marital task. Florence Courtenay observed in her 1922 book, *Physical Beauty: How to Develop and Preserve It,* that "Physical beauty is a definite part of the feminine sex appeal. And a happy marriage *depends largely* on a normal and happy sex appeal on the part of the woman and a corresponding sex interest on the part of the man." Women reorganized their priorities.

It was not just that they were encouraged to be more sexual. They had been raised in homes that reflected new familial patterns and that cultivated in them expectations of intimacy and emotional fulfillment. For our purposes, what is most important about this change is that overt sexuality—the kind once associated with disreputable women—became part of the middle-class woman's currency and, in conjunction with this, new, more potent pressures were put on her to match prevailing physical standards.[24]

The model wife was now supposed to be the athletic, intellectual, and competitive equal of her husband. She was supposed to be his companion, befitting the new concept of "companionate marriage" that had been introduced by experts. The concept seemed eminently suited to the newly emancipated woman and, in fact, proved an ideal way to integrate her into the structure of the family. But it also meant that the desirable body would be slim and almost boyish, with sexual differentiation minimized. The young woman did not want a body that resonated with images of a mature, maternal woman, but rather one of a young companion-lover, full of the vibrant youthful energy of the flapper. If in the past a young married woman could swell gracefully into matronly contours and not compromise her charms, in the twenties she no longer had this luxury. Now she had to keep the slender attractiveness of her courting days. As one journalist acidly observed, a new popular book might easily have been entitled, *Fat or How I Lost My Husband.*[25]

The new styles, athleticism, and exposure of the body may have given women an exhilarating sense of freedom, but they had to pay a price for it. Their body measurements and weight became critical to judgments about their attractiveness. It was no coincidence that the first rudimentary Miss America contest, with contestants in bathing suits, was held in 1921 or that the winner's measurements have been carefully preserved.

And of course, with slenderness and the importance of measurement came dieting. This was especially true now that modern clothes had done away with most mechanical aids and undergarments. Instead, women had to diet or internalize, as scholar Valerie Steele put it, the constraints of the corset. Thin women who didn't meet the Junoesque ideal of the Belle Epoque had had the option of padding themselves, even though this was regarded as an unfortunate compromise. But with the twenties styles, the unfashionably plump had nowhere to hide nor any way to reform their extra flesh: Dieting was the only option.

The change was dramatic because, in essence, the new, revealing styles and the emphasis on the exact details of the body were blurring the distinction between private and public life, between private and public self. Corsets and voluminous skirts had kept the public and the private self quite separate, and they served as aids to woman as a "public" spectacle. What she was underneath did not affect her public presentation. Flesh remained a private affair—a fact underlined by the popular euphemism for male and female genitals: one's "privates." But with the new styles and the new willingness to scrutinize what was exposed, the private body came closer to the surface and, in essence, became part of public life.

We can speculate further about why slenderness and a rather androgynous look came into fashion just when female clothing became so revealing and when respectable women, rather suddenly, proclaimed their sexuality. Perhaps the bosom and hips could be emphasized tastefully in the previous era precisely because women were presumed to be sexually innocent. If the civilizing process entailed either refining or hiding in private "animal-like functions," the elaboration of sexual differentiations were safe and civilized precisely because the woman who exhibited them was not overtly sexual in other ways. The suggestiveness of her clothing and shape were simultaneously denied by her demureness and presumably unsexual nature. On the other hand, when women became more overtly sexual and exposed more of their bodies, this kind of amplitude might seem, in a sense, too blatant. Suppression of curves and of secondary sexual characteristics perhaps suggested that their sexuality was still under control, still subject to internal restraints, still "civilized." In some sense, their eroticism thus remained private, undisplayed. Certainly the vamp, even while she was supposedly thin because she was consumed by the intensity of her passions, remained absolute mistress over her sexuality. She used it to manipulate men, to exert power over them.[26]

A number of factors made this first powerful slenderness craze more widespread than any before it. Fashion standards were beginning to influence a wider audience. Postwar prosperity allowed more and more women to heed fashion's message, and that message was everywhere in the emerging mass media. Newspapers, magazines, and the fledgling film industry informed an ever-widening audience about current trends. The increasing availability of affordable, ready-made clothing also contributed to this dissemination and reinforced the growing notion of "standard" sizes and "normal" women. If standardized clothing didn't directly create an urge for slenderness, it did create a desire to meet whatever fashionable ideal happened to be in vogue. Traditionally, a woman had sewn her own dresses or had employed a seamstress who designed them to fit her particular shape, but now the woman had to fit the dress.

Indeed, every facet of life that affected women and their perceptions of themselves was becoming consolidated, industrialized, and commercialized. The new beauty industry was among the most potent forces. Paradoxically, along with "natural," "liberating" styles came a new acceptance of "unnatural" beauty aids like makeup. While the rich had always had their private hairdressers, manicurists, and cosmeticians, the middle classes generally had made do with home beauty aids whose ingredients could be bought from the druggist or the general store. But in the 1890s these services started being offered to the general public by enterprising specialists who opened their own shops and charged reasonable prices. After the War, this industry expanded. It made fashion available to more women, and it helped spread new concepts about beauty. The burgeoning advertising industry promoted the idea that any woman could transform herself into the fashionable ideal. Fashion had always issued this message, but in the twenties, there were some new themes. The heated debate so prevalent in the nineteenth-century women's press about how much beauty should come from inside, and so be natural, and how much a matter of artificiality all but disappeared. In part because of the new image of women, it was accepted that art—or science—were to be freely used.

In fact, science had come to the aid of beauty. The new array of cosmetics, hair treatments, skin creams, powders, and other paraphernalia were touted as being the result of scientific investigation and/or invention. As a result, they commanded some of the prestige and respect people then associated with science. More importantly, this association stimulated the belief that women had the ability to improve their appearance. Just as science manipulated nature for human needs, so it gave women the tools to create their own beauty. In the twenties *Vogue* assured it readers that at least 25 percent of a woman's loveliness was due to her intelligent use of these aids. Beauty no longer came just from within, from a noble spirit and a pure heart. At least in part, it could be manufactured. Another line between private and public, inner and outer, was blurred.[27]

Science came to the aid of dieters, too, and this period saw the emergence of two of the essential and enduring props of diet obsession: the scale and the calorie. Called by Christine Herrick, in her 1917 book, *Lose Weight and Be Well,* "a materialized conscience," the new home scale provided an impartial, scientific way to know the truth about how you looked. The numbers, of course, were abstractions, but gradually these abstractions would seem more real than how one actually looked. With nutrition emerging as a science, food became increasingly anatomized by researchers, and among the elements to be seriously calculated were calories. Counting calories was touted as "the scientific system of weight control." Dr. Lulu Hunt Peters, who became the era's best-known female physician, also wrote the first best-selling weight-loss book, *Diet and Health, with Key to the Calories,* in 1917. Her advice sounds depressingly contemporary. Start with a fast, she advised, and then proceed to 1,200 calories a day. After the fat was shed, the reducer was to start the "Maintenance Diet," and Dr. Peters sternly admonished that calorie counting had to continue for the rest of the reducer's life. In 1923 the *Delineator* introduced the concept of calories to its readers and emphasized, "If you want to reduce, you must count calories."[28]

One important effect of this new nutritional knowledge was that women now believed they *could* control their weight. Dr. Morris Fishbein, editor of the

Journal of the American Medical Association, underlined the impact of the new science of nutrition. "Before establishing our modern knowledge about diet," he wrote in 1934, "it was taken for granted that the shape anyone might have had been conferred on him by a wise Providence, and that the best one could do would be to make the best of it." This, it appeared, was no longer true. Now, Dr. Fishbein continued, "every woman knows that she can, with suitable modifications of her diet and by the proper use of exercise, cause the pounds to pass away." Scientific knowledge had given women new power to shape their figures, or so they thought.[29]

But it wasn't easy to follow the caloric recommendations, not when the number of calories believed necessary to sustain a dieter's life kept getting lower and lower. Dr. Peters had insisted on 1,200 calories. In 1928 physicians began advocating very low-calorie diets for those who were severely obese— 600–750 calories. Ten years later the diet recommended for this group was down to 400 calories a day. But physicians had been pre-empted by the fashion conscious. The most popular diet of the era was the Hollywood 18-day diet, and it consisted of only 585 calories a day, derived from grapefruits, oranges, melba toast, green vegetables, and hard-boiled eggs. It apparently had the same wild popularity as the Scarsdale diet in its day. It was so widely followed that restaurants offered all its meals and hostesses checked with dinner guests to find which day of the diet they were on so they could serve the appropriate meal. If the calorie counting didn't work, or if it seemed too complicated a task, women took another tack—the zero-calorie solution—and tried fasting altogether. Many women, however, like journalist Barbara Ueland, took the middle ground—meals made up of lettuce, black coffee, and cigarettes.

Along with the low-calorie diets came the negative effects we now associate with dieting: emotional and physiological problems, and a cyclical treadmill of weight loss and gain. Women complained of irritability, fatigue, and melancholy, and more serious problems also seemed to be emerging. As early as 1930 Ueland reported that many doctors were concerned because some young women reduced "so fiercely that they will never be able to have children." They may have been suffering from amenorrhea, but it is not clear whether this was becoming a general problem. Six years later, a writer in *Fortune* Magazine lightly referred to another dieting practice that has become serious in our own day: purging by laxative use or by vomiting. He explained that "there is the system whereby you eat but do not feed. Usual practice in this case is to use an emetic right after your meal, but tickling the throat with a finger or feather will empty the stomach just as efficiently." He claimed this was one of "[the] eating systems that have captured the American mind," but he did not seem very alarmed about it. Emetics had been used freely to cure illness and gastrointestinal pains for centuries, and modern medicine was only slowly eradicating this practice. And constipation—often defined as less than one or even two bowel movements daily—was considered extremely unhealthy in this period, so laxative use was not seen as abuse. In any case, constipation was a recognized disadvantage of dieting, and diet tips often explained how to avoid it. In 1924 the *Literary Digest* cautioned reducers that "constipation is apt to prove a serious menace when the amount of food eaten is so materially decreased, and bulk will prove to be of great value here." Casting ahead to our own times were rumors of Hollywood starlets dying from excessive dieting, and in 1939 psychiatrist J. A. Ryle noted that the number of cases of anorexia nervosa had increased in the postwar years, a phenomenon he attributed to "the spread of the slimming fashion" and to "the more emotional lives of the younger generation."[30]

Although the slenderness craze of 1919–1935 seems remarkably similar to our own, and although it introduced many of the ideas we cherish today, it was emphatically different from our own craze, even at its zenith. This was a period of transition, and the craze did not create the hysteria or the terrible effects on women that we know today. The positive associations with plumpness were too recent and too well entrenched to be easily eradicated.

Slimness is a relative term. Certainly the slimness favored by the generation of the twenties and early thirties never approximated that favored by our own. The weights advocated by insurance companies were the actual average weights of their policyholders—not some mythic, ideal weights. And they were higher than any used between 1942–43 and today. For instance, a woman aged twenty-five who was 5′5″ (with 1- to 2-inch heels on) was advised to weigh between 121 and 141 pounds. In the 1959 table her "desirable" weight went down to 111–119 if she were small-framed, and to 116–130 if she were medium-framed. Furthermore, it was generally accepted that people gained weight as they aged. This gain was considered normal, and the insurance charts raised the desirable weight with age. Hence, they suggested that the same 5′5″ woman (with shoes on) should weigh 121 pounds at the age of twenty-five and 141 pounds at the age of sixty. It was gains in excess of these that caused alarm, although already in the mid-twenties some experts were advising adults not to continue to gain once they reached the age of forty.[31]

It wasn't just health officials who advocated body dimensions larger than those we now prefer. Even the fashionable weights of the period were much higher than ours. And for all the talk about narrower hips, the hips remained, ideally, substantially larger than anything we would consider acceptable. In 1922 the beauty writer Florence Courtenay explained that the ideal figure was a "lithe, well-rounded form, graceful yet not so plump as to be called voluptuous." Quite specifically, she recommended that a 5′3″ woman have measurements of 28.8–24.7–35.2 and weigh 119 pounds. If the bust measurement seems impossibly small, we must remember that the breasts were usually bound. Miss Courtenay went on to say that a 5′7″ woman should weigh 148 pounds.[32]

This seemed to be the body size of the beauties of the day. In 1922 and 1923, Mary Campbell reigned as Miss America, and she was 5′7″ and weighed a healthy 140 pounds. The same was true for the beloved actresses of the decade, such as Gloria Swanson, Clara Bow, and Billie Dove, who may have been slimmer than the actresses of the turn of the century, but who nonetheless could boast the same fullness as the Miss Americas. Ziegfeld chose the girls for his famous Follies, which lasted between 1907 and 1931, for their beautiful figures. He liked them bustier than the fashionable ideal and chose young women with 36" busts, 26" waists, and hips that were a solid 38".[33]

Nor did models resemble their anorexic modern counterparts. In the thirties, for the first time, photographs replaced fashion drawings in the women's magazines. The drawings had portrayed impossibly slender, elongated women whose bodies were eight times the length of their heads, though normal proportions are only six times the length of the head. The photographed models present a startling contrast to these drawings. They seem short-legged and plump, especially those in bathing suits.

In short, the standards of slenderness were not as extreme as ours, and the cult of slimness did not have the monolithic character it has today. Though more women were enfranchised into the fashion-beauty nexus, the democratization and standardization of beauty had only just begun. Competing regional, local, and ethnic standards were still powerful. And though beauty was increasingly being defined in terms of superficial physical characteristics, the idea that beauty came from other, inner qualities was still pervasive. Furthermore, there were still fashion categories for different ages. Lady Troubridge's lament that "no one is allowed to be middle-aged" reflected the beginning of a trend to set up youth as the only kind of beauty. But, although the wife-companion model of the twenties was blurring the distinctions between courting girl and married woman, there were still comfortable places in society—and in the hierarchy of beauty—for the matronly body.[34]

The imperative to be slim was not comprehensive because it was attacked from many quarters. Even Paul Poiret, when he found the style he had helped create leading to this slenderer form, expressed some regret. He recalled his lover, Raymonde, who had been voluptuous, "[as] they made them at that time," and observed that had he known such charms "were on the point of disappearing, perhaps [I] would have taken better advantage of them." American critics insisted that Europeans did not follow the craze, that, as Dr. Fishbein wrote in 1934, "the French women never succumbed to the craze for emaciation as did their American sisters." And many men apparently objected. In 1930 journalist Barbara Ueland wrote that "husbands and men in general all over the world seem to be exercised about it." Men preferred women with flesh on their bones. For somewhat different reasons, many cultural authorities also objected to the sinuous flapper image and styles. Respectable middle-class people, church leaders, and many educators, dismayed by this youth culture and all it represented, vehemently criticized the new fashions and the body that went with them.[35]

Beauty experts also set limits to fashionable slimness. They praised slenderness, but they abhorred a body that was close to the bone. Although the women's magazines and diet-aid ads concentrated on overweight women, they also gave considerable thought and space to the underweight woman. In January, 1922, the popular beauty expert, Susanna Cocroft, ran an ad in *Good Housekeeping* in which she promised, "You Can Weigh Exactly What You Should" with her services, and she included the testimonials of a woman who had lost 70 pounds and of another who had gained 30 pounds. *Good Housekeeping* ran an article in September, 1924, which clearly presumed thinness was an undesirable condition. It appealed to all readers, "whether you are thin, fat, or that comfortable state just between the two extremes . . . ." In 1930 a *Vogue* ad described "the most envied women today. To be sure," it read, "they are slim, but you would never think of calling them thin. Rounded slenderness seems to describe them perfectly." No one wanted to be skeletal.[36]

Though the medical profession and nutritionists were often prominent apologists for the cult of slimness, not all of them endorsed it either. Certainly there was no concerted campaign to urge Americans to lose weight as was to occur in subsequent decades. As late as 1946 Dr. Frederick Stare of the Harvard School of Public Health complained that he had seldom heard "a nutritionist give any attention to ideal weights as part of nutrition education," and he insisted that "the disregard of the impairment of health by consuming too many calories has been the single big defect in nutrition education." It was neglected largely because medical opinion still had not arrived at any consensus about the merits or dangers of fat. In 1926 Dr. Woods Hutchinson, a former president of the AMA, wrote that he was "puzzled" by "this present onslaught upon one of the most peaceable, useful, and law-abiding of our tissues"—fat. It would be hard to find a starker contrast to current attitudes. But if medical opinion was still divided about the necessity of sticking to the weight charts, it was in agreement that too thin was unhealthy. Low weight was still associated with dread diseases like TB and pneumonia, and in the popular press, many specialists criticized the inadequate diets women followed and the low weight they set as goals. In general, excessive thinness was still seen as a symptom of disorders that undermined the appetite, such as illness, worry, or a jittery temperament.[37]

During this period observers were disturbed by the fact that young women and even adolescents were trying to reduce, whereas in our day we all but snatch the food from their mouths. In 1926 Dr. Hutchinson reported that no one objected to mature women trying to "bring back within conventional limits and standards a liberality of outline which is either burdensome or unbecoming," but when it became clear that young girls were trying to reduce, "a storm of protest came rumbling up from every quarter." It was unquestioningly believed that young people needed a little extra padding. Even the 1907 insurance report contended that until a person was twenty-five, "an overweight not to exceed 110 percent of the standard . . . seems to indicate a certain hypernutrition and robustness of physique that is favorable to subsequent life." In 1931 Dr. Alonzo Taylor, a firm believer in the insurance-company statistics, nonetheless explained that some overweight was an asset until an individual was thirty- or even forty-years old, and only then did it become a liability.[38]

Physicians worried that young people who were underweight could not resist disease. They also worried about other effects dieting might have on growth. Dr. Hutchinson argued that young people needed "a special margin of adipose to grow on—a boost, so to speak, like the extra slap on the back when wishing them many happy returns of the day." In 1926 Dr. L. F. Barker of Johns Hopkins praised girls who were reducing because "they are exhibiting a willingness to curb their natural appetites for food and candy and for the fattening things of life for the sake of an ideal." In 1930, however, he was also warning that "the deliberate underfeeding by young girls and young women . . . is becoming a menace not only to the present, but to future generations." Directors of physical education programs worried because young female dieters were "below par in health and vigor." Even worse, some nutritionists and doctors reported that many reducing girls suffered from "nervous breakdowns." "Growing girls," these authorities emphasized, "need all the nourishment they can get at regular intervals during the day." Others feared lack of nourishment could affect the brain and impair girls' ability to do schoolwork. In brief, young women who tried to diet had to contend with the ominous, often vehement warnings of many authorities—and parents—who were absolutely opposed to the fad.[39]

Furthermore, many were still not convinced that people could totally control their body size. Their objections can be seen partially as a reaction against the modern trend toward uniform standards of body size and beauty, but there were also scientific reasons, in particular, heredity. In the twenties, America's leading eugenicist, Charles Davenport, proposed that fatness was a dominant genetic trait. Ueland reported in 1930 that a conference of physicians and dieticians "condemned the boyish form. They said all women seem to be trying to pour themselves into one mold which cannot possibly be done until, as Oliver Wendell Holmes said, we are able to 'select our ancestors with much greater care.' No matter what the diet, a Pecheron cannot be a race horse." And there was metabolism. Some people just seemed to burn calories faster than others. This idea was further endorsed by the theory of *luxuskonsumption,* first advanced by the German nutritionist, R. O. Neumann, at the turn of the century. Through meticulous studies of himself, he discovered that when overfed, his body spontaneously started burning extra calories and so kept its weight relatively stable. Just the reverse occurred with underfeeding: His metabolic rate slowed down to conserve calories. American researchers discounted this theory in 1931 (though it would be revived in the seventies), in part because they had difficulty duplicating the results, and also, perhaps, because they could not accept the idea that the mathematical equation, 3,500 calories equals a pound of fat, was incorrect. In discarding the theory, experts put the body even more firmly on the mechanical model of a machine that burned energy at a steady and predictable rate.[40]

There were also the glands. If metabolic explanations for overweight lost favor, glandular ones became more widely accepted, in part because of the rising prestige of endocrinology. They remained dominant until the forties and seemed to explain excessive thinness as well as excessive overweight. After 1914, when Morris Simmond discovered that tumors in the anterior pituitary caused loss of appetite and weight loss, anorexia nervosa became confused with Simmond's Disease, and the gland-weight link seemed even more convincing. Like anorexia, obesity was seen as a symptom of glandular abnormality. Many of the obese, like the anorexics, simply could not be held responsible for their weight. The problem was their glands, not their willpower. Even if obesity was an abnormality, in this period, at least, that abnormality was often seen as something the overweight person could not control.[41]

In terms of direct responses to human beings, more scorn was heaped on those who tried hard to be fashionably thin than on those who overate. Hilde Bruch's recent angry indictment of "thin fat people" who keep themselves chronically undernourished and exhibit the ill effects of such undernourishment just to be fashionably thin, were common in this early phase of the diet syndrome. The extremes of fashion were still being checked and countered by other social authorities and institutions.[42]

Furthermore, modern science and dehumanizing trends notwithstanding, food still retained its nurturing associations, attitudes that were bolstered in this period by growing knowledge about the nature and crucial importance of vitamins and minerals. In contrast to our supplement-popping age, most people were still expected to get these substances from the actual food they ate. Even calories were not considered inherently bad. They were seen as a vital source of energy. As always, advertisers appealed to the biases of consumers, and in 1922 the Florida Citrus Exchange promoted oranges with the promise that they were "rich in calories" and contained a "wealth of vitamins." In 1924 the California Prune and Apricot Growers' Exchange glowingly advertised that a pound of prunes "contained 1,300 energizing calories."[43]

This first significant thinness craze persisted well into the thirties, even though the Great Depression had hit, and soup kitchens filled with the hungry crowded the urban landscape. Mannish tailored suits replaced the twenties silhouette, and some women heaved a sigh of relief, thinking that the "revenge of thin women" was finally spent. But the figure under the clothes was still supposed to be slender. Nonetheless, by 1932 the craze was beginning to subside. All the conditions that had helped foster it were changing: the youthful rebellion, the emphasis on youth, and above all, the sense of financial security. In a nation gripped by depression and then war, with threats of food shortages and with rationing, overweight could hardly loom as a serious problem. The *Reader's Guide to Periodical Literature,* an index of the articles published in major magazines, gives evidence of this change. Between 1919 and 1932 it listed about eight articles a year devoted to "corpulence," an eigh-

teenth-century term used for obesity and overweight, which the Guide persisted in using until 1977. After 1932 the average dropped to two a year, and
between 1937 and 1945 there were even fewer. Already in 1939 one psychiatrist
wrote with relief that "the slimming fashion is now happily on the wane." And
Vogue was running articles on "How Not to Be So Thin."[44]

In retrospect, it is difficult to tell whether these national crises simply
interrupted the diet craze, or whether the craze itself had been only a superficial event. Most likely, it had affected only the upper strata of the population
and young women, especially those in urban areas, and had not penetrated
deeply into grass-roots America. The criticisms of it reflected deeply ingrained
ideas that checked its spread. And how much it had really spread remains
questionable. As late as 1944 a Gallup poll revealed that eight out of ten
housewives did not know the difference between a vitamin and a calorie—and
this of course was a crucial distinction, for vitamins were good and calories
bad for those who wanted to reduce. Dieting in this earlier period was a
fashionable game. It had not penetrated the national psyche as it would after
World War II.[45]

If overt concern about slenderness and dieting had subsided, they still
remained important issues in American life and firmly established lower
weight standards for succeeding generations. When *Harper's Bazaar* published
an article entitled "Reducing with Meat" in 1943 (the middle of the War), the
issue sold out and the diet had to be reprinted. And the glamorous starlets of
the thirties and forties continued to be slim, in some cases even slimmer than
their twenties' forebears. Greta Garbo, Ingrid Bergman, and Joan Crawford
all had a slenderness we can still admire today—but they certainly were not
skinny. Their bones did not show through their skin. By the mid-forties the
ideal female shape altered again, at least in the new and wildly popular pinup
posters. The ideal figure again resembled an hourglass with full hips, a small
waist, and a newly accentuated bust. The "sweater girl" had come into vogue.
She was slender, but she had curves and sweetly rounded flesh. Betty Grable
was the most celebrated pinup during World War II, but her figure looks
decidedly old-fashioned to modern eyes. Her famous legs are lusciously round
and sexy; they do not resemble the lean, long, muscled legs we admire today.

Despite the apparent relaxation of concern about overweight, certain elements were already converging that would cause a resurgence of diet-mania
in the fifties, among them the revised tables of the Metropolitan Life Insurance
Company and the promulgation of ideal weight standards, the seeming defeat
of the glandular and metabolic theories of weight gain, new histologic discoveries about fat as a tissue, and the rise of psychiatric explanations for weight
problems. These changing perceptions of overweight converged with other
developments, and together they laid the groundwork for the onslaught that
would be unleashed in 1950, when the real war on fat began.

Preference Becomes Prejudice: The War on Fat Begins, 1950–1960

Rather suddenly, after World War II, interest in weight loss crescendoed, penetrating more deeply into the culture and into the daily lives of ordinary Americans. For more than fifty years, ambivalent attitudes about weight had coexisted, but now, the pendulum swung firmly to one side. The preference for slenderness was transmuted into a profound abhorrence of fat. The "Age of Caloric Anxiety" began as the culture of slimming emerged.

The pivotal year was 1951. In the *Reader's Guide to Periodical Literature,* the number of articles on "corpulence" rose to ten immediately after the war, and between 1949 and 1951 it rose to fourteen. But in the following two years, it suddenly zoomed to fifty-four. This radical jump proved more than an anomaly. The number stayed equally high between 1953 and 1955, and then leapt to sixty-six between 1955 and 1957. Articles indexed under "weight" were no longer about weights and measures. In 1955–57, all fourteen entries were specifically about body weight, such as *Today's Health* January, 1956, article, "Is Your Weight Normal?" Body weight was becoming Americans' most important measure, a way to gauge health, beauty, and character.

Although cookbooks and recipe columns multiplied in response to the new abundance and affordability of domestic and foreign foods, and the culinary arts were considered more and more essential to femininity (a 1950 *Vogue* article even insinuated that women who didn't cook well were "nervous, unstable types" who would probably end up on a psychiatrist's couch), diet became a major preoccupation. The sudden avalanche of diets reflected Americans' new dilemma: how to eat well without getting fat. In the years 1951–53

103

and 1955–57, the number of articles on "diet" in the popular press trebled, reaching a spectacular high of ninety-seven, and, as with "weight," the word was being redefined to mean—almost exclusively—reduction.

With even greater intensity than in previous decades, diet lore consisted of refurbished traditional methods and popular—and frequently fantastic—reworking of medical and scientific research. This popularization and bastardization of scientific studies would bedevil all food and weight beliefs for the next thirty-five years. In 1959 the *New York Times Magazine* reported that the public's demand for diet advice was so intense that editors and writers "systematically ransack medical and nutrition journals for new developments."[1]

They found many. In June, 1956, professional gourmet and freelance writer Roy de Groot waxed ecstatic in a *Look* article about the "Revolutionary Rockefeller Diet" that had helped him shed 45 of his 281 pounds. The diet was based on a low-protein experiment conducted by Dr. Vincent P. Dole of the highly respected Rockefeller Institute for Medical Research. Appalled to find his experimental diet popularized, Dr. Dole immediately wrote a letter of explanation to the *Journal of the AMA* and reported that, aside from the possible dangers of such a regimen, the diet had not yet proved successful for curing obesity. Two months later the *Ladies' Home Journal* and *Vogue* popularized research with dextrose, an ingredient commonly used in infants' formula. Druggists were stunned to find their supplies of dextrose, which usually languished on the shelves, suddenly being swooped up by eager buyers. Other fads had less respectable sources. Periodically, members of the medical profession would inveigh against the dangers and ineffectiveness of fad diets, but there seemed no end to the public's desperation and gullibility when it came to weight loss.[2]

Though it never questioned the premise of dieting, the popular press occasionally did its part to stem the tide of fad diets, and urged would-be dieters to follow balanced eating plans that curtailed the quantity but not the quality of food eaten and that reduced weight sensibly and slowly. In November, 1956, *McCall's* ran an article entitled "Why Fad Diets Fail," and in 1959 *Life* exposed "The Wasteful, Phony, Crash Dieting Craze." *Life* lamented that none of the best-selling regimens were written by physicians, a vacuum that would be filled two years later when Dr. Herman Taller published his phenomenally successful book, *Calories Don't Count.* His high-fat diet, and the scientific justifications he gave for it, proved upsetting to health and nutrition professionals. Because he was a doctor, it seemed that the medical profession endorsed his scheme and so lent it credibility—even though the AMA did not consider it a "healthy" way to lose weight. Dr. Taller's authorship revealed that members of the medical profession might not be above entering the increasingly lucrative diet fray. This was the start of the ambiguous phenomenon we know today: doctors either writing, or lending their names to, books advocating highly questionable eating regimens.[3]

But even the most respected, medically approved diets of the time were, like today's counterparts, an odd mixture of fact and fantasy. It was universally held that all carbohydrates, whether simple or complex, were the culprit in weight gain. Yet this dictum, ardently as it was believed in the fifties, is today being reversed and endorsed with equal fervor.

The book trade also reflected emerging diet-mania, although only two diet books made it to the nonfiction best-seller lists in the fifties: Gaylord Hauser's *Look Younger, Live Longer* (#3 in 1950, #1 in 1951) and the *Better Homes and Gardens Diet Book* (#6 in 1955). Hauser's book was a mixture of health-food cant and weight-reduction lore. Enthusiastically supported by luminaries like Greta Garbo, Hauser advocated the liberal use of five "wonder foods": skimmed milk, brewer's yeast, wheat germ, yogurt, and blackstrap molasses. Health-food-store owners, accustomed to their small, fringe clientele, were stunned to find their sales suddenly increasing as Hauser's book sales approached the 500,000 mark. In subsequent years, more diet books graced bookstore shelves, though the "health-food" cant of Hauser and others disappeared from them, and by 1959, the *New York Times Magazine* noted with some astonishment that ninety-two diet books were in print. (By 1983 there would be almost four times this number.)[4]

Along with the diets came that now-common feature of American life: diet foods. In 1952 the Borden Company reported with some amazement that sales of one of its least popular "health" products, nonfat dry milk, had leapt from 5 million pounds to 60 million pounds. In December, 1952, *Business Week* reported that "a new and moderately booming market has opened up": low-calorie, dietetic foods. Such foods had been around for years (saccharine since 1879), but they were bought primarily by diabetics and health-food devotees. Grocery stores and the newly emerging supermarkets hadn't even bothered to stock them because of low demand, slow turnover, and high prices. But after World War II the diet industry got underway, with the first sugarless ginger ale marketed in metropolitan New York in the spring of 1952, followed swiftly by Flotill Products' Tasti-Diet, a new line of dietetic foods that included eight canned fruits, eight puddings, two jellies, and three salad dressings. Flotill's energetic president, Tillie Lewis, actively advertised her new products and urged food retailers to set up sections devoted to such goods.[5]

Within four years, *Newsweek* was writing about the "Big Bulge in Profits" enjoyed by these fledgling companies. Only 50,000 cases of low-calorie soft drinks had sold in 1952; by 1955, 15 million cases were being sold by companies like Cott Low Calorie, No-Cal, and Less-Cal. Tillie Lewis, it appeared, had been prescient. *Newsweek* reported in 1956 that "hardly a supermarket worthy of its supertitle can get along nowadays without a dietary-foods department."[6]

A seemingly ultimate form of low-calorie substitute appeared in 1959 with the introduction of the total food Metrecal. This one-meal liquid, which bore a startling resemblance to baby formula, reduced the dieter to a single, infantile choice in foodstuffs, the first of many such painless plans. Mead & Johnson, the pharmaceutical company that marketed Metrecal, saw its annual earnings go from $4 million in the late fifties to $13 million in 1960, the year after the product was released. Restaurants served it, movie and television stars raved about it, and *Time* magazine remarked on the "virulence of Metrecal fever." As with so many diet breakthroughs, however, the miracle was short-lived and, by 1962, Mead & Johnson's earnings dropped below even their pre-Metrecal days. Americans certainly hadn't given up on dieting. They were just out hunting for another breakthrough, another panacea.[7]

As Americans swapped their high-calorie goodies for low-calorie substitutes, traditional food industries began to feel the pinch and tried to fight back. Consumption of confectionary items had dropped from 18.4 pounds per capita in 1950 to 16.6 pounds in 1955; sugar sales slipped 4 percent between 1949 and 1955; and in 1955 the American Institute of Baking lamented that bread buying was on the decline, even though 200 baking companies were trying to market low-calorie loaves in 5,000 cities. Advertising wars began as each industry tried to defend its turf against the charge of "fattening"—a charge that was becoming equivalent to the kiss of death. By the late fifties, the American Sugar Refining Company planned to counter by investing $350,000 in an ad campaign that explained, "Three teaspoons of Domino sugar contain fewer calories than one-half of a medium grapefruit." The big soft-drink bottlers had still not entered the low-calorie market, but they encouraged an identification between their drinks and slenderness with ads and slogans like Pepsi-Cola's: "Aren't today's people wonderful? They're so wonderful to look at—these slender, handsome, active men and women of today . . . . "[8]

The entire food industry was beginning to be seen in terms of diet, but Americans did not simply rely on diets to control weight. They sought, too, to master their recalcitrant appetites, not with self-discipline but with scientific aid. Prescription and nonprescription appetite suppressants flooded the market. They ranged from the benign, candylike Ayds, whose sales quadrupled between 1949 and 1955, to amphetamines, which had first appeared in 1938 and whose dangers were not yet known. In 1952, 60,000 pounds of them were being produced annually in the United States, and women were using them freely for weight loss, with little objection from physicians who prescribed them regularly.[9]

Sales of other weight-loss aids also mushroomed in the 1950s. Bathroom-scale sales leapt 18 percent between 1955 and 1956 alone. The FDA and the U. S. Post Office scrambled to control the burgeoning mail-order trade in diet gimmicks. For those who felt in need of supervision, exercise salons and spas flourished. Although exercise still did not appeal overwhelmingly to the weight conscious, companies like Slenderella began luring would-be reducers by promising that machines would do their reducing for them. Slenderella opened its doors in 1951, and by 1959 it had seventy salons in fifty cities and grossed $20 million annually. And the decade's new medium joined forces with its new compulsion. Bonnie Prudden and Jack LaLanne led exercises on television, and LaLanne, who compared himself to evangelist Billy Graham ("He puts them into shape for the hereafter, and I get them fit for the here and now"), went from leading calisthenics on a local television show in San Francisco in 1951 to having the biggest national daytime show in 1960. The very well-heeled went to spas like the Golden Door or Elizabeth Arden's Maine Chance. Still other women began experimenting with group support as organizations devoted to weight loss came into being. TOPS (Take Off Pounds Sensibly) was founded in 1948 by Esther Manz, an overweight Milwaukee housewife who got the idea from an article on Alcoholics' Anonymous. By the early sixties, TOPS had grown from a club of three overweight friends into an organization with 2,481 chapters across the country and a combined weight loss of 374,061 pounds.[10]

If all these efforts failed, some turned to religion, for even God was slowly enlisted into the weight-loss crusade. One of the most stunning diet books of the decade, *Pray Your Weight Away* by the Reverend Charles W. Shedd, D.D., marked this change. Even the *New Republic,* which did not review diet books, could not help but comment about Reverend Shedd enlisting God's aid for such a secular and personal goal. In fact, Shedd's book inadvertently revealed how powerful the urge for slenderness was becoming and how axiomatic was the assumption that slenderness was the normal human condition. As the *New Republic* reviewer explained, Dr. Shedd equated "fat with sin . . . [and] tells us that God really made us all thin, except for the glandular cases, and that if our bodies really are to be temples of the Holy Spirit, we had best get them down to the size God intended." Associations between godliness and control of appetite were hardly new: Gluttony had been regarded as one of the Seven Deadly Sins since Early Christianity. What was radically new was that the "sin" had shifted from appetite to body size itself. Fatness was a worse sin than gluttony. Indeed, the glutton who stayed thin did not seem gluttonous. The idea that God had intended everyone to be a certain size—thin—allowed weight-loss efforts to be viewed as a holy quest, a fulfillment of God's design. Shedd prefigured a trend that would become more pronounced in the seventies, when evangelical religion became a vehicle for weight loss. He also underlined another, more crucial, turning point. Historically, religious leaders had been a counterfoil to the excesses of vanity and of fashion. But once slenderness was yoked to religious righteousness, the clergy would not protest nor caution when fashion standards became extreme.[11]

Why did Americans become more and more frantic about their weight in the 1950s, exhibiting compulsions that outlived any of the products meant to assuage them? We need to analyze the forces that created this compulsion because they are the primordial soup out of which our current obsession evolved. The women who dieted and popped diet pills, who bought the new dietetic products to store next to the new goodies provided by American abundance, and the men who groaned about their expanding waistlines were the parents and grandparents of the generation that turned dieting into a pathological disorder and eating right into a new religion.

As we saw in the previous chapter, between 1880 and 1920 a variety of profound cultural, aesthetic, and intellectual changes converged to turn the slender, streamlined body into the preferred body. These changes became more firmly entrenched and more familiar after World War II and set the stage for an intensification of this preference and for the development of new norms for body size and a newly focused attack on fat. A tightening alliance between aesthetic ideals and medical standards exacerbated the trend, which soon became an obsession for American women.

In the spring of 1947, in a Paris still suffering from wartime shortages of food and material, Christian Dior opened his doors and stunned the world with his New Look, bringing back an hourglass silhouette oddly reminiscent of the one Paul Poiret had banished forty years earlier. Yet there was a difference—this silhouette was as sharp, tailored, and tapered as a jet. Like Poiret, Dior was his own best spokesman: "I design clothes for flowerlike women with rounded shoulders, full feminine busts, and handspan waists above enormous spreading skirts . . . . I brought back the art of pleasing." *Vogue* immediately displayed the famous model, Centura, wearing Dior's new clothes; in June, *Life* head-lined, "Fashion Turmoil: Drastic New Styles Will Make Most Existing Clothes Obsolete"; and in August, *Time* called it a "revolution" and marveled that fashion was "going back to lines from which it had marched after World War I."[12]

The New Look caused a hoopla in part because *Life* was right. Even the most adroit seamstress couldn't alter the older styles with their squared, padded shoulders, their long, slim-hipped lines, their shorter hems, and their unemphasized waists, into the New Look. Women, on a mass scale, dumped their old wardrobes for new ones. (*Mademoiselle* advised them to send their castoffs to Europe where clothing was still desperately needed.) The New Look also caused a hoopla because *Time* had been right, too. Fashion did seem to be moving back to pre–World War I images of women. In a retrospective essay in 1950 *Vogue* described the thirties look of "manful padded shoulders" as giving the feeling that women "could carry a difficult world on them," and the forties' "frugal, spare silhouette" had conveyed a similar feeling. But now, suddenly, *softness, femininity,* and *flowerlike qualities* became the terms filling the fashion press. Rosie the Riveter gave way to June Cleaver, and the strong, lean-lined, worldly qualities of sirens like Greta Garbo and Marlene Dietrich were replaced by the sweet, curvaceous sexuality of Marilyn Monroe and Jayne Mansfield—who gave the icon of the pinup girl a new and glamorous reality— or by the elegant, cool composure of a Grace Kelly or a Suzy Parker.[13]

This new style was the catalyst for a renewed assault on fat, though contem-poraries at first thought otherwise. *Life,* for example, trumpeted the New Look with an article optimistically entitled, "Newest Styles Give Every Woman's Figure a Chance." Such optimism glimmered also because the fashionable ideal was not youthful, and it seemed likely that a more mature figure would go with a more mature ideal. In May, 1947, *Vogue* paid tribute to ripened beauty, featuring the twelve most-photographed models of the previous ten years, commenting that "these twelve share a look of non-adolescence, a look gained not so so much in being beautiful as [in] becoming so . . . . " In the same issue, it criticized women who tried to keep youthful looks: "Always a sad spectacle is the woman who, in her fifties, has managed to 'preserve' the beauty of her youth." The article concluded that "usually no woman can be said to dress faultlessly until she is beyond her first youth." Couturiers had always designed their clothing for the mature women of the world who were their clients, and Dior and Balenciega, the couture leaders of the fifties, were no exception.[14]

Yet, though the beauties of the day seem voluptuous to us now, contemporaries interpreted this look as a movement toward slenderness, and they were right. Certainly Dior's look did *not* give every figure a chance. The tiny waist was one catch, as it had been in the nineteenth century, and in 1948 *Mademoiselle* announced that "the pinched waist" had narrowed since its first appearance the previous year. In 1950 *Vogue* described the New Look as a "silhouette of flaring curves above lean lines." At the end of the decade Marilyn Maxwell, a former cover girl and a fashion editor and consultant, recalled that the Dior styles required such a slender body that "We wondered where we would get models who could fit into them. Then out of the woods came these slender nymphs without lungs and with very little of the flesh that keeps you alive." Top model Suzy Parker recalled that other models were always dieting and "living on codeine to keep up their energy. You never met a skinnier, meaner bunch of people."[15]

With the New Look came new rules of beauty, and slenderness was crucial. Beauty, *Vogue* explained in May, 1947, was made up of intangible qualities and physical facts. " . . . [T]he first step in the fact of beauty is figure. There is little camouflage and small excuse for an unpleasing shape." And in its article praising mature beauty, it reiterated that while looks, style, mentality, and everything else should change with maturity, the figure shouldn't: "A body not only slim but articulate is the consideration of any ageless-seeming woman. Doctor, diet, exercise and the massage table all play their parts." The stress on slimness was not just in articles about beauty. It could slip in anywhere. In 1948, when *Mademoiselle* asked what college men wanted in a girl, the answer was "the intelligence to develop a trim mind as well as a trim figure." *McCall's* gave its middle-class audiences a similar message. "Do Husbands Like Plump Wives?" it asked in its March, 1951, issue, and answered with a resounding no. Beatrice Gould, coeditor of the *Ladies' Home Journal,* instituted a program of finding successful women reducers around the country, and for more than two decades, their success stories were a regular feature in the magazine. It is not surprising, then, that in 1953 and 1954 Gallup polls, 45 percent of the women interviewed said they wanted to lose weight.[16]

Paradoxically, mid-decade witnessed the rise of fuller-figured celebrities such as Marilyn Monroe and other media stars, but it was also the time when the sheath dress and straight skirt took their places beside full skirts, and even greater emphasis was placed on slenderness. Fashions began to be described in terms of body size, as demonstrated by *Vogue*'s January, 1955, story on "Spring Suited Slenderness." By June, 1955, 49 percent of American women wanted to shed pounds, and the following year *Vogue* revealed how crucial body weight had become for a chic, rich look. It broke with long tradition—and elitism—by insisting that a good figure was even more basic than expensive clothes. "It's basic," the magazine explained, "even if you have the price of the Kohinoor diamond in your pocket—any fashion, regardless of cost, looks smarter on a good figure. And good figures vary, depending on build . . . but they never look overweight." Fashion was becoming more democratic as stylish beauty became as much a question of dietary restraint as of taste and money.[17]

The clothing industry translated these trends in practical terms. Clothing stores were stocking smaller sizes. "Twenty-five years ago," one dress-shop owner explained to *Newsweek* in 1956, "the smallest size we stocked was 12 or 14. Today it runs down to as small as size 6." Dresses advertised in the fashion magazines reflected this trend: Sizes in the late forties had usually been 10s to 18s, with occasional 8s. By the mid-50s, they were 8s with occasional 6s, and they went up to 14, sometimes 16, but rarely up to 18 or 20. To buy stylish clothes, the ordinary woman *had* to slim down.[18]

The urge for fashionable slenderness took a new turn in 1958 when rising hemlines brought increasing concentration on the figure and made the actual details of the body vitally important. Fashion rarely has left to chance or to nature's whims visible parts of the anatomy, especially parts of great sexual interest. They have traditionally had to meet certain standards. *Vogue* heralded rising hemlines in February, 1958, as an innovation "based on legs." It trilled that beautiful legs were the American woman's forte: "What the Grecian nose is to the Greeks, what the English complexion is to the English . . . well, that's what legs are in America. Only more so." But these weren't just any legs. They had to be "slender, shapely gams." Unfortunately, contrary to *Vogue*'s prattle, few American women had them naturally, so *Vogue* came to the rescue in its next issue, with advice about "how to have very good legs." And of course, weight loss was the key. "Usually," *Vogue* explained, "a leg case involves some general weight reduction; even five to ten pounds more than one's 'good' weight can have a discouraging way of settling about lazy leg muscles."[19]

A similar shift in fashion emphasis crucially affected figure consciousness: the glorification of the swimsuit. Swimsuits had been advertised for at least two decades in the fashion press, but it was only in 1958 that *Vogue* began to set standards for the "bathing-suit figure" and shifted attention from the suit to the body itself. It defined that figure as the one that "begins where the suit leaves off: the back, arms, thighs, calves—whatever can't be concealed." And it stressed that this exposure demanded a "degree of firmness that a passable dress figure might get by without." *Vogue* was introducing new standards and even a new vocabulary for the female figure. It explained to its readers the notion of "muscle tone" and its dreadful opposite: "The absence of muscle-tone, alas, has a name, too: flabbiness." Even slender women might not meet these new, stringent standards. The standards for public appearance, for the clothed body, were being applied to more private parts of the body.[20]

The fact that the women's press had begun to put extraordinary emphasis on slenderness does not explain why women took its precepts so much to heart. One reason is that in the fifties, the magazines and the couturiers had a power and an authority that would dissipate in later decades. For centuries, fashion had been based on the existence of a "structured society with a few privileged people worth emulating" at the top, as dress historian Kennedy Fraser aptly put it. Fashions in food, manners, entertainment, and clothing trickled down the social ladder to those eager to emulate the elite. For even though their membership changed with political and economic shifts, the elite were the arbiters of taste. If the rising tide of industrialization and democracy had besieged the citadel of fashion for more than a century, in the fifties, fashion was still structured in a rigid pyramid. The great French couturiers, Dior and Balenciega, ruled from its apex like absolute monarchs, their power consecrated by the elite women of the world—the aristocracy, the monied, and media celebrities—who chose them to design their clothing. The fashion press then publicized the styles: *Vogue* and *Harper's Bazaar* presumably for the wealthy who couldn't make it to the Paris showings, *Mademoiselle* for the debutante, collegiate set. From there, fashions and fashion information descended down the social hierarchy through magazines designed for the domestic middle classes, like *McCall's,* and through manufacturers who imitated the styles for the ready-to-wear department-store trade. And so the copying continued, down to the broad base of the social pyramid.[21]

The fashion magazines were particularly powerful in the fifties also because increasing upward mobility made a great mass of women anxious for advice about how to bring more graciousness into their lives. Magazines like *Vogue* could serve as guides for them. More crucially, in this era of de-mythologized, nonfigurative art, Hollywood and the fashion world—and especially the fashion photograph—had taken over from art the task of establishing the criteria of feminine beauty. The fifties has been called a decade of conformity. Certainly, in the world of fashion, there were clear standards and leadership. One look prevailed and women wanted to have it. And that look included slenderness.

They wanted to have it also because post-War abundance had helped democratize fashion far beyond the level it had reached in the twenties. For the first time, the average American woman had the time and money to play the fashion game. And as she reached out to fashion, it eagerly and profitably reached down to her. Magazines like *Vogue,* realizing that their survival depended on attracting a broader audience, began to appeal to a wider range of social classes. The commercial beauty industry, which had first emerged in the 1890s, now mushroomed into a vast commercial giant. Beauty aids and services once considered frivolous luxuries came to be seen as necessities. In 1957 alone, women spent a record $4 billion on them. They bought lipstick and—daringly—hair colorings; they went to charm schools and hair salons, all to remake themselves into stylish, poised beings. They could afford these luxuries because technological and organizational advances were making them affordable. As one mogul in the industry perceptively observed in 1958, "What we are selling is hope." It was the hope that a woman could make herself beautiful, that she could remake her appearance, her status, and even her personality. It was the hope that she could walk through the windows of the world *Vogue* presented, and join it.[22]

The democratization of fashion was not merely a vertical movement through the classes but also a horizontal movement in which the standards and looks of the urban centers spread out and effected a growing uniformity of behavior and dress. Local, regional, and ethnic differences were eroded further as Americans flocked to the cities and suburbs; as a vast network of highways was built and as cars, increasingly affordable, brought different areas closer together; as giant companies began to aim for national markets; as the mass media expanded; and as a generation of youngsters turned to television instead of to their elders for cultural cues. When the Miss America contest began appearing on television in 1954, Southerners, Northerners, Middle-Westerners, and Westerners were all there, looking pretty and pretty much the same, and boasting figures that hardly varied from body to body. It was the same body seen every day on billboards, television, at the movies, and in advertisements. It was, truly, Miss America.

As it spread these images, the media also performed another miracle of dissemination which made women believe they could resemble the beauty professionals. To attract a mass audience, they started trying to give the illusion that they were portraying average American women. When a woman watched glamorous movie stars or when she read *Vogue,* she saw women whom she wanted to resemble but whom she knew lived in a different universe than hers. She could dream of marrying the Prince of Monaco but knew the possibilities were small. But as the fashion magazines and other media reached for wider audiences, they tried to make the world they depicted and the standards they set seem more accessible. The television stars, the Miss Americas, movie actresses such as Doris Day and Sandra Dee, and even the Playboy Playmates dressed, behaved, and were put in settings and situations similar to those of normal, middle-class American girls and women. While the average housewife ironed or cooked, she could watch Harriet Nelson doing just what she was doing. The television stars seemed part of her world, as familiar in her kitchen as the neighbor next door. Miss America pageant directors demanded—and enforced—ladylike, wholesome qualities in contestants and portrayed them as ordinary college or high school girls who had been plucked out of their normal environments just for the event.[23]

The proliferation of popular magazines displaying the female figure reinforced larger trends. It dissipated the unsavoriness once associated with displaying the body for public judgment and with starkly physical criteria of beauty, and so encouraged "nice" middle-class girls to adopt these attitudes and behaviors. It also contributed to the standardization of images of beauty, accelerating the process *Vogue*'s Polly Devlin had associated with the films of the twenties. The ideal shifted away from the "recherché, the individual, and the singular toward a prototype that would appeal to mass audiences."[24]

The effect of this was that the looks of professional beauties now appeared to be the norm. Perfect teeth, skin, hair, features, and figures began to seem almost ordinary—and assets every woman could expect to have. Further advances in modern medicine, from orthodontia to prevention of diseases that left disfigurements, made such expectations seem reasonable. And the fashion industry kept promising that such looks could be bought or achieved through the skillful application of cosmetics and other beauty aids. Beauty itself ceased to be conceived as an exceptional, rare phenomenon. It was, in a sense, democratized. Women who noticed that they and few of their friends matched this norm were more likely to criticize their own and their friends' flaws than to conclude that the norm was not normal at all.

The pursuit of beauty and so, slenderness, also became more crucial in the fifties because new standards for the ideal woman emerged. In *The Feminine Mystique*, Betty Friedan documented both the demise of the ideal of an emancipated, self-reliant woman and women's flight back into the home. The mystique narrowed woman's socially sanctioned pursuits and her mental universe to romance, marriage, child-rearing, and homemaking. The hourglass figure indeed seemed to signal—or at least reinforce—a renewed differentiation between the sexes. A separate woman's culture and social life—volunteer committees, car pools, clubs—began to develop after the War. The women's press reflected this transformation. In the mid-forties, *Mademoiselle* regularly featured women who purposefully followed careers and gave serious thought to international events and who were to serve as models for readers. Alongside information on fashion were serious and thoughtful articles. Ten years later, the articles and images depicted suburban women concerned almost solely with their children and with beautifying their suburban homes and themselves.[25]

These changes affected women's concerns about their appearance, which occupied a larger share of their attention as their other interests narrowed and which were, indeed, a vital link to their principle goals. For most, these were marriage and children. Middle-class and upper-middle-class girls went to college to earn their "Mrs." along with their BA, and if they didn't walk out of their graduation ceremonies into wedding ceremonies, they were deemed failures and potential spinsters. Once they got their "Mrs.," they needed to hang on to it. They could do so only by cultivating their femininity, which largely involved staying attractive.

The fifties woman felt these pressures because the media—popular songs, films, and television shows—were mirroring social reality in their concentration on romantic courtship and family life. She indeed lived in a world of couples and families. The percentage of single American women over the age of fourteen dropped precipitously after World War II, from 24.3 percent in 1940 to an all-time low of 18.6 percent in 1957. The percentage of single men over the age of fourteen dropped even more precipitously, from 31.3 percent in 1940 to 24.5 percent in 1957. And women, like men, were marrying at ever-younger ages. In 1940 the median age of first marriage for males was 24.3 years; in 1957 it was 22.5 years. Women's median marriage age also dropped, from 21.5 years in 1940 to 20.3 years in 1957. And they were having scads of babies. After a century-long downward trend, the birthrate suddenly shot up as the baby-boom generation was delivered into the world. When women of the fifties worried about their appearance and their weight, and when they cautioned their daughters to do the same, they were responding to the social realities around them. Keeping fashionably attractive was an exciting new game, but it was also serious business for the business at hand: getting and staying married.[26]

But attention to appearance was more than a social strategy. America's rendition of Freudianism, which was popularized after the War, gave scientific authority—and even a sense of urgency—to the pursuit of beauty and to these other cultural developments. Women who exhibited aggressive traits, who opted for careers instead of marriage and childrearing, and who didn't prettify themselves were suspected of being psychologically maladjusted, victims of neurosis and "penis envy." The women's press was not alone in urging "femininity." The scientific community was establishing it as a standard of normal behavior. Fashion and fashion-consciousness were no longer viewed as surface concerns but rather as indispensable proof of normality. *Vogue* reflected this popularization and collusion when it glibly described as "clearly psychotic" women who didn't know how to "paint on" a presentable face.[27]

The feminine mystique and Freudianism—to which it owed much of its theoretical justification—redefined femininity in ways that heightened concerns not just about appearance in general, but about the undressed body in particular. Women were sexualized even further. Unlike the nineteenth century, when the distinctions drawn between masculinity and femininity stressed woman's asexual, spiritual nature, those of the mid-twentieth century downplayed both her intellectual and spiritual nature and stressed her sexuality.

Havelock Ellis's pioneering work after World War I had emphasized the importance of human sexuality, but Ellis's influence had been primarily among the young and the intellectuals. After World War II these ideas began to saturate the culture. From our vantage point, the fifties seem an era of remarkable sexual prudery and restraint, but in fact it was a time when these constraints loosened significantly. One study reported there were two-and-a-half times more references to sex in the media in 1960 than there had been in 1950. The decade opened with the Kinsey Report and closed with the sex-and-scandal-ridden novel, *Peyton Place.* [28]

Although historians have learned that the Victorians were less prudish than has generally been believed, the fact remains that prescriptively at least, control of sexual instincts had been elevated to the noblest of virtues and that, between the 1920s and 1950s, this value was inverted. Through the popularization of Freudianism, Americans had been introduced to the notion of the unconscious, to the danger of repressing instincts, and to the idea that infants and children as well as women had powerful erotic drives. Satisfying these drives did not become simply acceptable: it came to be viewed as essential to psychic health. It was in this context that even masturbation came to be regarded as normal and healthy and that the orgasm was restored to women. But this new belief did not encourage a simple matter-of-fact acceptance of sexuality like that prevalent in earlier centuries. Rather, it set up new expectations: Sexual fulfillment was viewed as the key to happiness. Sex consequently became more crucial even in conventional middle-class life. On the one hand, it enhanced marriage; on the other, the value of marriage itself was enhanced because it made sex possible and acceptable.

The body is, of course, the instrument for sex, and so tending to it also became an obligatory function. A woman who neglected it and her general appearance not only failed as a woman, she also jeopardized her ability to attract a man with whom she could realize sexual fulfillment, she threatened the development of her own sexuality and so her potential for happiness, and the very core of her womanliness—her sexuality—appeared to be abnormal. How her body looked and functioned became more central to her sense of inner worth. In this environment, the compulsion to have a pleasing figure became ever more intense. And more ammunition was added to the war on fat: A fat body came to be irrevocably associated with repressed or immature or perverse sexuality.

Men were spared these pressures to slim down. They did not have to alter their bodies continually to meet new standards because their clothing styles barely changed from decade to decade, and their ideal body size changed equally slowly. And men's clothing was concealing. It would have taken X-ray vision to penetrate through the period's wide-legged trousers and big jackets to see exactly how a man's body really looked. Not that men were indifferent to dress standards—they, too, were subject to powerful coercions that forced them to defer to the culture's dress code—but the corporate or professional suits were like somber uniforms which did not require the time, attention, and conscious choices that women's dress did and did not send the same multitude of complex messages. Male sartorial dullness may have been reinforced by another value: Not paying much attention to appearance (or not seeming to) was central to contemporary notions of masculinity. More fundamentally, men could not be sucked easily into dieting because of the persistent belief that a big, strong body was masculine and sexy. Even if it wasn't too strong, a big body gave the illusion of power and sexual vigor. These factors would have kept the slimming trend among men within the reasonable boundaries of the pre-War years had the health industry not entered the fray.[29]

Fashion is mutable, and slenderness might yet have remained a minor theme in our culture had it not been buttressed by a powerful movement from another quarter. Just four years after the New Look was unveiled, the health industry launched a massive campaign against overweight. No more was it merely ugly. It was lethal.

The instigator of this health campaign, which soon was also led by the health industry and medical community, was Louis I. Dublin of the Metropolitan Life Insurance Company. Dublin, a biologist, began working for Metropolitan in 1909 and rapidly became its "house intellectual and publicist." His career spanned almost six decades, and in his prolific output (more than 600 articles, papers, brochures, and speeches) he convinced a generation of physicians and Americans that overweight shortened life, that "We Are Digging Our Graves with Our Teeth"—as he vividly put it—and that "Obesity Is America's No. 1 Health Problem"—a phrase he first used in 1951.[30]

The insurance companies, and Dublin in particular, had been preaching the dangers of overweight for several decades, but they had not roused much enthusiastic support in the medical profession. This changed in 1951. In June of that year Dublin reported the results of his newest studies to an AMA symposium, and in October he addressed the sixtieth annual meeting of the Association of Life Insurance Medical Directors. These studies proved immensely persuasive. Dublin reported that the latest actuarial figures reconfirmed the correlation between overweight and higher mortality: Males with "marked obesity" had a mortality 70 percent above average-weight men while women's was 61 percent higher, and the "moderately obese" of both sexes had a mortality 42 percent above average. Much more striking was the fact that excess weight seemed to be taking a greater toll on American lives than it had previously. "There is some evidence," Dublin and his coauthors wrote, "that the excess mortality of overweights is greater now than in the past because death rates from diseases like pneumonia and tuberculosis, which were high among underweights, have declined sharply in recent decades."[31]

More striking still, Dublin overturned earlier notions about the benefits of some overweight for younger age groups. As late as 1940 Dublin had found, as had other insurance studies, that until the age of thirty, underweight correlated with a 16 percent *higher* rate of mortality. But in 1950 he revised this conclusion. Although his data continued to show decreasing mortality with higher weights in the fifteen- to nineteen-year-old age group, he now found that the reverse was true for the twenty- to thirty-year-old age group, and he argued that the protective effects of extra adipose tissue had been overvalued. In effect, Dublin was stripping fat of any positive functions, and he was lowering the age at which overweight became a problem.[32]

In doing so Dublin did more than just intensify the indictment against fat. He also gave new validity to the notion of "ideal weight." In 1923 insurance companies had developed this notion of a weight that correlated statistically with optimum life expectancy. In 1942 Dublin broke new ground with the publication of "Ideal Weights" for men, followed in 1943 by a similar list for women. Unlike earlier tables, these did not record average weights, but rather, weights everyone was to strive to achieve. Metropolitan explained that they were intended "to help people aim for a weight below the average for their height." These tables were based on the presumptions that there were weights that correlated with better health and longer life, that everyone ought to stay at these weights, and that what was average and so, normal, was not healthy.[33]

The medical profession had considered *obesity* an unhealthy and intractable condition for centuries, but it was always understood to be at the far end of the normal distribution curve for weight. Although Dublin's morbidity and mortality statistics were based on the extent to which people exceeded *average,* not ideal, weights—a fact not widely appreciated—he seemed to define over- weight as 10 percent above the ideal and obesity as 20–30 percent above it. In setting up a standard of normalcy that was well *below* average weights, Dublin in effect put more and more weight ranges under the umbrella of concern, and because of these redefinitions, turned both overweight and obesity into national epidemics. Average-weight people now were in the overweight, possibly even obese, category. *Overweight, obesity, plumpness, chubbiness,* and other terms, which once described very different sizes and had very different connotations, would begin to be used interchangeably as Dublin's views became more widely adopted. Americans would seem to be divided into only two groups—the fat and the thin.

But Dublin's new studies were a breakthrough in a far more important way as well. Demonstrating an association between overweight and higher mortal- ity did not prove that weight loss would reverse the pathogenic processes triggered by overweight. As late as 1947 Dr. Frederick Stare of the Harvard School of Public Health reported that the question as to "whether the treat- ment of obesity (that is, weight loss) produces favorable results or improved health and length of life," could not be answered. "So far as I know, this is a question that has not been given extensive study and for which there is no convincing evidence either way." Dublin's newest study unequivocally an- swered that question. Indeed, 2,300 of the policyholders in his sample had had to buy more expensive premiums because they were overweight, but they subsequently slimmed down enough to qualify for lower premiums. His data revealed that the slimmer's life expectancy returned virtually to that of some-one who had never been overweight; for one group of women, it was actually better than normal. As Dublin reported with surprising understatement, "The most encouraging feature of this study is the finding that weight loss improves the health outlook for overweight individuals." He seemed to have proved that dieting could indeed be a cure.[34]

Though Dublin's studies were based on statistical correlations, not on labo-ratory tests or scientific research, they soon came to be regarded as gospel. But statistics can be deceptive. Unfortunately, Dublin's studies both confirmed earlier life-insurance results and duplicated their flaws. These flaws reveal how much pre-existing prejudices informed research and conclusions and so helped the prejudice, thinner-is-healthier, take root.

Dublin's research was based on the experience of 25,998 men and 24,901 women who were insured between 1925 and 1934 and whose policy anniversa-ries occurred in 1950. Although the numbers were larger than in previous studies, the questionable methodology was identical. This was a self-selected population that tended to be of Northern European origin—a group that on the whole is inclined to be taller and leaner than other national and racial groups. In the early sixties, for example, the average (not ideal) weights of male MLIC policyholders were 9 to 10 pounds less than those for a larger national sample gathered by the U.S. government, and 3 to 4 pounds less for women. It was mere conjecture that the "ideal weight" for an Anglo-Saxon individual would also be ideal for someone of Mediterranean, Russian, African, or other stock.[35]

The policyholders were even a self-selected population of Anglo-Saxons; that is, they were not even representative of Anglo-Saxon health-weight rela-tionships precisely because buying life insurance was not the norm between 1925 and 1934. When in earlier decades, female policyholders had had mortal-ity rates higher than those in the nation at large, Dublin had astutely deduced that this was because the company did not actively recruit females, and so the women who purchased policies probably had been exceptional, possibly aware that they were not healthy. But Dublin never considered that the same might apply to his male policyholders, and especially to his overweight males who, since the turn of the century, had been considered high risks and so were not actively recruited and had to pay higher premiums. A healthy overweight person was simply less inclined to buy a life-insurance policy. In short, pre-existing prejudices probably skewed Dublin's sample so the data would indi-cate that lower-weight people were healthier and lived longer.

More damaging was the continued sloppiness in the collection and analysis of weight data. Applicants were weighed clothed and shod, with vague esti-mates made for how much the apparel weighed and how much shoes altered heights. In addition, a minimum of 20 percent of insurance applicants reported their own weights and heights—and in 1959, the Society of Actuaries found that self-reporters consistently under-reported their weights. Average-weight people under-reported by about 5 pounds, but among those who might qualify as overweight, the Society wrote, "the differential was quite sizeable, of the order of 10 pounds or more." A friendly family physician also was probably not above under-reporting weight to help a patient avoid a higher-priced premium. Consequently, many "overweights" probably ended up in the "normal" weight category. At least 20 percent of the raw data may have been incorrect, distorting the study results and biasing them in favor of lighter-weight people.[36]

Frequency of weighing remained the biggest methodological flaw. Policy-holders were still only weighed when they bought their premiums and never reweighed unless they bought a new policy or reapplied to change their risk category. Yet, as numerous studies have confirmed, people gain weight as they age. Consequently, what policyholders weighed when they bought premiums in their twenties or thirties revealed very little about what they weighed when they died fifteen or twenty or twenty-five years later. Even those overweight individuals who had reduced and who formed the basis of Dublin's research coup had not been reweighed to determine whether they had kept their slimmer forms. Age and weight gain simply had not been factored into the MLIC studies.

This may account for the puzzling fact that Dublin concluded that everyone should weigh what was ideal for a twenty-five-year-old. This dictum, too, was based on statistics, not on biological research. It seems reasonable to assume that his study showed heavier people died earlier precisely because he did not factor in age or weight gains and losses. The chronic diseases are diseases of middle-age and beyond, and since older people tend to be heavier, the correlation was inevitable. In a sense, Dublin seemed to be confirming the fact that older people die more frequently than young ones.

The most damaging flaw in Dublin's conclusions came from a bias built into the study from its outset. At the turn of the century, insurance companies had determined that overweight correlated with premature mortality. When Dublin did his own studies, it was weight that he focused on, not other, possibly more important, variables. Furthermore, proof of a coincidence between two phenomena is not proof of a causal connection between them. For example, Dublin and others argued that mature-onset diabetes was caused by obesity. But with the disease, large amounts of insulin are released into the blood, and insulin is a lipogenic, that is, fat-producing, hormone. Overweight may have been a *symptom* of the disease, not its cause. And while weight reduction helps control diabetes, it does not prevent its occurrence. This confusion between symptom and cause would remain as troubling as the validity of statistical correlations. While epidemiological studies must indeed rely on such correlations, they are not always useful. For example, Dublin might also have found that people who lived in white houses had higher rates of premature mortality, but such an association would have no meaning.[37]

Nonetheless, the insurance companies, with Dublin and the MLIC in the lead, launched a massive campaign in 1950–51 to get Americans to lose weight. They had become a powerful and extremely wealthy industry, and they used their influence and the expanding media to get their message across. By December, 1952, *Business Week* reported that the public had been besieged with advertisements warning about the ill-effects of overweight, such as the picture of a stoutish, middle-aged man, his buttons popping from his spreading girth, gleefully bringing a full fork to his mouth. The caption above the picture read: "Lengthening His Waistline . . . Shortening His Lifeline." This and similar ads appeared throughout the media and were reinforced by feature articles, many of them written by Dublin himself. A *Reader's Digest* piece in July, 1952, was catchily titled, "Stop Killing Your Husband" (by overfeeding him). *Business Week* explained that "overweights aren't left alone for a minute," and attributed the sudden and surprising upsurge in sales of dietetic foods to the effectiveness of this campaign.[38]

But the insurance companies, no matter how massive their campaign and how compelling their statistics, could not have seared fear of fat into the American psyche without the endorsement of a medical profession enjoying immense prestige in what many have called its "Golden Age." Polls revealed physicians were held in more esteem than even Supreme Court Justices. In 1950 and early 1951 Dublin presented his results at medical conventions and in the most prestigious medical journals. The effect was stunning. The medical community did more than support Dublin's campaign; they helped lead it. As Dublin reported in October, 1951, the AMA, the Public Health Service, and "a number of medical and health agencies, both voluntary and official," had joined the campaign.[39]

Medical spokesmen deluged the professional and lay press with their pronouncements. In June, 1951, Dr. James Hundley of the National Institutes of Health declared that "high blood pressure, heart disease, diabetes and a shortened life span are all associated with obesity." The following November, in a *U. S. News & World Report* article entitled, "Danger of Being Too Fat," Dr. Hundley answered the question, "Is excess fat really dangerous?" with an emphatic, "There is no question about that. It is." "Obesity has replaced vitamin-deficiency diseases as the #1 nutrition problem in the United States today," Dr. W.H. Sebrell, Jr., Director of the National Institutes of Health, announced in 1952. The same year, Dr. Lester Breslow, Consultant to the President's Commission on the Health Needs of the Nation, made a similar proclamation and stressed that even "normal Americans" were so heavy that it "induces excessive mortality." He urged that all Americans strive for the weights deemed desirable by the MLIC. The press informed the lay public about the unsettling news in a barrage of articles, like the 1952 *New York Times* piece entitled, "Overweight: America's #1 Health Problem." For the rest of the decade, these dire warnings continued unabated. Scientists were unequivocal. Overweight shortened life. Dieting and weight reduction lengthened it. "Pleasingly plump" was not just unfashionable: It was deadly.[40]

It is important to recognize the flawed source of medical concern because it indicates how deep-seated was the prejudice against heaviness. Scientists did not endorse the campaign for weight loss because of independent research they were doing. They endorsed it because of the MLIC studies. Throughout the literature in the lay and professional press, experts always returned to the MLIC data for confirmation of their argument that overweight was bad. Dr. Hundley of the NIH was asked by *U. S. News* what effect obesity had on death rates. He answered, "The most widely accepted figures are those of Metropolitan Life . . . . " In his 1951 article in the *Journal of Public Health,* Dr. Breslow relied entirely on Dublin's studies to confirm his warning that overweight had become a major public-health issue. Dr. Jean Mayer of Harvard's School of Public Health similarly bowed to the authority of the MLIC. In a 1955 *Atlantic* piece, he wrote that "life insurance companies, and in particular, Dr. Louis Dublin, deserve great credit for having repeatedly called attention to the very serious risks which accompany obesity." He acknowledged that the causal links were not always clear but nonetheless concluded that "there is no doubt that Dr. Dublin and his associates have overwhelming evidence for their formidable indictment of obesity." And so the links were forged wherein obesity and overweight came to be regarded unequivocally as pathogenic, and through public communication networks and at the doctor's office, this information was passed on to the general public.[41]

The power of the MLIC findings was made startlingly clear by one of Dr. Breslow's own studies. Between 1952 and 1957 he and his co-researchers studied 3,992 San Francisco longshoremen. They were uniformly overweight: 360 of them were 40 percent above the MLIC standard; on the average, they were 17 percent above the standard. Dr. Breslow anticipated that they would have mortality statistics well above average. Just the reverse occurred. "There was a strikingly lower incidence of coronary and other mortality than was experienced by all California males in comparable age groups," *Science Digest* reported. Yet this did not lead to questioning if the dictum "overweight shortens life" was false. Instead, the researchers reported being "perplexed by their own data" and said they had to be "cautious about drawing conclusions." Future medical research would also be shaped by and filtered through the MLIC dogma.[42]

While some experts did question the reliability of Dublin's statistics and conclusions, they were few in number. Most were persuaded because they were overwhelmed by the sheer quantity of policyholders studied, by the length of time they were followed, and by the consistency of the data. A private and even public researcher would have been hard pressed to duplicate the time span and large population Dublin had at his disposal. They also saw the large profits enjoyed by the insurance companies and reasoned that if incorrect criteria had been used for policy issues, profits would be suffering. And the explosion of knowledge about nutrition in the first half of the century had already alerted them to the importance of diet for health. The transition from undernutrition to overnutrition was easy to make.

The medical community was persuaded also because Dublin's studies seemed to explain a paradox at the core of America's post-War health statistics. On the one hand, between 1900 and 1950 Americans' average life expectancy had risen by twenty years, from 50 to 70. Improved nutrition and sanitation, tighter regulations on occupational hazards, antibiotics, and control of childhood and infectious diseases—especially of the two biggest nineteenth-century killers, TB and pneumonia—had given America one of the best mortality statistics in the world. But in the over–forty-five category the statistics were disheartening. With the reduction in deaths caused by infectious diseases, deaths from cardiovascular and what were called renal diseases were soaring. By 1950 they seemed epidemic, claiming 60 percent of the population over forty-five. Heart disease had become the nation's leading cause of death. Dublin and others understood that the very improvements they applauded were partially responsible for this shift. Simply, more people were surviving to the age when degenerative diseases appeared, and more of them were surviving with disabilities caused by now-curable illnesses. Nonetheless, America's mortality statistics in the over–forty-five male group lagged behind those of other advanced countries. Dublin stressed this fact. As he announced in 1951, the "mortality among our elders is too high." His weight/mortality data seemed to explain why this was the case: Americans were too fat. As emaciating diseases like TB and pneumonia lost their virulence, and degenerative diseases took their place, the lean, not the plump, body easily came to be viewed as the healthiest body.[43]

Scientists could accept Dublin's findings also because, over the decades, histologic studies had been giving body fat itself a new, more dangerous character. By the turn of the century, it was no longer seen as an inert tissue, one that served both as cushion and fuel for the body, but rather as an active, constantly moving tissue. In the twenties, controversy reigned as to whether its activity was constructive, "peaceable and law-abiding," as Dr. Woods Hutchinson put it in 1926, or destructive, infiltrating and clogging organs and arteries. By the fifties, the menacing image of fat prevailed. The most menacing fat of all appeared to be cholesterol in the blood, and by the next decade it would seem as frightening as body fat itself. The presumption was that "excess" body fat, particularly in a full-grown adult, served no beneficial functions, and in fact was pathogenic—though no biological research explained why this might be so.[44]

The scientific community could join the campaign for weight reduction also because biological explanations for weight abnormalities were passing out of favor. Weight control began to be seen almost exclsively as an exogenous or mechanical problem of diet and exercise, not an endogenous or biological one.

In the early thirties metabolic explanations had been discredited, and by the early forties, the glandular theory had its critics. Researchers began making distinctions between the glandular disorder, Simmond's Disease, and true anorexia nervosa, which came to be categorized as a psychiatric disorder. The same happened with obesity. By 1947 research had shown that only about 1 in 200 obesity cases had glandular abnormalities. It began to seem that overeating alone caused obesity. The question then was why the obese overate. The new psychoanalytic theories seemed to provide the answer. In February, 1947, Dr. Charles S. Freed announced in *JAMA* that obesity was not caused by "glandular imbalance," but by emotional tensions such as "worry, fear and insecurity," which led to overeating. In October, 1947 Hilde Bruch, one of the leading authorities on obesity, reported with uncharacteristic harshness that the glandular theory was "tommyrot" and that "fatness is a psychosomatic condition; the blubbery patient belongs not in the gym but in the psychiatrist's office." The fat person's most salient characteristics were "insecurity and immaturity."[45]

These ideas became pervasive in the fifties. Overweight people did not have a problem with their body machinery—their metabolism, glands, or even genes—but with their appetites. While some explored the biochemical reasons for appetite going amuck, psychiatrists explored the deeper emotional reasons why people ate more than their bodies "needed"—for the underlying presumption was that a body only needed what would bring it to "ideal weight." By 1959 the *New York Times Magazine* reported that 90 percent of all obesity cases were caused by "psychogenic" problems. A year later, a *New York Times Magazine* piece explained that even heredity was rarely a cause for overweight. It accounted for only 10 percent of obesity cases. These new attitudes allowed the health community to endorse wholeheartedly the campaign for weight control through diet.[46]

This tendency to discard biological explanations and view weight problems solely as a matter of appetite and personal will had other, profound repercussions. Experts began to insist that everyone keep his or her weight at the prescribed "ideal" even when nature seemed to dictate otherwise. They were well aware that the natural course of events was for adults to continue to gain weight after the age of twenty-five, and in the nineteenth century, such gains were considered evidence of robust health. Not anymore. What was natural and normal was no longer seen as healthy. Experts warned adults to eat fewer calories as they hit their middle years in order to counter this tendency. In an *Atlantic Monthly* article in 1955 physiologist Dr. Jean Mayer explained that even if people managed to keep their weights stable, their fat-to-lean ratios still increased with age. His solution was even grimmer than that suggested by other experts. Americans ought to "stop . . . weight gain at the age of twenty-five and over the later years, slowly . . . *lose* weight," he explained. They were to *vieillir sec*—that is, "age dry"—a rather unappetizing notion. Although this advice didn't receive general backing in the fifties, it would in later decades.[47]

Nor were pregnant women spared the imperative to keep their weights down. They were advised to gain only 15 to 20 pounds. This caution originally derived from concern about a serious complication of pregnancy, toxemia, which causes edema or fluid retention and, as a result, weight gain. Once again, symptom was confused with cause. Physicians encouraged all pregnant women to keep their weight-gain low to avoid the disease. They also advocated little gain so that postpartum depression would not be exacerbated by a woman's bleak realization that even after delivery she still had ample pounds to lose. In their view, too, fat served no positive function. By the early seventies, medical research had shown that weight gain did not *cause* toxemia, but rather was a symptom of it. And it had shown that limiting the caloric intake of pregnant women could have adverse effects on the fetus, leading to greater likelihood of neonatal complications. But for the pregnant American woman in the fifties and sixties, weight gain and hearty appetite were no longer sanctioned by the culture, even though biology had programmed her to experience both.[48]

The genetic explanations for overweight were harder to dismiss. Experts were increasingly aware that some people were genetically predisposed to obesity or plumpness. Certainly such genetic tendencies had been the basis for animal breeding for centuries. But rather than give allowance for these tendencies, they urged the genetically predisposed to counter them by strict dieting. Even children were not exempt from this rule. Experts were alarmed by new studies which reconfirmed that overweight ran in families. With one obese parent, a child had a 40 percent chance of being obese; with two obese parents, the chances doubled. Experts concluded that this genetic tendency had to be controlled early in life. In 1959 *Newsweek* quoted Dr. Jean Mayer as saying, "A large majority of overweight people inherit their tendency to be fat." His prescription: "strict reducing programs for children of obese parents who develop unhealthy chubbiness in the early years." Even inherited characteristics of body size could not be accepted with equanimity.[49]

The dictum to be wary of childhood weight gain did not just apply to children of the obese. With the new definition of overweight, average Americans were considered too fat, so few families could be exempt from the caution. The obese youngster had been cause for alarm for several decades, but until the fifties it was presumed such youngsters were a rare exception, not the rule. In addition, it had generally been accepted that some extra adipose tissue augured well for health and growth. In the fifties Dr. Spock assured parents that some plumpness was common for seven- to twelve-year-olds and that it tended to disappear by the age of fifteen. But now, with the new definitions of overweight and obesity, and with the new awareness of how often this "overweight" persisted into adult years, overweight seemed a potential problem for all young Americans, especially those in puberty. The popular press was filled with articles about teenagers and preteenagers who had reduced successfully. In 1960 *Newsweek* warned about "Teenage Gluttons," and one expert, Dr. Stanley Garn, warned that even six-year-olds had to be kept from "[eating their] way into a premature grave at sixty, even if it means making life less joyous in the childhood period." In the fifties, average-weight or what we would call slightly plumpish children and teenagers were not the target of weight-loss campaigns, but even for them, weight gain and plumpness had begun to seem alarming. This decade produced a weight-conscious generation of children.[50]

The demise of the glandular theories and the ascendance of psychiatric explanations for obesity also gave scientific authority to the increasingly negative qualities associated with the fat person. Already in 1940 and 1942, Dr. William H. Sheldon of Harvard had argued that people could be divided into three main body types or what he called "somatypes"—the endomorph (basically stocky and fat), the mesomorph (muscular and well-proportioned), and the ectomorph (lean and long)—and he attributed certain characteristics to each. The endomorph was rather lazy, slow, and peaceful, made of "soft metal, which has not temper in it and will not take an edge . . . a certain flabbiness or lack of intensity in the mental and moral outlook." Psychiatric theory reinforced and expanded upon this negative imagery. By the late forties, any remaining positive associations with plumpness were stripped away. *Time* magazine undermined the old association between fat and good nature in a 1947 article entitled "Fat and Unhappy"; others charged that "Obesity Hides Insecurity"; and *Newsweek* remarked on the odd phenomenon that in the past, it had been believed that nervousness, tension, and worry caused thinness, while now, they were believed to cause fatness. The human body was still the same and these were still undesirable traits, but now they were being shifted onto what had become the unattractive body type.

The psychiatric model added other, more pejorative, associations with overweight. The overweight also seemed immature and infantile, riddled with unresolved psychic conflicts. Such ideas quickly invaded mainstream America. In the fifties, Dear Abby received an angry letter from a woman who had been given the name of a psychiatrist because she was overweight. "Now, Abby," she wrote, "I am not crazy, I am just a little overweight. Have you ever heard anything so insulting?" Abby's response was that a psychiatrist might be helpful. Evidently, insults were the fate of the fat.[51]

The new theories left overweight people bereft of any excuse for their fatness. Body weight had become solely a question of personal habits, of diet and exercise—that is of psychic health and personal self-control. With this theory, a man or woman could only blame themselves if they were fat, and very possibly, learn to hate themselves if their body size did not fall within established norms. Certainly, they could no longer blame their bodies for their deviation from the new norm.

Another effect of the new ideas about weight was the establishment of new standards about its causes—diet and appetite. "Healthy" appetite was no longer defined by how much one ate but rather by how much one weighed. The body was seen as a finely calibrated combustion engine that should weigh a certain amount, and scientists issued recommendations about exactly how many calories, calibrated to age, height, and activity levels, were needed to achieve this goal. Researchers and the National Academy of Sciences' Food and Nutrition Board, mobilized originally to determine ideal diets for World War II soldiers, applied their expertise to peacetime conditions. The idea crystallized that the amount of calories people needed could be determined by the relationship between their body weight and height. Quite simply, the more overweight someone was, the fewer calories he or she should consume. The popular notion was emerging that people did not need much caloric fuel to function effectively and cheerfully, especially if they were overweight.[52]

Attitudes toward appetite changed. It came to be seen as the troubling instinct of the age. With the psychoanalytic model of overweight, it was presumed that people overate, not because of pleasure or hunger or biological promptings, but rather because of unsatisfied emotional needs or because of oral cravings that stemmed from unresolved conflicts. Psychoanalysts like Hilde Bruch had observed such pathology in many of their obese patients. But in the fifties, this diagnosis ceased to be applied only to severely obese people. It was applied to all those average Americans who were above "ideal" weight. Robust appetite, when attached to a robust body, was no longer seen as evidence of a healthy delight with food but instead as a rather unsavory symptom of neuroses and infantile longings. This model set up some paradoxical associations. The overfed body was, strangely, an empty body, one plagued with emotional needs that food would never satisfy. In this construct, food was abstracted beyond even a scientific quantity of calories and nutrients. It had been abstracted into an emotional symbol. It began to be viewed almost exclusively as nourishment for the troubled psyche, not the body. The person who "craved" a rich dessert or a calorie-laden meal did not really crave food. He or she craved emotional warmth, love, and self-respect, and food, it was argued, was used—in vain—as a substitute for these longings. The stomach and the palate were becoming irrelevant to food, and hunger itself ceased to be a trustworthy guide for eating.

The psychoanalytic model also reinforced powerfully the connection between sexual maladjustment and fatness. It wasn't just that the overweight woman neglected her appearance and so, manifested her underdeveloped femininity. For both sexes, the overeating that caused fatness was itself seen as a symptom of sexual immaturity or repression. Appetite for food became inextricably tangled up with the appetite for sex. But the sexual instinct came to be regarded as more powerful, more important, and more respectable than the instinct to please the palate or fill the stomach. In fact, it began to seem that these were not two distinct biological urges but rather one urge. Lust for culinary pleasure was merely a manifestation of a thwarted erotic drive.

The health industry was changing Americans' experience of food. Hunger, appetite, and satiety are produced as much by cultural conditioning and habit as by biological demands. If we are told that being full is healthy and produces a sense of well-being—that "after-dinner peace that passeth all understanding" as *Vogue* put it in 1947—we are likely to respond this way to sensations of fullness. If, on the other hand, we are told repeatedly that being full is unpleasant, gluttonous, and unhealthy, then we will respond very differently to the exact same meal and quantity of food. Few can resist these cultural values, particularly those who grow up with them. Paradoxically, just as Americans realized the dream of abundance and stood before a beautifully laden banquet table, they were ordered to taste only, never to feast.[53]

For this newly weight-conscious generation, the dining room table was becoming a battlefield on which instinct fought with civilization's demands. Appetite that produced a body larger than the new rigid standard was now considered a symptom of an "animal-like" drive that had not been civilized properly. The "overweight" body itself betrayed this failure of control and lack of good breeding. Well-bred young girls would prove most susceptible to this new standard. They would also prove most susceptible to eating disorders.

In a larger sense, the medical profession and the insurance companies were setting up new standards of normal body size, and these were similar to the standards being endorsed by psychology and fashion. Health authorities seemed to be endorsing the body ideal set up by fashion, even though fashionable weights were lower than healthy weights. In many instances, experts quite explicitly praised the new fashions for making Americans diet-conscious. In a 1955 *Atlantic Monthly* article, Dr. Jean Mayer praised the Dior look because it "has often succeeded where health education has failed." He did, however, caution that this tendency was not always desirable and warned that "the desire to achieve the figure of Lauren Bacall has led many girls in their teens and twenties to starve themselves into a state of physical weakness and headache."

But such admonitions and distinctions between fashionable and healthy weights were rare, and when invoked, were not put very strongly. Fashion and other popular magazines frequently interviewed the experts for tips on weight loss, and such cautions were noticeably absent. In February, 1956, *Vogue* interviewed the nation's foremost authorites about current diet research. No mention was made of women or girls who were trying to get down to the body dimensions of a Lauren Bacall. When *Vogue*'s interviewer asked about "women who could very well weigh 10 pounds more than they do but yet manage to control it," the experts did not suggest that such underweight was silly or potentially unhealthy, nor did they find anything amiss in the implication that such women were not "naturally" thin but instead "controlled" their impulse to eat. Dr. Jean Mayer responded that "they eat less, apparently because they are not hungry." No distinctions were being made between women who wanted to lose 5 to 10 pounds to get down to a low fashionable weight and women or men who needed to lose 50 to 100 pounds. As a result of this collusion, the medical establishment, like the religious, ceased perform-ing one of its most venerable functions: putting brakes on the extremes of fashion.[54]

It is not surprising that this collusion had its most powerful impact on women. Although the weight-loss campaign had initially been directed primar-ily at men because they were the ones who had the highest incidence of premature heart disease, polls repeatedly showed that women formed the vast majority of dieters. In 1954 Gallup found that twice as many women as men worried about their weights, and one in three of them dieted as opposed to one in seven men. Over the next seven years this pattern didn't change, despite the health campaign. In 1961, 72 percent of dieters were women, and 28 percent were men. And if men did diet for health reasons, women didn't. A 1959 Roper poll found that 66 percent of them dieted to "make their clothes fit better" or because they didn't want "to look heavy." In 1959 the *New York Times* reported that Americans had developed a "dieting neurosis" that was most powerful among women, not men.[55]

This collusion, however, also affected both sexes because, by giving scientific endorsement to pre-existing prejudices against the obese and overweight, it permitted both government and private employers to *require* employees to reduce—precisely because health, not attractiveness, seemed to be their mo-tive. By the end of the decade there was a spate of cases of employees' jobs or promotions being explicitly contingent on their success at losing weight.[56]

As always, the external world and the way it was perceived affected the internal world. The medical profession, and the nation as a whole, embraced the antifat campaign because they were responding to contemporary moral and social values and specific historical circumstances. At the root of the condemnation of fatness and overeating was concern about the effects of America's growing prosperity and technology. In the largest sense, the panic about fat was a reaction to modernization.

Although Americans had not gotten appreciably fatter over the century, there was a general presumption that post-War plenty and ease would make them so and thus would aggravate the epidemic of degenerative diseases. Americans seemed to be developing a "fatogenic" society. Post-War prosper-ity, with all the changes it wrought, was precisely what made medical and national leaders lead the campaign against overweight; it was also why weight loss became a widespread cultural concern only in the 1950s. Historical condi-tions were ripe for its emergence. Certainly, health and government officials could not have led a campaign against overweight during the previous twenty years—the Depression and the War years—even though it was in this period that the dangers of overweight were becoming more firmly established. A problem with abundance simply would not have seemed plausible, nor would it have been a sensible political issue.

Abundance and prosperity were not the only changes taking place. Food shopping and storage habits were transformed. Formerly, the middle-class housewife had walked to the store, bringing back only what she could carry and store in what was usually a small pantry. But the automobile, the supermarket, larger kitchens, and the availability of refrigerators and home freezers changed all that. Now the housewife could drive to the new supermarket, fill her cart with foods packaged in large containers, load them in her car, and then store them in her new freezer, large refrigerator, or ample suburban pantry. The housewife didn't bring home a pint of ice-cream anymore; she returned with a gallon or half gallon container of it. The problem with this new culinary security was underlined in 1961 by Dr. S. W. Kalb, former nutrition chairman of the New Jersey Medical Society: "[The housewife] buys a week's worth [of groceries] . . . and her family consumes it in four or five days." The opportunity, and the temptation, to overeat were becoming omnipresent.[57]

The sedentary habits spawned by modernization also alarmed experts. Underexercise was seen as the other cause of the "fatogenic" society, one that came to be stressed increasingly in the late fifties. Americans simply didn't have to expend much physical energy anymore. Increasing automation meant the farmer and manual laborer could be more productive with significantly less effort. The big shift from blue-collar to white-collar jobs meant that the American male spent his working hours sitting behind a desk instead of exerting himself physically. Shorter work weeks gave him the luxury of leisure time, but instead of spending that time chopping wood or playing sports, he spent it sitting in front of that marvelous new form of home entertainment: the television set. The automobile (especially with the rising numbers of two-car families) and labor-saving devices spared his wife caloric expenditure as well. Dr. Herman Pollack, chairman of the American Heart Association's Nutrition Committee, explained at a 1959 conference that "not too long ago [the American woman would have] . . . spent 240 calories scrubbing the family wash and another 50 calories hauling it on the line. Today, dumping the clothes in the automatic washer and tapping a button takes no more than 50 calories." Even America's youth seemed to suffer from the underexercise syndrome. Television was taking them off the playing fields, and as soon as they could, teenagers exchanged their bicycles for cars.[58]

National leaders and scientists were uneasy about the moral effects of these changes. Throughout the fifties, overweight, morality, and health themes kept intermingling. When Dr. James Hundley of the National Institutes of Health first publicized the problem of obesity in 1951, he called it "[a] luxury we cannot afford." It was, he argued, "a waste of our national resources not only in manpower but in food." These were political and moral, not health, judgments. In 1954 *Life* magazine unequivocally told its audience that "the uncompromising truth is that obesity is a result of gluttony"—a moral, not a scientific judgment. In 1956, quoting the experts, *Science Digest* proclaimed, "Obesity Blamed on Overbuying of Food"—the implication being both that obesity was common (largely because of the new definition of it) and that culinary self-indulgence was the reason for it. Two years later the same magazine headlined, "Overweight? Blame Our Soft, Lazy Way of Life."[59]

This moral concern had many sources. The Depression remained a vivid and painful collective memory, one that would last for several decades. There seemed to be a fear that if the new prosperity were misused, a debacle might ensue like that which follwed the prosperous twenties. This nagging distrust of the new plenty reinforced other deep-rooted concerns. Since the late nineteenth century there had been a persistent worry that America's traditional elite was getting soft, losing the moral fiber and physical strength that had helped it settle the nation, and that this softness was allowing new immigrant groups and the lower classes to displace it. In the early twentieth century, people like Theodore Roosevelt had stressed the importance of cultivating the "manly arts" to combat this trend. Now, in the mid-twentieth century, with the middle classes beginning to enjoy luxuries once reserved for the elite, there was concern that the backbone of the whole nation might be weakening. This caused special panic as the Cold War got under way. Competition with Russia heated up, and keeping Americans morally and physically fit, especially American children, seemed essential if that battle was to be won.

These political concerns also reflected complex historical prejudices. The leading Western nations had been concerned about the "rise of the masses"—about the political, economic, and cultural consequences of democratization—since the mid-nineteenth century. Americans had become especially concerned about these developments in the 1880s when the rush of eastern and southern European immigration began and when the traditional elite found itself displaced by a rising tide of self-made men. By the 1950s it was clear that prosperity was democratizing even further the life-style once reserved for the upper classes, a view underlined by the increasingly common notion that prosperity was "democratizing obesity." Would "common" Americans be corrupted by this luxury? Would they know how to use their new leisure and money? Women's magazines helped "cultivate" the average American woman by instructing her about Paris fashions, about refined cooking, and about etiquette. The health industry seemed to be trying to perform a similar function: educating the middle and lower-middle classes about how to use restraint and selectiveness in the face of all this new abundance and ease. The campaign seemed to be part of the long historical process of educating and "civilizing" the masses.

This bias was revealed quite clearly by the weight-loss diets advocated in the fifties. Although scientists knew that carbohydrates and proteins had the same number of calories per gram and that only fat was "more fattening" (with twice the number of calories per gram), the diet dicta of the period ruled out complex carbohydrates and encouraged meals of protein, vegetables, fruit, and low-fat milk products. Yet complex carbohydrates, particularly starches like bread, potatoes, pasta, and rice, had long been the dietary staples of most lower-class and ethnic groups. They became the verboten foods of the period, with the stigma of fattening added to their stigma of being lower-class. Milk had not been common in the European or American lower-class diet, and both meat and (in urban America) fresh vegetables and fruits were expensive. In short, the type of meal advocated was that typical of America's educated classes. Only the cautions about dietary fats and sweet desserts seemed to cross class boundaries.

At the root of the new body standard, we can also glimpse the persistence of a prejudice that had been operative in the twenties. When they set up an ideal or healthy body type, health officials did not choose the stocky build typical of southern or eastern European immigrants or of peasants—even though peasants were popularly believed to be strong and durable. Instead, they chose the lean, long look that aesthetics had established as ideal, a look associated with America's blue bloods and with European aristocrats. It was the body of the racehorse, not the workhorse. It was the look America's better-educated groups already were trying to achieve. In its 1951 polls Gallup was struck by the fact that the better educated a person was, the more he or she wanted to lose weight. The more educated were, also, on the whole, the more affluent and were more responsive to fashion's dictates. Granted, Dublin's statistics had led him to endorse this body type, but the fact that it was associated with the elite no doubt helped others, even the medical profession, accept Dublin's conclusions. Had he come up with a short, stocky standard, the medical profession may have been less credulous.[60]

How much even Louis Dublin was influenced by these prejudices is indicated by his list of reasons why people should reduce. As early as August, 1952, in the MLIC's *Statistical Bulletin,* Dublin wrote about the "Handicaps of Overweight." After listing the usual health "penalties" of overweight, he went on to detail the "handicaps" it imposed in the personal life of individuals: Employers preferred normal-weight job applicants; children ostracized obese youngsters; the obese girl's chances for marriage were poorer than her thinner rivals'; and, echoing the new psychological theories, "the fat person is not always the jolly individual he is pictured to be. His overweight is sometimes a manifestation of his feeling of inadequacy." In short, Dublin was justifying his dictum that people reduce on the basis of pre-existing cultural preferences, not on the basis of health. The overweight faced these handicaps, not because they seemed unhealthy, but because others preferred "normal-weight" individuals. It was comparable to saying someone should avoid a disease not because it is unhealthy but because others don't like its symptoms. Dublin may have been describing accurately the experience of obese people, but he had redefined both *obesity* and *overweight* so that they no longer referred to abnormal body sizes but rather, to average body sizes. Influenced by a fashionable preference, he had given scientific justification to it. Physicians shared this cultural bias, and it made them, too, less critical of the MLIC data. In a curiously circular dynamic, an aesthetic taste for slenderness had influenced health standards, and these health standards, in turn, spread and intensified the quest for slenderness.[61]

These larger concerns may also explain the surprisingly facile acceptance of an association between abundance, overweight, and degenerative diseases whose causes were still unknown. Americans had witnessed the sharp drop in mortality from infectious disease and the spectacular rise of mortality from cardiovascular and other diseases. The primary difference they saw between the past and the present, and between themselves and other nations with better mortality rates for the middle-aged, was the rising tide of affluence, culinary abundance, and the decline of physical labor. It all seemed simple and straight-forward—suspiciously so. Susan Sontag trenchantly observed that when the cause of a disease is unknown, the illness becomes a metaphor for other cultural concerns and conflicts. This had occurred with tuberculosis in an era when it causes were unknown: The same seemed to be happening with heart disease, cancer, and the other killers of the mid-twentieth century.[62]

In another curiously circular dynamic, vast numbers of Americans re-sponded to the cultural command to slim down precisely because of their increasing affluence and leisure. They could conceive of emulating the upper classes because, for the first time, they had the money and leisure to do so. Historian J. H. Plumb described how, over the previous two centuries, the "acquisition of increased leisure, combined with a modest affluence in a rising social class, has usually led to a desire for self-improvement," a desire reflected in an increased demand for books, education, music, sporting goods, health care and for what was fashionable in clothing as well as cooking and interior decorating. In short, it was the democratization of what formerly had been aristocratic culture. The pursuit of these activities trickled down the social ladder as more and more classes could afford them, and eventually turned leisure activities into a vital commercial industry. In the nineteenth century, but even more in mid-twentieth-century America, this trickling erupted into a veritable flood, and fueled the emergence of a mass, urban-based culture. Self-improvement and social betterment became preeminent goals, a phenome-non underlined by Americans' new urge to "keep up with the Joneses." A vastly greater number of Americans was now responsive to the messages being peddled by cultural authorities. And, one message peddled with increasing fervor was that slender was best.[63]

Faith in the efficacy of diet persisted through the fifties and, indeed, through to the eighties, even though considerable evidence showed its premises might be seriously flawed. It wasn't as easy to get Americans to shed weight or to keep it off as had been expected. What had begun as a fairly straightforward proposition, getting Americans to reduce their caloric intake, had boomer-anged into a complicated problem. Diets didn't seem to work. Reviewing the results of weight-reduction programs conducted between 1939 and 1951, psy-chiatrist Albert J. Stunkard concluded that "[the] results of treatment for obesity are remarkably similar and remarkably poor . . . . " By the early sixties

Dr. Philip White of the AMA's Council on Food and Nutrition had to confess the embarrassing truth that overweight was "a public-health problem without a public-health solution." Psychiatrists and psychologists were making no better headway in isolating the etiology of overweight. They could not find any one psychological profile or explanation for the overweight "neurotics". Other research was throwing uncomfortable doubts on even the overeating/overweight equation. Instead of causing a rethinking of basic premises about overweight, these problems simply led to more funding for more research.[64]

All the ingredients for the diet-mania that we know today had emerged in the 1950s. But still, there were significant differences. Many authorities still tried to buck the trend—something they would not do again until the alarm about eating disorders. In July, 1955, *Woman's Home Companion* reported that "Teenage Dieting Has the Experts Worried." Hilde Bruch published *The Importance of Overweight* in 1957 and balked about the new orthodoxy. She was one of the few who objected to the erection of a rigid standard of body size and who doubted the validity of the MLIC's findings. "The fact is," she wrote, "that some people function at their best with a relatively greater amount of fat tissue . . . . " She re-emphasized that nature makes people in different sizes and mused how odd it was that Americans, of all people, should try to impose one body form on everyone. "It is an amazing paradox," she wrote, "that our culture, with its great flexibility and liberal ideas, attempts to superimpose one form of body build on those whom nature has endowed differently." Even the AMA was stunned by the diet-mania that had taken root in America. Its exhortation that people eat more moderately had not produced thinner Americans. Instead, it had produced a "dieting neurosis" that many AMA members criticized.[65]

Some criticized the unpleasantly puritanical and scientific attitude toward food. In 1960 in the *Nation,* David Cort railed against the "pompous sadism" of the diet advisers and claimed it reflected the "prescriber's anti-social disapproval of other people having any fun." He reminded his readers of a well-known truth that authorities seemed hell-bent on turning into an abnormal sin: "One of the major anticipations that keeps many people going is the next meal; it is a large part of what they mean by happiness and they should not lightly be deprived of it." Hilde Bruch, in more sober and clinical terms, pointed out that eating is a great satisfaction to most people, and even if some used food as a "sedative" or a neurotic crutch, it certainly was a relatively harmless one. Outbursts like these, unashamedly justifying the joys of eating and denouncing the guilt increasingly being attached to it, would become scarce in the next decades.[66]

Food had only begun to lose its innocence. There was no "panic in the pantry" yet. Although researchers had already begun to explore whether specific foods—sugar, fats, cholesterol—caused heart disease and whether additives caused cancer, their work was still in the preliminary stages. Americans still weren't terrified that their food supply and their eating habits were lethal. The only problem was that they ate too much. At its worst, food was a sedative or a drug, not because of any quality in the food itself but because of the eater's psychological problems. A 1950s mother might be accused of overfeeding her family; she was not yet accused of poisoning it. "Healthy" eating involved merely a calorie count, not a Ph.D. in nutrition.

Neither was there yet an epidemic of St. Vitus's dance. Adult Americans left sports and exercise to their children and to the pros. Although Jean Mayer and some other experts emphasized the importance of exercise for weight control, few experts advocated it. In 1951, when *U. S. News* asked Dr. Hundley about the value of exercise for weight loss, he replied it was "of very little value." It was generally believed that exercise spurred appetite, "and the result is that you eat as much as you burn up," Hundley explained. Even worse, the numbers didn't add up. "You have to walk thirty-five miles to burn up a pound of fat," claimed Hundley, and that seemed like an unreasonable task for anyone. By the late fifties, Jean Mayer had helped persuade many that exercise was important for both weight loss and to prevent heart disease. "Exercise has been too long neglected as part of the method of reducing," Mayer declared in 1956. Even so, the exercise advocated was modest: fifteen knee bends and a two-mile walk a day, *Newsweek* reported experts advising.[67]

Furthermore, in the fifties, fashion was still more a matter of clothes than of the figures underneath them. Until 1958, and even for a long time after, clothing, not body shape, dominated the fashion pages. True, a woman was incessantly reminded that she should be slender, but the magazines did not prescribe how each detail of her anatomy should look. When in 1948 *Mademoiselle* listed the beauty preparations of the bride, all it had to say about the bride's figure was, "Oh, of course it's divine, one of the things that first made Harry notice you." Such reassurances would disappear from the fashion press in later decades. But even in the fifties fashion had not yet passed any decrees about thighs, hips, breasts, behinds, and arms and wouldn't begin to do so until 1958, when *Vogue* started to set standards about legs and about the bathing-suit figure. There was no reason for women to agonize about every detail of their anatomies. No one was setting specific standards about them.[68]

And fashion, though becoming more rigorous, was still kind to women. It was still a handmaiden of Beauty. It still provided tools for the ordinary, flawed figure to look good. Women relied on girdles, on the cut and fabric of clothes, not just on diet, to shape their forms. The women's press was filled with ads that promised girdles and bras would help out where nature had failed. Girdle sales soared to all-time highs as women donned them to mold their recalcitrant flesh. This underwear was quite modern. It molded the body with elastic instead of encasing it in a cage of whalebone or cane, but still it managed to tame the figure. The lines and the fabrics of 1950s fashion still allowed for a certain amount of internal manipulation and construction. In later decades, diaphanous fabrics and relaxed cuts would require a perfectly kept body underneath them to look good—and a body unaided by girdle or corset. The woman of the fifties was spared the agonies of her successors.

Girls and women did not seem to suffer from the distorted body images that would become so common in later decades. True, psychologist Sidney Jourard found in the 1950s that women were less satisfied than men about the way they looked. They wanted to lose weight, to have smaller waists and hips, and to change their breast size—the overriding female body issue of the 1950s—but these preoccupations did not produce the self-loathing that would become so common later.[69]

Even more importantly, Americans had not been persuaded completely that abundance and overweight were unhealthy and dangerous. This was a complacent age, and Americans were basking in the glow of their newfound plenty and well-being. Even after the media blitz about heart disease, they were not convinced that it was frightening. In a 1939 Gallup poll, 76 percent of the sample listed cancer as the worst disease; only 9 percent listed heart trouble. In 1965, twenty-six years later, public response was similar. Sixty-two percent listed cancer as the worst illness; only 9 percent listed heart trouble. People believed that overweight shortened life—they just didn't believe it shortened life very much, the makers of Metrecal found after conducting extensive interviews in the late fifties and early sixties. "Most people think it shortens life by maybe five minutes," one researcher concluded. He added that their personal experience did not convince them that overweight caused premature deaths because "there is no *visible threat* that people are dying of overeating."[70]

And it was difficult to transform deeply held beliefs about food and body size. As late as 1964 Dr. Ernest Dichter, once referred to as the "Führer" of motivation researchers, observed that it was difficult to persuade Americans to diet and lose weight for several reasons. They still didn't trust their affluence, he suggested, and feared that an economic depression and deprivation could reappear suddenly, snatching from them their newfound bounty. And they resisted diet advice because they didn't like the idea that someone wanted to take goods away from them. Even more, Dr. Dichter astutely commented, "there's something unnatural about dieting," especially amidst plenty, especially because eating remained such a private, family-based, emotional, and sensual pleasure. More trenchantly, Dichter remarked that people still had an almost subconscious fear of leanness. They equated it with illness and death and with an unpleasant asceticism: "A lean guy doesn't celebrate any orgies." Men also equated it with impotence (though they also equated obesity with impotence), and Dr. Dichter made the observation, startling to our ears, that "if you could convince people, specifically men, that the lean person is sexually more potent . . . dieting might be universally followed." He added, however, that "people just don't believe [that] being overweight makes you impotent." Certinly, within ten years, it would be generally accepted that an overweight man was less sexy and less potent than one at his "ideal" weight.[71]

Another difference between the fifties and subsequent decades was that the standard of slenderness was not as rigid as it would become. The styles of teenagers' clothes were still differentiated fom those of mature women, who consequently did not have to have the bodies of eighteen-year-old girls. High-fashion models and movie stars like Lauren Bacall were flanked by more fully fleshed beauties like Ava Gardener, Elizabeth Taylor, Jane Russell, the teenage idol Sandra Dee, and, of course, the legendary Marilyn Monroe. If our ideal of beauty today is long and lean like a thoroughbred, the ideal in the fifties included both this type and one that was soft, cuddly, and kittenish.

But the most crucial difference between this time and our own is that the standard of slenderness was not as extreme. The "ideal" weights of the MLIC tables were several pounds more than they would be after 1959, when they were issued as "desirable" weights. And certainly, fashionable slenderness had not yet approached the skinniness prized in subsequent decades. Although a woman's figure was increasingly being described by her dress size, that size was usually a perfect 10 or 12 or 7 or 9, not a 4, 3, 2, or 1 as would be the case later. The ideal woman still had some graspable flesh on her. Her bones were not supposed to show. Marilyn Monroe weighed 122 pounds in her famous nude calendar pose and probably quite a bit more when she starred in films like *Some Like It Hot.*

The Miss Americas still had flesh on their bones, too, though less than in the 1940s. In 1954 the average contestant weighed 121 pounds and measured 5'6.1"—about 13 pounds less than the national average, and just a little less than the MLIC's ideal weights. That same year, the reigning Miss America, Evelyn Ay, measured 5'8" and weighed 132 pounds; in 1957 the crown went to Marion McKnight, who was 5'5" and weighed 120 pounds. Yet in the three years between 1980 and 1983, the average weight for a 5'8" contestant was 117 pounds—15 pounds less than Miss Ay—and the average weight for a 5'5" contestant was 108.5 pounds—almost 12 pounds less than Miss McKnight. Even *Playboy,* in its first issue, showed women with flesh on their frames. It included candid photos of cavorting nude California girls who had hips and buttocks that were full and even dimpled. Their behinds undoubtedly jiggled and wiggled when they walked. The ideal was slimmer than it had been in the forties, but it was not yet skinny. Americans, especially American women, wanted to be slim, but what they meant by slimness was different than what we mean today.[72]

In the fifties, preference had turned into prejudice; in the sixties, it evolved into myth. The standard of slenderness got thinner and the war against fat escalated.

7

Prejudice Becomes Myth: 1960–1970

Developments in the fifties had created the culture of slimming and an atmosphere in which the urge and standards for slenderness could become more extreme. They did. New developments in the sixties gave added momentum to the trend. The decade opened with the glamorous Kennedy presidency, and the impeccably refined Jacqueline Kennedy emerged as one of a number of attenuated female ideals. It closed with the cultural chaos caused by the youthful rebels of the counterculture and their increasingly militant demands for an end to the war in Vietnam and for liberation—political, social, personal, and sexual. Among the values this upheaval seared into the national psyche were that youth was the only desirable stage of life and youthfulness the most desirable quality of those over thirty. Weight loss came to be seen as the key to perpetuating and recapturing both. Slenderness gathered a romantic nimbus inseparable from the growing cult of youth, making Americans' quest for thinness more insistent. It also became more difficult, as both medical and fashionable standards of body size became ever-thinner. By the end of the decade, an emaciated seventeen-year-old girl, Twiggy, was our fashion and aesthetic ideal.

The tensions of the era could have made body weight seem a minor issue, but they did not. The steady growth of the weight-loss industry attested to Americans' growing urge, in the jargon of the era, to "take inches off." The magazines kept issuing a steady stream of diets, publishing about thirty each year. The book trade also reflected this crescendoing interest. In 1959 ninety-two diet books were in print; by 1973 *Newsweek* reported that "several hundred" cluttered bookstore shelves, many of them now endorsed or written by doctors. The decade began with the smashing success of Dr. Taller's 1961 book, *Calories Don't Count* (a refurbished version of a high-fat diet that originated in Germany in the 1880s) and closed with the equally successful high-protein, water-gagging regimen of the *Doctor's Quick Weight Loss Diet* (1968) by Dr. Irwin Stillman. Its sales reached the 5-million mark within a few years.[1]

The diet-food industry burst beyond its modest beginnings. Metrecal found a competitor in Pet Milk's Sego, and their combined sales amounted to $450 million a year by 1965. Alternatives to high-calorie foods kept appearing, from nondairy creamers to the spectacularly successful diet sodas Tab and Diet-Rite. With the change in American food attitudes, many seemed no longer to want food that did the job—provided energy through calories—or harbored the dangers—chief among them, fat—that food did. Calories were no longer even equated with energy but rather with sluggish fat. In 1962 40 percent of American families were using "lo-cal" products; eight years later, 70 percent of them were.[2]

Lo-cal food did not interfere with the parallel growth of fantastic weight-loss gimmicks, most of which were sold over the counter or through the mails. There were obesity-removing creams, reducing pills, and dubious contraptions like Relaxacisors and Jack Feather's rubber belts, which purportedly took "inches off." Six-hundred thousand of these were sold before the government intervened in 1971. Government officials estimated that diet hucksters were bilking the nation out of anywhere from $250 million to $1 billion a year.[3]

Reducers also still expected modern medicine to find a solution to their weight problems, and diet doctors—and prescriptions for diuretics and diet pills—proliferated. By 1970 ten billion amphetamine pills were produced annually and, as a *Life* article revealed in 1968, many doctors prescribed them without even examining the patient. Amphetamines, which were supposed to dampen appetite, seemed to be a socially sanctioned addiction, despite the warnings of many experts. Not until 1972 did the government begin to bear down on amphetamine production and prescriptions. In the 1960s "speed" was just one more medical miracle that was supposed to cure eaters of their fat.[4]

Group dieting also surged in popularity. Many health agencies began "anticoronary" clubs for middle-aged men who needed to reduce, start exercising, and lower their fat intake. These clubs grew and received enthusiastic endorsement from the medical community, even after research showed they did not produce more permanent weight loss than other methods. The ranks of TOPS reached 60,000, and it found itself with many imitators. In 1960 three Los Angeles housewives started Overeaters' Anonymous, modeled on Alcoholics' Anonymous and dedicated to the idea that overeating was a compulsion that could never be cured but only controlled through strong doses of spiritual aid. Three years later another housewife, Jean Nidetch, started Weight Watchers, which also relied on evangelical fervor, group support, and peer pressure. Weight Watchers' revenues jumped from $160,000 in 1964 to $8 million in 1970. Other group organizations also sprouted up: Diet Control Centers in 1968, Appetite Control Centers in 1969. Women formed the bulk of members in all of these organizations: in the sixties OA was 95 percent female; TOPS 98 percent. In this decade of change, one thing hadn't—women were still the ones caught up in the rage for slenderness.[5]

The rise of these group organizations reflected the growing faith in group therapy, which was developed in the forties, as a psychotherapeutic method, and the growing frustration of the overweight who found traditional diet aids simply weren't effective. In OA we also see emerging the idea that people could be addicted to food, that their compulsion to eat could be similar to alcoholics' or gamblers' self-destructive, compulsive behavior. The group method also pointed to a new trend toward public, therapy-oriented, confession about weight and eating problems, but when these groups were formed, such eating problems presumably occurred only among the significantly overweight, not among the general population. This presumption would change rapidly in the next two decades.

Most significant from our perspective, exercise entered the picture as an important adjunct to diet. Exercise gurus such as Jack LaLanne started to appear on television, carrying their message into the homes of millions of women viewers, while growing health and fitness concerns began to urge exercise for men, too.[6]

Following the cultural rhythms that had been intensifying since the turn of the century, in the sixties, the web of beliefs condemning fatness grew more deeply entrenched, and official panic mounted about the "overweight society." Thinness was redefined as ever-thinner, and still more people found themselves outside the boundaries of the sanctioned norms.

Once again, the insurance industry led the way by setting up new standards. Louis Dublin had helped launch a research project by the Society of Actuaries which pooled the data of twenty-six American and Canadian insurance companies. They ended up with an unprecedented sample of 4,900,000 policyholders and carefully examined the relationships between body weights and mortality, and between blood pressure and mortality. This research culminated in Dublin's crowning achievement, the massive *Build and Blood Pressure Study* (BBPS), published in 1959. Its results became medical gospel and were included in medical textbooks and in all discussions about American health.[7]

The results unequivocally reconfirmed that the risk of premature death increased linearly with the degree of overweight. This was hardly news. What was new was that "healthy" weights apparently were even lower than had been believed. As a result, the MLIC changed its "ideal weights" to the milder "desirable weights"—but the mildness was deceptive. "Desirable weights" were lower than "ideal weights," and they were 10 to 15 percent below average weights. Once again, by fiat, the percentage of Americans categorized as fat suddenly grew. Several million Americans who had gone to sleep secure that their weights were in the healthy range awoke one morning to find that they, too, had a weight problem.

Dublin and the Society of Actuaries had not just lowered weight standards. In their massive study, they consistently repeated that being somewhat underweight was always healthier, effectively removing any sense that people could be too thin. As Dr. C. S. Chlouverakis put it in the *Journal of Obesity and Bariatric Medicine,* the insurance company data "would suggest that the goal of every individual would be to be as thin as possible"—a deduction that spread among the general public.[8]

Not only were optimum weights getting lower, but, according to MLIC data, Americans were also getting heavier. Or at least men were. Short men had gained about 5 pounds compared to their counterparts in similar studies conducted in 1885–1900 and 1909–1927, and average-height men had gained 1 to 3 pounds. Tall men had gained less. But women, more responsive to the previous decade's weight-loss campaigns, were getting lighter. Twenty-five-year-olds were 5 to 6 pounds lighter, and women thirty-five to fifty-five were generally 2 to 4 pounds lighter. This fact did not dispel the fear that American abundance was dangerous. Rather, it validated the idea that weight loss could be achieved through diet, and women's weights still caused concern. Because "desirable weights" were lower, the average woman was still heavier than she was supposed to be.[9]

The BBPS had all the flaws of previous insurance studies, particularly the sloppy methods for collecting weight and mortality data. Dublin believed he had answered his earlier critics because the new sample was more representative of the population at large and because the MLIC had adjusted "desirable weights" according to whether one had a small, medium, or large frame, but the BBPS was the first of the insurance studies to be published in its entirety, and some experts found more serious flaws. Many objected because there were no criteria to measure different body builds. Others objected that the statistical correlations still shed no light on whether obesity was actually a *cause* of mortality or merely another *symptom* of a body type prone to premature death. Dr. Jean Mayer noted that the study merely showed "a lanky, not very muscular body type is associated with a longer-than-average life expectancy."[10]

Furthermore, the BBPS data had been based on how much people were above *average,* not desirable, weights, and yet throughout the professional and lay literature, the refrain was, "Overweight is defined as body weight in excess of desirable weight." This confusion may explain why Dr. Philip White, the AMA's Director of Food and Nutrition, reported that there "is a definite school of thought that it isn't until a person gets 30 or 40 percent above his desirable weight that you begin to see enough difference in the mortality and morbidity rates to be worrisome." A more startling revelation appeared in the *New England Journal of Medicine* in 1966: A reassessment of the BBPS data showed there actually was no significant excess of mortality until individuals reached a level of "extreme obesity." Much of the panic seemed to be unwarranted. Other problems in the BBPS would become more apparent later, such as the short time policyholders were followed—an average of 7.8 years—and the small number of policies actually terminated by death—barely 3 percent.[11]

These weaknesses did not stem the tidal wave of opinion endorsing the new MLIC dicta. Few physicians demurred, and many prestigious experts, journalist Peter Wyden found, not only recommended weight loss to their patients and the public but also tried to become somewhat underweight themselves, struggling against what in a different era would have been viewed as a trivial 3 or 4 pounds.[12]

Most other authorities also embraced the findings. More funding was funneled into obesity research, and the federal government committed itself to the campaign against overweight even more energetically than in the previous decade. During 1961–62, the U. S. Public Health Service (USPHS) began to conduct its own height-weight studies of the U. S. population, acknowledging its debt to the insurance companies for bringing attention to the importance of body weight. In 1966 the USPHS published *Obesity and Health;* in 1969 there was a special White House Conference on Food, Nutrition, and Health. The conference report opened with an adamant echo of the BBPS position. "Obesity is a real health problem," it declared. "Mortality rates from lung, heart, and circulatory diseases are higher for the obese person . . . . " When government hearings on American nutrition were conducted in 1968–69, their original purpose was to examine the extent of hunger in "the other America" that Michael Harrington had suddenly brought to public attention, but, paradoxically, congressmen and expert witnesses alike constantly found themselves drawn back, as though mesmerized by it, to the problem of obesity in the general population.[13]

The government's height-weight studies added to the mounting panic about overweight because they indicated that the epidemic was even more serious than the MLIC had suggested. Average weights of uninsured Americans were higher than those of insured Americans, and they were gaining more than the insured population: Since 1912 men had gained 1 to 5 pounds, women 2 to 6 pounds. Officials deduced that 25 to 45 percent of adults over thirty were at least 20 percent overweight—up from both the estimated 20 percent in 1933 and the 1950's estimate of 25 percent. More disturbing, if the data included adults over thirty who were 5 percent or more overweight, the estimates could reach 90 percent. The huge gap between what Americans were supposed to weigh and what they actually weighed was getting wider, and threatened to get wider still. Dr. Oral Kline, Assistant Commissioner for Science of the Food and Drug Administration, echoed a widespread fear: "The nation could become so overweight that we won't be able to move."[14]

One potent reason this spectre caused panic was because of the link between obesity and heart disease. The country's main killer, heart disease claimed more than twice as many lives as the second major cause of death, cancer, and among its principal victims were men in their working prime. Yet even an educated group like corporate executives were ignoring the health dicta to lose weight. Executive Health Examiners evaluated 18,000 top-level executives a year and found that 93 percent of them were overweight.[15]

The mounting concern also expanded to include children. Frustrated by the poor success of weight-loss programs, experts reasoned that the only solution was to avoid weight gain altogether. But at what age did fat become so stubbornly fixed on the human frame? Experts began glancing down the age column, and studies began appearing in 1960 which indicated that the plumpness of childhood was never lost. One frequently cited study had revealed that 84 percent of the boys and 82 percent of the girls who were overweight in grade school remained overweight as adults. Even the plumpness of childhood now seemed sinister. In the sudden spate of summer camps for overweight children, in the frequent warnings from pediatricians and the women's press, and in the attitudes of teachers and parents, children learned that for them, too, fat was dangerous. A generation was being reared to fear flesh and appetite.[16]

Along with the lower weight standards came renewed faith that body weight was a matter of personal discipline and eating habits. The psychogenic explanation for overweight had been a caveat in this model because, although it too discounted natural variations in physique and appetite by presuming that everyone should be a certain body size, it also presumed that weight was not entirely a matter of conscious control but rather the result of unconscious drives. This explanation became somewhat suspect in the sixties, as more researchers reported that no consistent psychological profile could be associated with obesity. As early as 1957 psychiatrist Harold Kaplan and clinical psychologist Helen Kaplan had reviewed the literature on obesity and concluded that "almost all conceivable psychological impulses and conflicts have been accused of causing overeating, and many symbolic meanings have been assigned to food." They did not, however, discard the neurotic explanation for obesity but instead rather weakly concluded that "*any* emotional conflict may eventually result in the symptom of overeating," a belief that remained firmly embedded in both popular and professional psychology.[17]

A few years later psychiatrist Albert Stunkard's research further undermined the psychogenic explanations. Using the Midtown Manhattan Study, which had evaluated the prevalence of neurosis in an urban population, Stunkard analyzed the correlation between neurosis and overweight. He found none. Instead, he and his associates found that obesity correlated with socioeconomic status (SES). Thirty percent of the women in the lowest SES group were obese as opposed to 16 percent in the middle group, and a mere 5 percent in the upper group. For men, the correlates were less pronounced, though similar. Even more startling, when they were upwardly mobile, women were thinner: Only 12 percent of those moving up in class were obese, as opposed to 22 percent of those falling down the socioeconomic ladder. Stunkard surmised that among the lowest SES group, female obesity was normal and so acceptable, while among higher groups it was both abnormal and a social liability, which made higher-SES women work harder at controlling their eating and conse-quently, their weight—a presumption confirmed by later data which showed that though the upper and upper-middle classes comprised only 11 percent of the population, they included 24 percent of the nation's dieters. Stunkard's findings made psychological and physiological causes of overweight seem min-imal compared to the impact of cultural standards and so contributed to the shift toward viewing weight almost exclusively as a matter of conscious self-control.[18]

Paralleling the downward trend in weight standards came ever-lower esti-mations of how many calories people needed. The National Academy of Sciences lowered its caloric recommendations in 1957, again in 1963, and again in 1968, when it suggested that a 154-pound twenty-two-year-old male of average size needed 2,800 calories daily, and a similar woman of 127 pounds needed only 2,000 calories daily. Although experts kept revising the assump-tion that adults needed fewer calories with each passing decade—evidence that what human caloric needs actually were remained an unresolved issue—some adhered to it because, as one researcher explained, the decline in metabolic rate with age "is of such magnitude that obesity and overweight can be produced in subjects of normal weight as they grow older by not changing exercise or eating habits." Overweight people were advised to follow more deprivatory regimes, consuming only about half the calories of normal-weight individuals, and the obese in supervised programs were put on 400- and even zero-calorie diets.[19]

One result of the new medical trends was that the fattish body ceased to be regarded as a better nourished body. In the government hearings in 1966, experts kept referring to obesity as a form of "malnutrition"—a term loaded with negative connotations. Since the twenties malnutrition had been associated with nutritional-deficiency diseases and with poverty, dirt, and ignorance. The term also reflected a new and growing prejudice. While later studies revealed that some obese people, particularly poor ones, did not get enough essential nutrients, the presumption that this was also true of the comfortable, over-weight, middle classes was hardly justified. The paradoxical conviction grew that the fat body was somehow an undernourished, vulgar, and ignorant body.

This cluster of beliefs was endlessly and frenetically pushed upon the public, with not a hint of the doubts that troubled some experts. As usual, the medical and insurance communities were only part of a larger fabric constraining the weight-conscious. To understand how the prejudice against fat turned into a myth about thinness in the sixties, we must look at fashion, for it was fashion, in its largest sense, that wed youth and thinness and turned them into an American mythology. Oddly enough, in their romantic dismissal of all that was middle-aged, middle-class, and middle-American, the decade's social and fashion revolutionaries endorsed "Establishment" prejudices about body size. What emerged was a philosophy in which youth was all, and thinness guaran-teed youth.

* * *

Fashion does not exist in a vacuum. It came to romanticize and adulate youth for demographic and economic reasons. In the sixties we can again see those circumstances that created slender ideals in the 1830s and 1920s: a period of social and cultural upheaval, redefinitions of the role of women, and an expanding economy. But the revolution spawned in the sixties proved more extreme and far-reaching than its predecessors, in part because it was endorsed so thoroughly by other cultural developments and institutions.

The election of John F. Kennedy was the formal inception of America's youth-oriented cultural swing. Kennedy, at forty-three the youngest man ever elected president, set a tone of youthful idealism and vigor, and history and demographics supplied him with a responsive population. On the one hand, there were the growing numbers of Americans enjoying longer life spans. Since 1947 concern had mounted about how this development might hurt American society and, as more Americans lived longer, the solution seemed to be to prolong youth and to encourage youthfulness in middle age.[20]

On the other hand, and much more influential, the first wave of the 71 million babies of the post-War baby boom began to come of age in 1960. By their sheer bulk, they were destined to dominate the culture. When they became consumers in the sixties American businesses and advertisers focused on them and mobilized to tap the vast, affluent market they formed. In doing so, they mythologized and glamorized the "Pepsi Generation." And this pampered, media-nourished group, so full of high personal expectations, herded together in high schools and colleges, formed its own subculture and, Narcissislike, also idealized its own youthful image.

Their numbers and their confidence, born of a stable world, gave the attack they unleashed on that world tremendous potence, causing a cultural upheaval far greater than that of the 1920s. In the late fifties east-coast college students started reviving hootenannies and folk music, which had seemed "pinko" during the McCarthy era, and they started participating in civil rights marches. In the mid-sixties, whether as flower children or drugged psychedelic mystics, SDSers or Stalinists, would-be rock stars or community organizers, Weathermen or Black Panther sympathizers, this generation turned its back on its own middle-class culture, charging that America did not live up to its own ideals. They were united by their exhilarating belief that they could create a better world and by their contempt for the "Establishment." They rebelled against American politics and policies, against all forms of repression and oppression, against materialism and commercialism, against the war in Vietnam, against middle-class morals and values like the work ethic, against all traditional authority, and against everything else connected to what they perceived to be the "corrupt" and spiritually stagnant edifice of American society.[21]

The young were reinforced by a new cultural leadership, the "culturati," made up of bohemians and artists, painters, photographers, writers, journalists, the creators of experimental theater and underground movies. Together, these groups upended the old structure of high culture, and through wild experimentation, kept pushing beyond acceptable boundaries, only to cross the new boundaries they had barely established.

As one perception collapsed into another, middle-class and middle-aged—thirty-years old or more—became synonymous, and a middle-aged body became as repellent as a middle-aged mentality. Together they were a form of living death. The "ugly American" was invariably a fat American. Thinness and youthfulness became identical notions in the popular imagination.

The world of fashion, reeling from the impact of the counterculture, quickly adapted, and some of the rebels entered the fashion world to begin change from the inside. Fashion had to respond to the young. They had the buying power, and yet they scorned fashion traditions. In the fifties, as bobby-soxers, they had formed their own dress subculture but had still dutifully followed the lead of their elders, and fashion had been what trickled down from Paris and from the wealthy social elite. Jackie Kennedy was the last representative of that group to embody the fashion ideal. By the mid-sixties the young weren't buying the clothes or following the rules set by *Vogue,* the French couturiers, or their elders. The pyramidic structure of fashion came tumbling down. Fashion was thoroughly democratized—even revolutionized. Styles were set, not by the elite but by "the street." This revolution had been brewing since the fifties, when the democratization of fashion had allowed the middle classes to imitate the elite more ably. But now, the fashion impulse itself came from below, from upstart designers who took their cues from the working classes, from beatnik and avant garde artists, and from the pop teen culture, who aimed specifically at the popular market—like the phenomenally successful Mary Quant—and from the young, who set their own styles.[22]

The media acknowledged that the young were taking over the cultural role of the elite, nowhere more explicitly than in *Vogue*'s 1963 piece, "The New Upper Class, the Kids." The young undermined the traditional impulses behind fashion: declaring wealth, status, and acceptance in genteel society. The expense of clothing no longer had much cachet: Wendy Vanderbilt posed proudly for *Time* in one of her "favorite" evening dresses from the boutique Paraphernalia. Cost: $26. Poverty had become chic. The young even rebelled against traditional shopping patterns by shunning big department stores and going instead to small boutiques or to secondhand clothing stores.[23]

Fashion arbiters like *Vogue* were unsettled. They had lost control of fashion, lost their grip on its language and rules, and there was no single look anymore. The young dressed in jeans and cowboy hats, in granny dresses and other prizes they dug up in secondhand stores, in the miniskirts of the young designers, in the traditional garb of Third World countries that did not yet seem to use machines to make clothing, in the uniforms of revolutionaries, or in the wild psychedelic styles that coexisted with the "natural" look of those who simply scorned attention to dress and appearance. The media and the beauty industry tried to bring coherence to the "creative anarchy" unleashed by the young. They grasped firmly the two ideals beneath the new looks—youthfulness and slenderness—and pushed them.

In 1963 *Vogue* boldly announced that youth was where fashion began. "There's a new girl on the scene," it proclaimed. She "looks right as a young animal. She's probably eighteen or thereabouts. That's where the fashion-wave begins." By 1967 *Vogue* was splaying across its pages models of startling thinness and immaturity, like Twiggy and Edie Sedgwick. It no longer set up sophisticated society women for readers to emulate, but rather, these barely mature girls. Youth was not perceived simply as an age, however. It was a state of being and therefore theoretically accessible to anyone. Fashion's views about stopping the clock and arresting age had striking parallels with the dicta of the medical community.[24]

Along with this adulation of youth came increasingly girlish, prepubescently revealing clothes. Skirts became as short and skimpy as those once worn by youngsters. *Vogue* supported these immodest styles, though not without some initial protest. In 1959 the magazine said no to the French bikini, but by 1964 America's own designer, Rudi Gernreich, had stunned the fashion world with his topless suit. The same happened with shorter skirts. In 1962 *Vogue* said no to the shorter hemlines coming from Paris, but by 1964 it had to capitulate. The British Invasion that changed rock and roll in America also brought mod styles, and hems began to rise all over the country. *Time* reported in 1967 that skirts went from the "micro-mini to the micro-micro to the 'Oh my God,' and the 'Hello Officer.' " Tops kept getting skimpier too, and with the emerging lust for freedom and physical comfort, slips, girdles, and even bras were blithely discarded, leaving adult women with little-girl outerwear—and little girl underwear. Little stood between a woman's naked body and the eyes of the world. By 1969 *Time* was marveling over the "nude look," which included see-through blouses and even pants and loosely crocheted dresses with no linings. Even those who did not wear these styles found their bodies more exposed. The little dresses were made of ever-softer fabrics that revealed rather than shaped the figure, and they were to be worn more tightly than ever before. In 1965 *Vogue* advised its readers to get clothing that "fits the way new clothes are meant to fit. It's a size smaller than you would have worn last year."[25]

These changes signaled a redefinition of femininity. No longer sedate and elegantly remote, the ideal woman now looked young and behaved youthfully. She was energetic, tomboyishly active, and irreverent. Even the language of the fashion press became energized. So did the more compelling, nonverbal, images. A 1963 *Vogue* article, "Sporting a New Breed of Fashion," pictured a purebred Arabian horse leaping forward from behind the model. What was a horse doing in a fashion magazine? A lot. With the horse, *Vogue* had found a perfect visual symbol for the new ideal woman, and it appeared and reappeared for the next fifteen years. A covert sexual element was part of the message, but a vigorous, sleek animal was also a distillation of all the qualities the new woman sought. It had breeding—class and impeccable pedigree—mixed with a wild freedom. It was natural and unspoiled, and it had energy, speed, and grace. The fashion models were also caught in motion. They began cavorting and leaping in ways once suitable only for youngsters. By 1969 the motorcycle was as popular a visual image as the horse, and *Vogue* heralded "The Girl in the Driver's Seat." She was described this way: "Wind in her hair, spark in her eye, steel in her spine—you know the type: living's her thing. . . . Petrol doesn't power her, her own vitality does." Such was the ideal girl-woman of the sixties, and the prototype of the liberated woman of the seventies.[26]

This assault on conventional femininity was reinforced by the emergent women's movement. Betty Friedan's *The Feminine Mystique* (1963), with its scathing indictment of the domestic trap into which women had fallen, found a receptive audience in the rebellious sixties. Friedan and others were also preoccupied with female energy and argued that women's unused abilities and repressed creative energy caused the pervasive malaise found among housewifes—and their overweight. They, too, conjured an image of vitality, of a woman who irreverently crossed the sexual-role barriers.

The sense of liberation and sexual freedom in the new styles may have been exhilarating, but they had a nasty effect on women's relationships with their bodies. *Vogue* began to focus on the body as much as on clothes, in part because there was little they could dictate with the anarchic styles, but mostly because if the body was exposed, it had to meet certain standards. When hems had started rising in 1958, *Vogue* had felt it necessary to let women know what their legs should look like and how to get them to look that way. When the bikini came out in 1959, *Vogue* warned they were not for everybody. "One must be young, beautifully toned in the muscle department . . . and blessed with a naturally spare but unbony figure—long lines, no angles." As styles became ever more revealing, such standards began to be applied to everyday wear, not just beachwear. The overwhelming importance now given to details of the anatomy was underlined by *Vogue*'s January, 1965, issue. The magazine had begun dedicating each January issue to an item of dress that would be a thematic focus for the year. But the "Year of the Hat" and "The Year of the Blouse" were startlingly followed in 1965 by the "Year of the Body." The magazine declared: "The body is the great new fashion power, the premise of every look named for fame . . . . "—a declaration that cast its shadow well into the 1980s.[27]

With freedom as a mandate, action as a symbol, and clothes pubescently revealing, thinness became ever more crucial. A slender body was a must for the little-girl styles and for the energetic image. For in the sixties, when so many cultural beliefs were being overturned, the association between a stream-lined form and kinetic potential remained inviolate. But the slenderness fashion extolled was far thinner than "healthy" slimness—*Mademoiselle* scoffed that "healthy" weights were suitable only for girls "trying out for a ladies' wrestling team"—but one standard colored another, and as "healthy" weights dropped, fashionable weights plunged. The crisp, aristocratic lines of Jackie Kennedy shrunk into the meagerness of Twiggy who, when she hit the fashion pages in 1967, stood at 5'7.5" and weighed a mere 91 pounds.[28]

As usual, aesthetic ideals were bound up with questions of sex, morality, and behavior, and these were transformed by the movement for sexual liberation. The sixties' youth seemed to be taking the neo-Freudianism of their parents to its logical conclusion in their demand for "free love," for sexual fulfillment without the constraints of marriage or of emotional commitments. ("Are We the Last Married Generation?" *McCall's* plaintively asked in 1969.) Virginity was an embarrassment, promiscuity a legitimate form of play. Fashion's emphasis on the body reflected, and was powerfully reinforced by, the drive toward sexual freedom.[29]

The young called for sexual liberation because they believed their sexual desires—and their bodies—were as innocent and harmless as those of a healthy young animal. This romance with nature spawned new expectations about the body. It was to be proudly exposed. Public nudity or seminudity began to be seen as a form of therapy or as proof that one had cast off prudish, middle-class "hang-ups." In dramatic productions like the rock musical *Hair,* in fashion photography, and on the screen, nudity became increasingly common. *Vogue* celebrated this emergence "from our Victorian past" in a 1967 article encouraging the new "pride of body" and enthused that " . . . in the meagerest bikini, we lie in the sun, as secure in the decency and cleanliness of our skin as a child." Women were seduced into expecting the kind of body they could be proud of, one that, when stripped, would look as taut and smooth as a child's.[30]

The idealization of a childish, prepubescent body in an age of sexual freedom seems, on the surface, somewhat paradoxical. Perhaps, America's prudish heritage prohibited the exposure of true adult nakedness. And certainly, a childish body symbolized the younger generation's faith in innocent sexuality. In addition, for all the era's celebration of naturalness, fashion generally abhors an undressed look. Traditionally, it had disguised flaws natural to the naked body and had also signaled that one had prepared for public presentation. But now, near-nakedness was now a form of dress.

The slenderness of this decade also had a political element to it. In the midst of plenty, of overkill, even of overproduction, Twiggy and her many imitators symbolized an indifference to abundance, a careless nonchalance about it. On another level, this unencumbered body symbolized a person not weighted down by stored-up baggage—physical, material, or emotional. It was the body of the romantic gamin cherished by the youth of the period.

More directly, Twiggy's skinniness was merely an extreme of a fashionable trend in the sixties, itself an age of extremism. Fashion tends to operate by these internal dynamics. A special feature appears, rather quickly goes to extremes, and then is abandoned, or remains as an understated vestige before it disappears. The Twiggy phenomenon was unique, not because it was a fashion extreme, but because it was an extreme of body shape itself, not of the clothes that covered the body.

Twiggy's popularity reflected the intermingling of the world of fashion and the new culturati in art. Modern art was moving further away from figurative representation and toward minimalism. In 1967, the year of Twiggy, *Vogue* was also praising the linear sculptures of Giacometti. In the same issue in which *Life* introduced Twiggy, it ran an article on artist Ad Reinhardt who, it explained, was a "Master of the Minimal." And though *Life* did not make the connection, it seemed that Twiggy was mistress of the minimal. The dehumanization in art was paralleled by the dehumanization in fashion.[31]

There was some resistance to the emaciated Twiggy look. Many sex idols still had curves, such as Brigette Bardot and Jane Fonda (when she appeared in *Barbarella* in 1968). The Miss Americas of the sixties remained stubbornly like their fifties' counterparts, in deliberate rejection of the radicalism associated with the Twiggy look. The contestants' hair stayed in bouffants, and their average heights hovered between 5'6" and 5'6.5", their weights between 118 and 120—almost 30 pounds more than Twiggy. In fact, by 1970 the pageant seemed so anachronistic that journalist Frank Deford wrote a history of it, convinced he was writing its obituary.[32]

Some in the counterculture also rejected the skinny look as another "Madison Avenue" predilection, especially the "flower children" who had opted for a preindustrial rural life-style and who celebrated a fertile Earth-Mother image. Many who initially resisted the "Twiggy look" found their resistance eroded. In embracing Twiggy, the fashion magazines shrewdly bridged the gap between themselves and the chaotic counterculture, inviting the young rebels to accept them.

As always, on its journey from the genuinely young to the beauty professionals, slender consciousness traveled to the middle-class, middle-aged housewife who came to imitate, in diluted form, the fashions and aesthetics of the time. Even *Ladies' Home Journal,* that bastion of the middle-class homemaker, announced in 1966 that the once-sacrosanct rule that styles vary with age, was now defunct: "Dress your age once meant look your age, too. New Definition: Forget your age. Every age is the right age for today's fashions." As though to prove its point, another issue showed a grandmother, mother, and teenage daughter all wearing the same minidress. Fashion could not have encapsulated more perfectly the health industry's dictum that everyone maintain the body size of a twenty-five-year-old.[33]

The cruelest—and ultimately most damaging—aspect of fashion's lust for slenderness was its insistence that women could achieve it, regardless of their genes or age. In the fifties *Vogue* had assured women they could go out and buy beauty. In the sixties it assured them that "body beautifulness is get-able.

Just as a dress is something subject to choice, so, within reason, is body chic."
It promised that "the figure everyone needs for fashion" could be achieved
through sensible diet, exercise, and above all, "will power."[34]

Vogue, of course, was merely repeating medical "truisms." When it celebrated slenderness and slenderness's ability to preserve youthfulness, it simply
put in fashion language what the medical profession had been saying for more
than a decade. When it assured women they could almost resemble a Twiggy,
regardless of their age and genes, it was spouting a self-help formula dear to
Americans and endorsing what the health industry was saying. When it celebrated Twiggy as an ideal, it merely gave a fashionable stamp to the medical
dictum, "thinner is better," and it confirmed that one could never be too thin.
And in this articulate union—and deadly alliance—the prejudice of the past
became the myth of the future. Weight loss beckoned as a form of self-
transformation and as a bridge over the generation gap.

Women were assaulted on all sides by the imperative—and the promise—of
slenderness. As the mass media grew increasingly pervasive, as greater affluence further commercialized leisure—making more Americans eager for self-
improvement and for public badges of it—this assault became more powerful.
Albert Stunkard's study of the relationship between social status and obesity
underscored how intimately they were intertwined. And, as always, external
standards were internalized. Women were being persuaded to expect a perfect
body, and they knew how much more central bodily appearance had become
in the scale of human values. But when they compared themselves to the steady
stream of ever-thinner, more undressed public images, few escaped feeling fat
and misshapen. Many began to see their own bodies as shameful grotesqueries.

Teenagers and young adults were especially susceptible to this reaction.
They were growing up in an era when traditional authorities and values were
being undermined, and so the influence of the media and of their peer groups
was particularly potent, unchecked by competing values. Studies of high-
school girls in 1966 and 1969 revealed that the percentage of those who
thought they were too fat had risen from 50 percent to 80 percent—though
in the latter group, only 15 percent were overweight by medical standards.
When asked if they thought they were more attractive than other girls, they
answered yes only if they weighed 85 to 94 percent of the average—or below.
Other studies suggested such thinness did not appeal to boys. When asked to
choose their ideal female silhouette, girls tended to choose extreme ectomorphs
(long and slender) while boys tended to choose curvier, endomorphic silhouettes. Girls clearly were trying to meet an ideal of beauty independent of
standards boys conveyed to them.[35]

When these young women saw Twiggy, they had no reason to reject her as
a too-thin ideal. They had grown up hearing the indictments of overweight,
watching their parents, especially their mothers, diet. They had absorbed all
the pejorative, humiliating qualities their culture associated with "fatness."

They had no collective memory of a time when plumpness was equated with robust health or with sexuality.

Tragically, these years are a particularly vulnerable period for the development of body self-concepts. Hilde Bruch and Albert Stunkard had found that people who were obese during adolescence and later reached a normal body weight never lost the feeling that they were fat. Middle-aged adults who had become heavier in their mature years never exhibited the psychological pain, the distorted body image, or the self-loathing of those who suffered adolescent obesity. Yet a whole generation of girls was growing up with a body standard that was impossibly thin, and it was against this standard that they measured themselves.[36]

This generation was also fertile soil for the rise of eating disorders because of perceptions about what caused overweight. Studies of teenagers indicated that boys believed their overweight was caused by muscles, while girls invariably attributed theirs to fat. Fat, of course, had potent negative connotations, while muscles did not. In addition, boys believed their weight was a reflection of their exercise habits while girls believed theirs was solely a function of their eating habits. Parents subtly, or not so subtly, reinforced these attitudes. Researchers found that parents urged boys to eat, regardless of their weight, while they did so with daughters only if they were relatively thin. Our culture enforced the belief that boys always needed to eat but that girls did not; that boys lost weight through exercise while girls lost it through dieting. These girls became our current generation of trapped women.

Two other themes emerged from the "fat-phobia" and the cultural chaos of the sixties: the importance of exercise and the importance of a "healthy" diet. In the fifties very few experts recommended exercise for weight loss because of the deeply rooted belief that it increased appetite and so caused weight gain. But many who surveyed the "fatogenic" society felt that underexercising was as much a problem as overeating, and their views were articulated increasingly in the sixties. Dr. Jean Mayer, head of Harvard's School of Public Health, played a leading role in the emerging exercise campaign, one similar to that played by Louis Dublin in the fifties' weight-loss campaign.[37]

Mayer originally investigated why appetite mechanisms became "deranged" and led to overeating and so, obesity, but he discovered that many Americans were eating the recommended number of calories for their age and yet still were gaining weight. A series of studies he did of rodent and human populations convinced him that appetite was "a sensible and reliable mechanism for keeping weight stable"—*if* the subject maintained "normal activity levels." In his most startling study, he reported that obese high-school girls did not necessarily eat more than their slender peers—shocking evidence that many overweight people were perfectly honest when they said they ate like birds but still gained—and he argued that their weight differences were caused by their different activity levels. In slow-motion replays of the girls playing at sports, he demonstrated that the obese exerted themselves far less than their normal-weight counterparts. He thus confirmed what many had already suspected: Exercise was a crucial determinant of body weight.[38]

Mayer deduced that recommended calorie intakes produced overweight because they had been based on a pre–push-button era. He argued that mod-ernization made Americans far more sedentary than their predecessors, and so they burned fewer calories and disrupted appetite mechanisms that were dependent on "normal activity levels." He hastened to add that he was not suggesting adults were not busy, only that they were not physically exerting themselves. "I am convinced," he wrote in 1968, "that inactivity is the most important factor explaining the frequency of 'creeping' overweight in modern societies."[39]

Mayer was quick to point out that his idea was hardly new. For decades scientists had calibrated recommended calorie intakes with activity levels. Animal breeders, too, had known that a sedentary animal fattened up more quickly than an active one. Mayer's position was new because he revealed how much exercise had been neglected in the overweight equation, how much the inactivity of modern Americans had been underestimated, how much inac-tivity disrupted appetite mechanisms, and because he laid to rest the fifties' prejudices against exercise. He showed that while extra exercise did increase the appetites of the very active, it actually depressed the appetites of the formerly sedentary, and he showed that moderate exercise indeed helped burn calories.

Authorities were excited by Mayer's research. It seemed to answer the troubling question of why Americans weren't losing weight. Exercise was initially advocated because it helped with weight loss, but Mayer and others were finding that it also might have some independent vascular benefits. Some studies suggested that more active people had lower rates of heart disease (although this, too, remained speculative: the authors of the best-known study retracted their conclusions three years after publication, though they con-tinued to be widely cited), and others suggested that high serum cholesterol levels, believed to be a risk factor in heart disease, could be lowered through exercise.[40]

There were other, subtler reasons exercise was advocated. Though a greater number of men were gaining weight, and men suffered more frequently from heart disease, they generally were unwilling to diet. An aura of femininity clung to dieting, and the old associations between successful masculinity and hearty appetite persisted. Exercise was a weight-loss technique that could appeal to men. And if men viewed dieting as an adjunct to exercise, then its feminine associations would be diluted. In addition, many researchers had found what motivational researcher Dr. Dichter had guessed: People preferred being able to act on a problem. Exercise was just such a positive act, while dieting was a prescription *not* to do something.[41]

But getting people to exercise looked like it might be as difficult a task as getting them to diet. When journalist Peter Wyden researched the problem of overweight in 1965, he found the experts frustrated. They had a "vague hope" that people could be persuaded somehow to burn off excess calories by "plunging into a national orgy of folkdancing, swimming, and taking families for wholesome walks around the subdivision" or that "sports could be made more interesting." Another official put it more trenchantly and prophetically: "Somebody is going to have to make it fashionable to get some exercise."[42]

The experts did not leave Americans' exercise habits to chance and their work began another front of diet intensification that paralleled those reinforced by fashion and society. Campaigns stepped up to fight overeating *and* underexercising. Insurance companies issued publications like *Metropolitan Life's Exercise Guide* (1966), and the government poured money into its own efforts. The President's Council on Physical Fitness for Youth was changed into the National Council on Physical Fitness to include adults, and it published a 35-cent smash hit, *Adult Physical Fitness: A Program for Men and Women* in 1964, which advocated the moderate exercise Mayer had recommended and insisted that "even the elderly, the inactive, and the overweight can perform these exercises." The popular press besieged the public with articles about the importance of exercise, and their number leapt from twenty-seven between 1959 and 1961 to fifty-seven between 1963 and 1965. They ranged from "Physical Fitness on the New Frontier" to the hopeful "Best Diet Is Exercise" by the prolific Jean Mayer. In 1965 the first chart of the number of calories burned by different exercises was published—a prototype of those that would be cherished in later decades. And the food industries hit hardest by the diet ethic eagerly promoted this weight-control technique, which took some of the onus off their products.

The weight-loss/exercise campaigners received help from unexpected quarters in 1967 when the coach of the University of Oregon's track team, Bill Bowerman, published *Jogging* and shared the exciting news that you didn't have to be college-aged to run around a track. His book stimulated a shift toward more strenuous exercise, and, most importantly, introduced a sport that was indeed "more interesting." By the end of the year, *U. S. News* announced, "Jogging for Health and Heart. It's Catching On." The trend gained momentum, especially when Kenneth Cooper's *Aerobics* appeared in 1968 and gave exercisers a method for measuring their exertion: their pulse rates. By the end of the sixties it had become axiomatic that to lose weight, one should diet *and* exercise, and that to avoid heart disease, one should do the same. In 1969 *Forbes* proclaimed to its business audience that "It's Not Just Overeating That's Killing Us. It's Underexercising, Too"—another article by Jean Mayer. When, the following year, *Fortune* asked "Why Are They Running, Stretching, Starving?" it could answer unequivocally that American businessmen had been terrified into it by the spectre of heart disease.[43]

They also had been coerced into it. Both government and civilian authorities absorbed and enforced the diet/exercise dicta. A 1963 army regulation stated that officers "whose usefulness to the service is substantially affected by failure to achieve and maintain desirable weight levels" might lose promotions or even be discharged. The navy and the air force followed suit. Their presumptions reflected the new prejudices of the era—that people could and should weigh a prescribed amount—and the new myth of the era—that overweight by MLIC standards could hurt performance.[44]

Civilian industries brought the campaign into the workplace largely because of fear of heart disease. In 1970 *Fortune* outlined the unofficial and semiofficial tactics used to keep executives streamlined. Managers kept a vigilant eye on subordinates' weights and some "[wrote] blunt memos to subordinates to warn they [were] becoming noticeably plump." Many corporations gave top executives study leaves with the understanding that they were also to lose weight while they were away. Some businesses tried incentives that combined monetary bait and the good-natured enthusiasm of a pep club, such as Lowe's Inc., of Cassopolis, Michigan, which began the ICATLYC (I Can't Afford to Lose You Club) and offered a yearly bonus to employees who lost weight and kept it off. In accordance with the truisms coming from health officials, the company's president was sure this expense would be balanced by the savings because, *Time* reported in 1969, he figured that "for every executive who keels over too soon, the company must spend twice his annual salary training a replacement."[45]

In many U. S. corporations, the war against overweight did not remain so informal but was officially institutionalized. NASA paved the way in 1965 when it began an elaborate program to monitor its Washington D.C. staff for possible heart disease and set up a fully equipped gymnasium and exercise room. Its success inspired other major U. S. corporations to do the same. Overweight no longer compromised just health and looks. Now it could threaten job security and promotions. Body weight had become another measure of job competence. And now, company executives could interfere with what had once been private, individual matters: body size and eating habits. The cultural forces demanding thinness, restraint of appetite, and exercise had become exceedingly powerful.

Historically, Americans had had other bouts of exercise fever, but the one that began in the sixties grew out of the same panic about modernity that had spawned the campaign against overweight. Throughout the sixties the popular press echoed the fears expressed by health officials and social commentators: that America's technical advances and affluence could be its undoing. America was in a crisis of transition. As automation invaded the home and workplace, it appeared that human exertion—and even jobs and the work ethic itself—might become obsolete. In 1964 Dr. Richard Bellman of the Rand Corporation was predicting that in twenty-five years, 98 percent of all American goods and services would be produced by just 2 percent of the population. The unnerving notion of a "workless world" seeped into serious and popular discussions, causing panic about an evermore sedentary and aimless population. "The Task Ahead: How to Take Life Easy," Ernest Havemann entitled his *Life* article in 1964. Already, with increasingly shorter working hours, ordinary citizens seemed to have more leisure time than they knew what to do with.[46]

It was not just technology that was pushing us into a new, physically lazy mode of life. It was also greed and lack of self-restraint. At the root of Mayer's and others' critiques of underexercising and overeating was a larger, moral indictment of the consumer society. Mayer angrily wrote that "we sacrifice fitness, looks and often our health to the 'need' for automobiles, and the beauty of our landscape to roads and pollution, again for the sake of quicker transportation or mass availability of cheap goods." Such disgust pervaded most official discussions of the overweight problem. But this critique posed a difficult problem. How could officials condemn overconsumption when the health of the American economy was based on it? On many levels, exercise seemed to resolve this ticklish dilemma. Overproduction had become a threat to America's well-being; excessive waste—such as fat—one of its ugliest by-products. Exercise seemed ideal, not just as a healthy antidote to mechanization, but also as a way, metaphorically, to put the excess to good use and so not pay the price for it.[47]

These were the theoretical underpinnings for the insistence on exercise, but, as always, people were not lured to it because of grim formulations but because it had become fashionable. Physical fitness was really brought to national attention by President Kennedy, who established the Council on Physical Fitness and integrated its precepts into the school system, and who sought to revitalize America by reviving the "manly arts." More importantly, the public was treated to pictures of the Kennedy clan romping at football, sailing, skiing, tennis, and just walking on the beach. Suddenly, fitness had the luster of Kennedy's Camelot, another triumph of empowered youth.

The exercise advocates in fact got indirect support from the "empowered youth" of the counterculture who, while they scorned fashionable ideals, also rejected the gluttonous, automated, consumer society. This critique and their romance with a "return to nature" allowed them to endorse exercise as a form of moral and political action. Their romance with childlike qualities and their insistence that these be retained throughout adulthood also paved the way for exercise—play—to be an acceptable feature of adult life.

Initially, the exercise ethic did not affect women as deeply as men. In the early sixties fashion magazines began promoting exercise as a way to tone up the body for the new, baring styles, not for fun or health. *Vogue* did not even pretend that exercise was fun, and knowing full well that women found it tedious, recommended that readers try more "interesting" and meaningful routines like Tai Chi and yoga, which were conveniently yoked to the demands of beauty.[48]

Even if *Vogue* didn't gush over the joys of exercise (visible signs of exertion and muscles were still unerotic, unfeminine), its visual and verbal imagery, as we have seen, became increasingly action prone and paved the way for exercising women and exercise itself to be glamorized. The youth movement's romance with "nature" and with the natural body and its functions—as opposed to the overcivilized body—and feminists' strident attacks on the "lady" all conspired to make exertion and perspiring, even sweating, acceptable for women. And, in any case, women were lured increasingly by the halcyon promise that exercise might make them thinner.

The third front of weight consciousness that began in the sixties and expanded in the seventies was "healthy" food. In the fifties the only worry about America's food supply had been its abundance, but, in the sixties, concern mounted that it was also physically and "spiritually" dangerous.

Initially, this concern was prompted by scientists who followed up on statistical evidence of a link between excess blood cholesterol levels and heart disease. The waxy substance, cholesterol, seemed to be deposited on arterial walls where it accumulated, blocked blood flow to the heart, and so triggered heart attacks. Researchers theorized that fatty and/or high-cholesterol foods caused excessive serum cholesterol, a theory that could explain the epidemic of heart disease. It wasn't so much that Americans were eating more calories but rather that the treasured culinary luxury, fat, no longer comprised only 33.6 percent of the average diet as it had in 1920: In 1956 it comprised 41.4 percent. Fat, the most calorically dense food, was no longer condemned just for being fattening. It loomed as an independent cause of heart disease.[49]

As in the exercise campaign, the anticholesterol campaign had an eminent spokesman: physiologist and nutritionist, Ancel Keys. Keys had roundly criticized the BBPS and the MLIC because his own research had shown that the only physiological variable predictive of heart disease was a high cholesterol level. Weight was irrelevant. Keys's later international studies also suggested that rates of coronary death correlated with the amount of fat in the diet. In 1950 Dr. Lawrence Kinsell had discovered that polyunsaturated fats *lowered* blood cholesterol levels, monosaturated fats left them unaffected, and saturated (animal) fats raised them. This data was coordinated, and many began to urge Americans to reduce their fat and cholesterol intake and to make sure they consumed more polyunsaturated than saturated fat (known as the *P/S ratio*).

This advice roused considerable controversy. Some doubted the correlation between heart disease and high cholesterol. Others questioned whether high-fat/cholesterol diets actually had much to do with blood cholesterol levels. New international studies suggested they might not. Comparisons of Swiss Alpine villagers and Basel residents showed that although the villagers daily consumed 30 percent more saturated fat and 1,000 more calories than the Basel residents, they had lower cholesterol levels. (Dr. Jean Mayer attributed the difference to the villagers' more active life-style—another reason he endorsed exercise.) Others pointed out that the human liver could produce three times more cholesterol per day than Americans consumed in food. Was diet really the culprit? Still others claimed Keys was minimizing other risks for heart disease, from family history, to smoking, to overweight, to hypertension, to inactivity.[50]

But before these issues could be properly debated in scientific circles, the dictum was absorbed in the popular consciousness in a pattern that became typical of other "health-food" advice. In December, 1960, the American Heart Association (AHA) cautiously endorsed these dietary changes but only for people who had other high-risk factors for heart disease, and it warned that people should not expect too much from such dietary shifts. There still was no "final proof" that such changes would prevent heart disease. But just a month later *Time* did a cover story on Ancel Keys and turned the strange term, *cholesterol,* into a household word and a household nemesis. The magazine did not mention the AHA qualifications, and since it focused on Keys rather than on the issues, the controversies received only one sentence.[51]

Quite possibly, Americans would have been alarmed only briefly about cholesterol, except for another facet of American life: advertising. People who didn't read magazines certainly couldn't miss the ads. In August, 1962, the AMA also endorsed the cautious AHA recommendation, and advertisers had a field day. They promoted their foods by using choice phrases from the official pronouncements and by grossly inflating the "health" claims. The AMA, alarmed by how its modest recommendation was being commercially exploited and abused (by vegetable-oil producers among others), officially condemned the new "food fad" and warned that the "anti-fat, anti-cholesterol fad is not just foolish and futile, [but also] risky." Immediately, the American Dairy Association, already hard hit by the public's panic about cholesterol, ran ads to reprint this "new and very important statement." Nutrition issues had become a commercial merry-go-round, and public confusion and passions mounted.

For our purposes, what is most important about the cholesterol issue is how much it grew out of and exacerbated "fat-phobia." Throughout this book, I have argued that medical judgments and the direction of scientific research are often shaped by larger cultural values. Certainly this was the case with fat in the twentieth century. In part, the cholesterol panic was one of its by-products. American abundance and overeating had already been blamed for the epidemic of heart disease, and it seemed perfectly logical that the content of diet was also a cause, especially fat because it is the most tasty and most caloric food—and because a generation of scientists was predisposed to be suspicious of fat and to minimize or deny any positive functions it might serve. It was easy to transfer the guilt from fat on the body to fat in food. Even Keys, who did not think overweight was the main cause of heart disease, told *Time* that he had a "personal distaste for obesity," which he found "disgusting," and that the recommended dietary shifts would be beneficial because they helped with weight loss. He had even more contempt for the weak will that presumably produced obesity, and it was apparent that the self-discipline required to diet was also required to avoid fatty foods. Journalist Peter Wyden angrily observed that Americans weren't trying to lower their cholesterol because "it was fat that made most foods taste good, and taste—not fear of disease—rules the American appetite." While it seems sensible that taste should rule appetite, in the antioverweight climate, this resistance just seemed further proof of Americans' unruly appetites. The cholesterol dicta merely expanded the attack on fat. Fat in our food now seemed as lethal as body fat, and now we also had to worry about fat *in* our bodies where we couldn't even see it.[52]

The cholesterol scare was part of a larger, less official indictment of America's food habits. Initially, the fears about modernization that spawned the exercise crusade also spawned new concerns about food. Increasing commercialization and industrialization of America's food supply seemed potentially dangerous. In 1958 Congress passed the controversial Delaney Clause, which required the FDA to check all new additives for their possible carcinogenic effects, and in 1962 Rachel Carson published *Silent Spring*, which exposed the extent to which Americans were contaminating their environment. The counterculture youth turned Adelle Davis into a nutrition guru, and her 1954 book, *Let's Eat Right to Keep Fit*, grew increasingly popular in the sixties. She condemned the modern medical establishment for its ignorance about nutrition and about the impact of nutrition on health, and she warned against all the "unnaturally" grown and processed foods of modern societies. In the sixties only the FDA, fringe health-food devotees, and the counterculture youth considered these to be vital issues, but they surged into the mainstream of American life in the seventies.

Such concerns were not new to America. In the 1830s Sylvester Graham had launched a health-food movement that had persisted in varying forms, and the counterculture's repudiation of "unnatural" processed foods paralleled many of Graham's presumptions. To return to "natural" homemade foods was to return to better, unadulterated nutrition, to personal control over food, and to food that was filled with the love of the person who made it. The counterculture's passion for "natural" foods was also part of their rejection of anything machine-made, mass-produced, and profitable to big business. It was part of their attack on the Establishment and on the habits of their parents, and as such, was as much a political as a health statement.[53]

The alternative food systems that developed—from organic food to Zen macrobiotics (MB), which at its highest stage was a near-starvation rice regimen—all shared certain basic premises. Chief among them was that what you ate affected your spiritual and mental state, a conviction that inspired much of the dietary experimentation. Michio Kushi, the disciple of George Oshawa who invented MB, argued that the "dialectic of world peace is through diet." The quest for spiritual transcendence and for an end to war seemed to end up in the kitchen. Another cherished premise was that most illness sprang from poor eating habits. To a generation that had grown up hearing how America's culinary abundance was dangerous because it caused obesity and so heart disease, it was easy to make the logical jump that food caused health or disease and that American habits were unhealthy. And finally, all these food systems presumed not only that you would feel better if you ate healthfully, but also that you would *look* better. Certainly you wouldn't be fat. Even the most spiritually-rooted of the diets, MB, was touted by some of its adherents for its "drastic" weight-reducing effects. When *Newsweek* covered the MB craze in 1965, it found abhorrence of fatness, gluttony, and the Establishment inextricably mixed with the search for transcendent purity. One macrobiote claimed MB "helps you leave the Great American Deception which is a self-deluding stimulus that makes you content in a kind of fat, disgusting way."[54]

In the sixties fat *was* perceived as disgusting, and so were those who suffered from it. Researchers began to document the growing prejudice against the obese. In 1966 G. L. Maddox and other researchers concluded that "Americans regard obesity as a socially deviant form of physical disability." Unsettling data confirmed that in competition for jobs and promotions, the overweight were at a significant disadvantage, a fact underlined by Metrecal's 1965 ad, "Not one of the top 50 U. S. corporations has a fat president." Jean Mayer and H. Canning found that overweight adolescents had fewer acceptances at the colleges of their choice than did their thinner competitors, even though their qualifications were often identical. They speculated that this disadvantage was caused by the unconscious prejudices of either the teachers who wrote recommendations or of college interviewers. More disturbing still, researchers found this prejudice among physicians, who described their obese patients as "more weak-willed, ugly, and awkward" than other patients. As with other cultural values, this one was passed on to children. Studies revealed that negative associations with overweight appeared by age four and hardened by age seven, and that overweight youngsters were shunned by their peers.[55]

Most tragically of all, the overweight absorbed these cultural estimates as self-estimates, and learned to hate themselves. When Jean Nidetch started her informal gatherings of overweight friends, she found them too ashamed to admit they splurged and snacked, especially in front of the slender nutritionists who usually ran reducing programs, which may explain why the diet clubs became so popular. Erving Goffman has argued that stigmatized groups are cut off from society and tend to associate with their "own kind"—those who share their stigma—for support and acceptance as well as for "instruction in the tricks of the trade," that is, how to get along in a hostile environment. The fat were now just such a stigmatized group, and diet clubs brought them together and appointed formerly fat leaders, who could better understand and sympathize with their plight.

The overweight women's shame about their eating habits was understandable in the sixties when respected authorities were pronouncing that the fat had no physiological need for food. In this liberal era, hunger was the only urge that was not to be generously gratified, and "overeating"—whatever brought one above "desirable" weight—came to be viewed as a shameful, self-destructive act. Cultural attitudes toward appetite and food were revised as research continued to determine *why* people overate. Experts still believed that psychological problems, such as frustration, depression, or insecurity, were at the root of overweight. These were all expressions of emotional neediness—a quality that most Americans found deplorable. Or they insisted that people overate because they had been raised in families with "unhealthy" food attitudes. *Time* summed up the experts' views in 1961: "Some families place undue emphasis on food: conversations center around it and rich delicacies are offered as rewards, withheld as punishments." More disturbing, cardiologist Norman Joliffe explained, "The child gains the feeling that food is the purpose of life." The presumptions were that this necessity of life and sensual pleasure, food, should not be eagerly anticipated or be a focus in life, and that if people loved to eat and regularly overate, they would not do anything else worthwhile. In a sense, eating would consume the eater. All those historical figures who had been both "gluttonous" and made a mark on history—including St. Thomas Aquinas, Montaigne, King Henry VIII, Louis XIV, Mendel, Samuel Johnson, and former President Taft—quietly faded from memory.[56]

So troublesome had the question of appetite become that studies were conducted to analyze what had once been self-evident, but no longer was: the relationship between mood and hunger. In 1965 research was begun that revealed that as hunger intensified, mood became more negative (depressed, apathetic, irritable, tense), but that as hunger was satisfied, mood became more positive (cheerful and calm), which led some researchers to the tautological conclusion that negative mood aggravated weight problems. Quite simply, it was no longer taken for granted that hungry people weren't particularly happy people or that even people with normal weights tended to get irritable waiting for their next meal, or that eating and a satisfied stomach produced pleasurable feelings. Scientists and others were stripping biological validity from these reactions.[57]

Experts could argue that overeating was a "disgusting" self-indulgence because they believed satisfying appetite too generously caused heart disease. The cruel trap, however, was that even ordinary nongluttons seemed to fall into the gluttonous category, now that gluttony was defined by body weight, the MLIO's chart of desirable weights had been revised downward, and fashion endorsed a virtually emaciated ideal.

Hilde Bruch dared protest against the trend, arguing that yes, indeed, eating could be a great solace in life and that it wasn't so terrible a solace. Certainly it was better than suicide, murder, drug addiction, alcoholism, or other ways people might handle their problems. She even dared insist that in many cases, people could function well *only* with an ample diet and with padding well above "desirable weight." Only in Bruch's steady good sense do wefindany defense of the pleasure and innocence of food and of overeating.[58]

The prejudice against fat had another side that helped escalate diet-mania: a myth about what slenderizing would bring to the formerly fat. The romance of self-transformation had been a theme in diet literature for decades, but it took on new vitality in the sixties. Health officials and fashion spokespeople turned reducing into a fountain of youth, a way to stave off aging and recapture youthful vitality, happiness, and beauty. Fashion proclaimed the undeniable. Slenderness could make one part of the sexually charged world of the "beautiful people." But more was going on. Scientists began investigating which character traits differentiated the fat and the thin, and the very questions they raised revealed how deep-rooted the prejudice against fat had become. The slender were considered quicker, more competent, better adjusted, and more disciplined and moral than the fat. A 1967 study concluded that being overweight did not affect IQ or college board scores—but the very question presumed there might be relationship between body weight, intelligence, and performance. The myth developed that slimming could bring all these cherished qualities.[59]

Popular and some professional psychologists took this notion one step further. As long as the belief prevailed that everyone could reach the "ideal" body size, then it was also possible to argue that everyone had a thin person within—a beautiful, sexy, intelligent, exciting person just waiting to burst forth. Dr. Theodore Isaac Rubin, formerly president of the American Institute for Psychoanalysis, gave medical endorsement and also a very original twist to this notion. He argued that many overweight people were fat not because unconscious problems caused overeating, but because unconsciously, they actually were afraid of being thin. He explained that "to some, being less than what they were—substantial—is as bad as losing a leg. Fatness has a resigned quality, an anaesthetizing effect, but at least it's familiar. By contrast, a sudden feeling of aliveness can be terrifying." To give an example of Rubin's theory, *Newsweek* quoted Jean W., a housewife who had lost 50 pounds. She had been afraid of losing it. "You don't know what the person is like under all this fat. She might turn into a sensuous woman who leaves her husband," she explained, and added, "Furthermore, losing weight and having people compliment you puts pressure and responsibility on you—and we fat people don't like responsibility."[60]

The presumptions in Rubin's and Jean W.'s comments are heartrending and underscore the new mythology. Rubin himself was a "formerly fat" psychiatrist, yet he didn't question for a moment that thinness brought "a sudden feeling of aliveness" so intense that it was terrifying. Jean W. was convinced fat people didn't like responsibility and were rarely complimented. She also believed a 50-pound weight loss would change her so much that she might find her fat self had chosen the wrong mate and the wrong life for the real person within, the thin person. In the sixties, such notions were rampant. But thin had gotten so much thinner that few were left who didn't think they had a weight problem. And women, fretting over only 5 to 25 pounds, believed, too, with a sickening certainty, that those pounds were keeping them from happiness, self-fulfillment, self-respect, and romance.

Again, Bruch and Stunkard were among the few who, after years of experience with obese patients, protested against this trend toward mythification. They argued that many negative traits associated with overweight, such as lethargy and depression, were not inherent traits but rather a result of the prejudice the overweight experienced. They pointed out that dieting was not always an uplifting experience, nor suitable for everyone. For many, it induced depression and severe emotional reactions. And Bruch argued that the inflated hopes about what thinness would bring could prove disastrous. Many people stuck to diets and reached their weight goals, only to find they were no different than they had been before. They had the same problems, the same personalities, the same abilities, the same jobs, and the same families as before. All that was different was their weight. It was lower. They were filled with despair and disappointment—and often soared back up to their prediet poundage. Bruch scolded that "we should stop going around reaching unreality." She prophetically added, "We are being rushed into a pathology that is no pathology." She recommended dieters expect only one thing from weight loss: weight loss. It was a bleak suggestion. If thinning brought none of its glorious benefits, why do it?[61]

Bruch has been one of the most influential, respected, and prolific experts on psychology and weight, but sadly, her sage insights had little effect in the sixties outside scientific circles. The urgency to become thin had become much too powerful, the official indictment of fatness too rigid and pervasive, and the glamorous, romantic allure surrounding it too magnetic. Most of all, the myth of self-transformation through weight loss was too precious to be relinquished. Bruch was crying in the wilderness. She couldn't puncture America's new romantic myth. The groundwork was laid for myth to become obsession.

III

MYTH BECOMES OBSESSION: 1970–1980

8

The Health/Exercise Ethic Emerges

The extremes of the sixties did not end in the seventies, at least not for Americans' fat-phobia. Social and economic developments and new scientific theories reinforced our deepening obsession and made it expand to include the last exempt age group, infants and toddlers. They also made the imperative to be thin more exacting. Healthy was redefined. Now you had to be thin and fit, calipers in hand to decipher your fat-to-lean ratio. Beauty was redefined in a similar way. Thin wasn't good enough anymore. We learned that flab, and the worst blight of all, cellulite, could mar even the featherweight body. With these new standards, exercise edged from the wings into center stage as the cure for overweight and its new, more deadly variant, flab. By the end of the decade, Americans of all ages were in training. They wanted to be athletes, or at least look like athletes. Aesthetic, health, social, and moral values further intermeshed and reinforced one another, raising fat-phobia to a new pitch.

A fundamental difference between the seventies and the previous two decades was the emergence of health-consciousness as an ethical principle. The ethic was based on the deepening conviction that modernization threatened our individual, physical survival because of the life-style it spawned. We were overweight, underexercised, and sickly, corrupted by our technology and our food supply. We came to believe that the typical American diet—high in fat, salt, meat, and refined sugar—was not only fattening but also unhealthy in and of itself. We panicked about food processing that drained the nutrients out of food and new production techniques and additives that made our food dangerously carcinogenic. Because of the moral overtone thinness and fitness had now developed, we felt these dangers were lethal for our souls as well as our bodies.

But we also believed that we could change these habits, and that if we did, we would improve our health, our life expectancy, and our beauty. The quest for personal health became an American preoccupation, a fashionable passion of the pacesetters—the radical generation—who set the national tone and style. *Life-style* became the catchword of the decade. Alternative life-styles were extremely fashionable, and they invariably reflected the philosophy of the health ethic.

This ethic intensified the imperative to be slim, for avoiding overweight was one of its central tenets. We cannot understand the rise of eating disorders as a national epidemic, nor the rise of distorted body images among women, nor the frantic exercise/diet routines of even the most liberated of them without understanding the development of the health ethic. It formed the supportive background in which women's obsessions with their bodies and their weights flourished unchecked. It gave a new dignity and justification to their preoccupation with their figures and to their attitudes about food. It was the fundamental reason myth became obsession.

Psychiatrists and obesity experts Bruch and Stunkard commented separately on the rising concern about weight in 1973. "The condemnation of overweight appears to be on the increase," wrote Bruch, and Stunkard observed that "during the past twenty-five years, interest in weight reduction in our country has grown from a mild concern to an overriding preoccupation. At present, interest in obesity almost assumes the dimensions of a national neurosis." It was also evident in the vast growth of the weight-loss industry.[1]

Diet-mania mounted. The number of diet articles and books soared above their 1960s highs. Between 1968 and 1969, twenty-five diet articles were listed in the *Reader's Guide*. By 1978–79, the number had leapt to eighty-eight—a deceptively low figure since the *Guide* did not include the diet columns that were now regular magazine features nor the myriad diets that routinely appeared in more popular publications. Reflecting the pervasive and elaborate nature of weight consciousness, the diets' emphasis shifted from just weight loss to concerns such as longevity and well-being. Diet books inundated the public. In his publication for *Consumer Guide,* Theodore Berland evaluated more than one hundred published in the seventies, and he had only touched the tip of the iceberg. In 1973 the Senate Select Committee on Nutrition and Human Needs had turned up fifty-one new egg-and-grapefruit diets alone. *Dr. Atkins' Diet Revolution* (1972) made publishing history when 1 million hardback copies sold in just seven months. Officials, including the AMA's Council on Foods and Nutrition, were alarmed by the book's popularity and vehemently condemned its high-fat diet. Atkins's success also spurred them to begin trying, more energetically than in the past, to warn the public against the new avalanche of unhealthy and faddist diets. It seemed as if every new life-style, every fringe movement, had its contribution to make to the national weight-loss effort, from transactional analysis to hypnosis to meditation, and each was welcomed by a frantic and devouring public.[2]

Interest in exercise also soared. The number of articles about it in the popular press went from twenty in 1969–70 to sixty in 1978–79, and the percentage of adults who reported exercising regularly more than doubled from 21 percent in 1961 to 44 percent in 1977. Sales of exercise equipment mounted, reflecting those sports that had gripped the national imagination. Tennis and skiing were early leaders, but toward the end of the decade, jogging became pre-eminent. James Fixx's, *The Complete Book of Running* was a smashing success when it appeared in 1977: 1 million copies sold in the hardcover edition alone.[3]

Radical—and sometimes dangerous—methods for weight loss reflected both obsession about weight and changing attitudes to food. Fasting gained in popularity. In this diet- and health-conscious time, it offered the double advantage of weight loss with system purification. Americans had become so phobic about fat, the dangerous effects of food and its emotional meaning that they could easily buy the idea that not eating was healthier than eating, that somehow eating initiated dangerous bodily processes. Confusion reigned about the relationship of food to appetite, need to desire. This environment spawned opinions like that of fasting advocate, psychiatrist Allan Cott, who wrote in his 1977 book, *Fasting As a Way of Life,* "You will not be hungry. Any so-called hunger 'pains' are simply normal gastric contractions or stomach spasms. They represent the sensation of hunger rather than true hunger." Outlandish as this sounds, Cott was simply articulating embedded attitudes. Americans had been told something similar for more than two decades by highly reputable authorities. They had been told that their sensations of hunger represented the *desire* for food or for emotional gratification, not their *need* for nourishment. They had been encouraged to deny their need for food and to deny its emotional, sensual aspects.[4]

For those who had trouble fasting, there were semifasts that gave the dieter a vacation from food through liquid protein or formula diets. In a grim corollary, an estimated sixty deaths were caused by these semistarvation regimens, and by 1978 the U. S. Center for Disease Control cautioned against the use of formulas for more than two months. But Americans were undaunted. Better dead than fat.[5]

If most people didn't resort to these extreme measures, they still fervently sought ways to satisfy their appetites without paying any caloric costs. The low-calorie food industry burst beyond its 1960s levels as manufacturers expanded their brands of "lite" and diet foods. High-cholesterol and fattening foods could now be replaced with the likes of egg substitutes, "turkey dogs," and light beer (first introduced in 1953, though not successful until 1973). Weight Watchers began producing prepared frozen-diet dinners, which by 1978 accounted for about 20 percent of its $39 million revenues. By 1981 Nutri/System Weight Loss Centers, which dispensed dehydrated dietetic meals, had annual revenues of $48 million. Americans' mounting passion to exchange caloric for low-caloric foods translated into 10 percent growth per year for the diet-food industry, and a 20 percent growth per year for the diet soft-drink industry. By 1980 such foods amounted to almost 7 percent of all

U. S. food sales. But even these statistics don't convey the pervasiveness of the crescendoing diet lust. Caught on the defensive, advertisers of common foods performed sleights-of-hand, highlighting the low-calorie properties of their products: Mushrooms were promoted as "low calorie"; in 1980 Star-Kist ran a $12 million ad campaign for its water-packed tuna which promised, "Great taste, great for the waist." A profound change was brewing in America's food culture and food attitudes. Americans wanted food that wasn't quite food, the pleasure of eating without its consequences.[6]

The popularity of group dieting gained momentum. Almost 9 million people had been registered in Weight Watchers by 1977. The active membership of TOPS jumped from 60,000 in the mid-sixties to 336,000 in 1980. And the hosts of successful imitators multiplied; Diet Center, Inc. (with 3 million dieters served between 1970 and 1980), The Diet Workshop, Diet Control Centers, Appetite Control Centers, Weigh of Life, Compulsive Eating Re-education Group, Dieters Counseling Service, and a variety of small-scale, local variants. In 1980 a "Dieter's Referral Service" booklet listed more than eighty weight-loss programs in Manhattan alone.[7]

Even God was enlisted in the weight-loss crusade. The seventies witnessed the spectacular rise of evangelically inspired weight-loss groups and books. The Prayer-Diet Clubs of the fifties gave way to Overeaters' Victorious, the Workshop in Lenten Living, the 3D (for Diet, Discipline, and Discipleship), and the Jesus System for Weight Control. There were Frances Hunter's *God's Answer to Fat—Lose It!* (1976), Joan Cavanaugh's *More of Jesus and Less of Me* (1976), and C. S. Lovett's chillingly titled 1978 book, *Help Lord—The Devil Wants Me Fat!* in which he warned that the devil had cleverly found the best way to slip into people's lives—through seemingly "innocent" food. Such religious authorities did not try to brake Americans' passion for weight loss, but rather, wholeheartedly endorsed it. The profane quest for weight loss had become sacred, the virtuous—slim—body as crucial as a virtuous soul. Church leaders were officiating at the erection of a new sin—fatness—and of a new demonology, one connected solely with food. Such attitudes spilled over into secular society. Blue Shield's 1975 campaign for weight loss included one ad that pictured an obese male with bulging midriff, wrinkled trousers, and popping shirt buttons, accompanied by the caption, "When God created man, is this what He had in mind?"[8]

Despite frantic official efforts to quell misleading advertising and the spread of fantastic gimmicks for weight loss, both continued to mount. In 1973 Woodrow Wirsign, then president of the Better Business Bureau of Metropolitan New York, estimated that Americans would be "bilked out of" $2 to $10 billion by "medical quackery," including reducing machines, belts, creams, and pajamas, acupress and acupuncture, and ear stapling, all promising to help them take inches off—and all incapable of doing the job. Other, more modern, devices also hit the market in the seventies, such as the Diet Conscience, a battery-operated voice that berated you when you opened the refrigerator door

("Are you eating again? Shame on you! No wonder you look the way you do"); and the electronic diet fork with built-in lights that signaled to the eater when to eat (green light), how long to eat, and when to stop (red light). Comical as these devices may sound, for millions of purchasers they were deadly serious tools in the deadly serious fight against overweight. Americans' desperation was fueling their gullibility and their willingness to be abused and exploited.[9]

Despite the persistence and expansion of traditional methods for weight loss, two new techniques did appear in the seventies. An obsessed populace was matched by an obsessed and frustrated professional population. A medical miracle that would aid weight loss had not been discovered, and physicians desperately sought a way to cure gross obesity. In the early seventies they began more aggressive treatments for the massively obese: intestinal bypass surgery in which the intestines are severed and reconnected at the ileum, so that they bypass most of the small intestine, where nutrients are normally absorbed. The resulting "malabsorption syndrome" generally resulted in 100-pound weight losses. In 1983 Berland estimated that 50,000 people a year had the surgery. The bypass was fraught with life-threatening complications, and later in the decade the somewhat less dangerous procedures, gastric stapling and jaw wiring, were introduced. It should be stressed that physicians set increasingly rigid criteria about who qualified for such radical procedures, but the procedures nonetheless had profound symbolic implications. They seemed a violent punishment to the fat body, a forceful and crude way to manipulate the sins of appetite: enter the body and literally make the stomach smaller, shorten the intestine that let too much food get absorbed, physically clamp shut the mouths that would-be dieters couldn't keep shut by themselves. How many frustrated dieters hadn't wished they could do the same to themselves? The crudeness of these techniques bore a startling resemblance to the contraptions and surgery used by late-nineteenth-century physicians to keep youth from "self-abuse"—that is, masturbation. The late-twentieth-century procedures symbolized perfectly our culture's perception of modern instinctual ills: Our mouths were too wide, our stomachs too big, our very innards too greedy.[10]

The other new technique for weight loss was behavior modification. Despite its persistence, the classic model of psychological causes for obesity—conflict or neurotic neediness—continued to lose credibility at the same time that they often became more fantastic. But psychologists still believed that everyone was programmed to be slender and that the reason they weren't was because fat and thin people thought and ate differently. In the late sixties two researchers, working independently, came up with a simple and persuasive explanation for the differences and with what seemed to be a cure. In 1967 psychologist Richard Stuart published his remarkably successful method for treating obese patients. Using the behavioral model of experimental psychology, he had subjects record when, where, what, and under what circumstances they ate so they might identify the stimuli that triggered their eating. He then instructed them to change these patterns by keeping food only in the kitchen, eating only in one place, doing nothing else when they ate but eat, and chewing carefully. In essence, he tried to restrict eating, to keep it a self-contained, isolated activity.

Experts were stunned and excited by Stuart's remarkable success with this practical program, and their enthusiasm mounted when, the following year, social psychologist Stanley Schachter of Columbia University published the results of his own experiments. They provided a theoretical explanation for Stuart's success. He and his associates conducted a series of experiments which suggested that external cues, not internal conflicts or even sensations of hunger, caused fat people to eat. In contrast, thin people seemed to eat only in response to internal signals. For example, in one experiment, subjects were put in an isolated room with a supply of crackers and a prominent clock, which researchers secretly could speed up or slow down. Subjects were asked to perform some simple tasks while, unbeknownst to them, researchers fiddled with the clock. They found that the fat subjects ate crackers according to the clock—that is, they ate more if they thought it was past their dinnertime— while the thin subjects were not influenced by the time. It appeared that fat people were defenseless against external food cues and that what Stuart had done was to retrain them so that they either eliminated these cues or learned to resist them.[11]

The behavior modification approach became wildly popular because, at least for a while, it had a higher success rate than other weight-loss programs and because, like surgical intervention, it attacked the problem of appetite frontally. It did not require long, involved psychotherapy because it presumed that fattening eating habits were not a result of deep inner conflicts but rather a learned behavior that could be unlearned. By 1975 more than a hundred scholarly publications on the subject had appeared along with hundreds of books written by respected professionals, pop psychologists, and laymen who fervently spouted what amounted to a self-help philosophy.

Behavior modification theory did reconsecrate the American faith that individuals were absolutely responsible for their body size. Gluttonous and sedentary habits were the only reason the fat did not maintain "desirable weight." This reaffirmation put renewed pressure and renewed shame on those who did not conform to the narrow MLIC standard, and it made them ever more willing to accept punishment and abuse for their fatness.

Yet even in its mildest, most professional form, behavior modification insulted the dignity of adults. Its methods of re-education resembled child training systems. Mature, middle-aged people allowed themselves to be infantilized because their humiliating overweight was proof—both to themselves and to those treating them—that they needed this guidance.

Behavior modification also profoundly escalated the war on appetite and on food. Earlier psychological theories had presumed that food was a comfort for the emotionally disturbed, and the goal was to resolve the inner psychic conflicts that caused this dependence. The behaviorists instead tried to make sure food would not be regarded in this way. The prevailing attitude was underscored by one expert who scolded that "feeding has changed from a necessity to a form of pleasurable entertainment." *Feeding,* a term borrowed from zoology and animal husbandry, was now applied to humans precisely because it could be justified only as a necessity. Behaviorists and others were trying to strip food of its cultural richness, of its sacred, festive, sensual, artistic, and emotional associations much as, in another context, sex was being stripped of its traditional associations. Behavior modification gave renewed life to programs like Schick's which was developed in the 1940s to create avoidance to alcohol. In this program, the overweight paid to get electric shocks and other such punishments while they ate their favorite foods so that they would associate pain and discomfort with those pleasures—and cease to regard them as pleasures. In all its forms, the behavior modification approach essentially tried to distance people from food, to replace old food rituals with new, unevocative ones.[12]

The approach also encouraged and sanctioned obsessive, minute attention to eating habits, body weight and self-control—professionally endorsed codifications of the bizarre behavior exhibited by anorexics and bulemics. The behavior modification books advised reducers to keep a diary recording what they planned to eat before they ate and what they did eat, to chew slowly, to put their forks down after every other bite, to control hunger by finding other, distracting activities when the urge to eat hit. Mary Catherine and Robert Tyson, a physician and a psychologist, insisted, in their *Psychology of Successful Weight Control,* that " . . . you must regard the number on your scale as the most important number in your life." Americans were being encouraged to emulate the habits and attitudes of eating-disorder victims.[13]

Once again, the medical and insurance communities helped fuel the obsessive and expanding concern with weight. A comparison of the USPH's 1966 report, *Obesity and Health,* and the 1974 publications of the Senate Select Committee on Nutrition and Human Needs, reveals that beliefs about the dangers of overweight were becoming more deeply entrenched. Despite the firmness of its conclusion that overweight was bad, the 1966 publication acknowledged the inconclusive nature of information about overweight and about its causes and effects, and claimed only that obesity was "associated" with certain diseases. Such ambivalence disappeared from the published edition of the 1974 Senate hearings. Senator George McGovern headed this committee, and Dr. Jean Mayer was its general coordinator. Although many experts still presented data and raised questions that undermined the obesity-health links, the published testimony began with the unequivocal statement that "obesity is considered to be a contributor to many different disorders such as coronary heart disease, arthritis, pulmonary dysfunction, sleep disorders, social disability, and decreased ability to withstand trauma and surgery." And it unequivocally contended that weight loss would resolve these problems. "Many, if not all of these hazards to health can be decreased by weight reduction or by prevention of weight gain during childhood and middle age."[14]

The health and insurance communities and the government fed the growing panic with new perceptions, more rigorous standards, and a plethora of data, because the overweight problem seemed to be getting still worse. Metropolitan Life found dismal gains among policyholders. Between 1961–62 and 1972–73, both men and women had gained an average of 4 pounds at all heights. The federal government now also conducted its own regular height/weight studies, and its 1972–73 results were equally alarming. With only some exceptions, Americans were getting heavier, men by about 3 pounds, women by about 1 pound. Health officials' fears were being realized. Despite the two-decade campaign for weight control, the "fatogenic" society was winning.[15]

Cardiovascular disease was still the leading cause of death in the United States, and concern about it was at the heart of these fears. Experts testifying at the Senate committee hearings underlined the terrible cost of heart disease. One expert testified that in 1967 cardiovascular disease cost the nation $29.9 billion, and he estimated this cost would be substantially higher in 1974 because of inflation and the spread of expensive procedures like coronary bypass surgery. Even these figures didn't reveal the full cost of cardiovascular disease. Other experts observed that millions of Americans who suffered from mild forms of these illnesses had high rates of absenteeism and of early retirement. The government and other health officials had compelling reasons to step up the attack on overweight.[16]

Officials also made the attack more comprehensive. Suddenly, even infants and toddlers were drawn into the cycle. For centuries, a plump, robust baby had been considered a healthy baby. This was no longer true. Drs. Jules Hirsch and Jerome L. Knittle, highly esteemed researchers at the Rockefeller Institute, reported their discovery that "very obese" people not only had bigger fat cells than lean people, they also had more fat cells: 600 billion as opposed to 300 billion. Through their experiments with rats, they found that feeding patterns in infancy, when cell division occurred, caused *hyperplastic obesity*— that is, too many fat cells. Researchers extrapolated from the rodent experience and argued that, for the same reasons, the overfed human infant was doomed to a lifelong weight problem. Those extra cells would constantly crave filling, and the misfed infant would grow into a perpetually hungry, overweight adult. These findings seemed to explain why obese children so often grew into obese adults and why so many Americans couldn't control their appetites: Their excess fat cells wouldn't let them. This heartening theory implied there was a long-term cure for America's leading health problem. Fat adults still might be difficult to treat, but the new generation could be spared the agonies of its overweight parents.[17]

The enthusiasm with which the professional and lay public greeted this theory in 1970 was matched only by the alacrity with which action was taken.

By 1973 scores of articles had appeared in the lay and scholarly press disseminating the new information. "Fat Babies Grow into Fat People," the ever-popular and prolific Dr. Jean Mayer wrote in *Family Health.* "When to Start Dieting? At Birth," *Medical World News* told its readers in September, 1973. Nutritionists scrambled to revise their standards about infant feeding, and pediatricians revised their image of what constituted a healthy baby. "The plump, healthy-looking infant has long been considered the hallmark of good mothering," *Medical World News* commented. "The concept that maximum growth of the infant is not synonymous with optimum growth requires a reorientation in our approach to public health and nutritional education." That reorientation was under way. Acceptable body size for infants suddenly got thinner, paralleling the trends for adult weights.[18]

Women didn't miss the message. Highly sensitized to experts' advice about how to rear their children, mothers—who in any case were already terrified of fat and who had already been blamed for the chubbiness of schoolage children—began to worry when their babies thrived too much. By 1981 a prominent pediatrician noted that "obesity is said to be the major pediatric nutritional problem today," and he observed that "many families request advice in an effort to prevent the development of obesity in children at one and two years of age." Older children got the same message. Teachers spread the word to their students, and the connection between overeating, overweight, and disease entered high-school biology textbooks.[19]

Weight-loss books for younger and younger children began to appear. James Marshall's *Yummers* came out in 1972 for children in second grade and below, and so did Mary Lynn Salot's *100 Hamburgers: The Getting Thin Book,* written for overweight preschoolers. As historian Hillel Schwartz astutely pointed out, all these books had one underlying message: "Fat children start toward thinness only when they take control of their lives . . . . Their new thinness is the curious badge of maturity." Children now were being given the same message as adults—and the same opportunities. Summer camps for fat children proliferated: Weight Watchers reported that between 1969 and 1979, twelve hundred children had attended its summer camps.[20]

Only a few experts questioned the validity of Hirsch's and Knittle's theory, though their objections would eventually prevail. Some protested that childhood build predicted adult build only after the first year of life, or after the fifth year. Hilde Bruch once again resisted the new orthodoxy. She pointed out that it was almost impossible to "overfeed" a child, especially an infant or toddler. Any parent who had tried to do so knew what a losing—and emotionally costly—battle it was. She also cautioned that the excess number of fat cells Hirsch had described were exceedingly rare and usually occurred in people who were so fat that they appeared as "fat" people in circuses or freak shows. Others pointed out that although approximately 80 percent of obese children became obese adults, only 30 percent of overweight adults reported having been overweight as children, so infant feeding seemed irrelevant. Still others cautioned against extrapolating from rodent to human biology. Dr. D. B. Cheek pointed out that the adipose history of rats and humans is quite different: Fat deposition in rats is delayed until just before puberty, while in humans it begins three to four weeks before birth and reaches its maximum velocity at twelve months. The most damaging criticism highlighted the extent to which this new explanation still begged the question of whether it was nature (genes) or nurture (eating habits) that caused obesity. Many insisted that genes determined quantity of fat cells, not infant feeding habits.[21]

The theory incorporated a number of curious premises. Its proponents maintained that children should not carry "extra" fat, not because of its effects on childhood health but because of what it boded for adult health. In accordance with the decades-long suspicion of fat, they presumed even infant fat served no purpose. In an earlier era, it had been considered vital to help youngsters fight off and survive childhood diseases, but now antibiotics fulfilled that function. It had also been regarded as essential to healthy growth. Now, it seemed to have no legitimate functions left. Across the board, many theorists apparently were also abandoning the belief that anything resembling "natural" appetite existed. If even newborn babies, still ignorant of cultural standards, didn't eat primarily in response to hunger, then who did? Was "natural" appetite a myth?

The scientific community exacerbated weight concerns by introducing a new element into the weight calculations of the decade, one that both grew from and fueled the health/exercise ethic. Where "weight" had previously been considered a single entity, and people were urged to adhere to ever-lower standards of normality, now suddenly it was a complex mass, made up of new elements we had to control and be obsessed by: lean and fat body mass.

This new standard had its origins in various criticisms of the MLIC weight standard. Since the fifties many health authorities, Jean Mayer prominent among them, had stressed that how much people weighed wasn't the important factor; how much fat they had on their bodies was. The danger was excess fat, not large bones and muscles. In the fifties and sixties Mayer and others had demonstrated that many athletes weighed more than their "desirable weight," but they certainly didn't have extra stores of adipose tissue. Their higher scale readings came from well-developed bone and muscle, and it seemed unreasonable that a fit, muscled body was unhealthy or that it could lead to heart disease and other ailments. Furthermore, Ancel Keys and Mayer had objected to the MLIC's vagueness about "frame size." Some people had bulkier builds than others, and there was no way their "desirable weights" could be the same. To solve these problems, Mayer recommended that calipers be used to measure the proportion of people's fat. This alone could give an accurate indication of whether people, whatever their weights, were burdened with excess flesh. By the 1970s the Public Health Service was doing caliper and/or scale weight measurements. Calipers screened the hefty, fit athletes who might otherwise seem overweight, and most distressingly, apparently thin people who really didn't have a developed muscle on their bodies.[22]

This new standard instilled more panic and paranoia about weight. Quality—as well as quantity—suddenly mattered, and sedentary office workers blessed with natural slimness suddenly found themselves "on the hook." They might be slim but they weren't healthy. And the poor woman who kept herself stylishly thin through chronic dieting now learned she might not measure up. She might not weigh much, and she might look great in clothes, but any wiggle on her meager form, any trace of cellulite—the dimpled fat often found on women's thighs and buttocks—or of a bulge betrayed the awful truth: She was carrying unseemly, unhealthy, and unsightly fat. She was thin—but she was fat. *Leanness,* soon to be called *fitness,* became the new ideal standard. The war against body fat had escalated.

As always, the new standard made its way into the health, beauty, and fashion worlds, and into the popular press, and Americans were deluged with new measurements and new methodologies. How much fat was good, how much bad? Figures were bandied about as scientists and would-be experts tried to find the exact "healthy" proportions. The many numbers that constituted ideal weight now were joined by those that constituted ideal fat-to-lean ratios. Several experts pointed out that the average healthy twenty-year-old woman had 28.7 percent body fat while the average sixty-year-old woman had 41.5 percent. This shift in ratio was also true for men. The average twenty-year-old man had 11 percent body fat; the average fifty-year-old had 25.8 percent. But, just as with ideal weight, so with ideal fat proportions: Lower was always better. By the late seventies experts and self-proclaimed experts were spreading a host of ideal percentages, and they were all low. In his *Fit or Fat,* the ever-popular Covert Bailey authoritatively claimed that the maximum healthy percentage of fat for men was 15 percent, for women 22 percent. He conceded that his own measurements of "thousands" had revealed that most men averaged 23 percent fat, most women 36 percent. But he then declared what we had been hearing for decades about weight: Just because you were normal did not mean you were healthy.[23]

The ideology of fat percentages was identical to that about weight. Fat, like extra weight, served no healthy function. The lower you were—in fat percentages and on the scales—the healthier you were. And, as with weight, experts and the public believed everyone should try to fight the natural tendency to increase fat stores with age. Well aware of this tendency, but denying, as so many did, its validity, Jean Mayer explained that "even in the active individual, however, age inexorably infiltrates existing tissue with fat," and he recommended that we try to buck this trend. In the seventies no one even questioned whether this weight/fat gain was not only normal (they knew it was) but also healthy. Paradoxically, despite the era's reverence for everything "natural," this generation believed, unquestioningly, that in this case, nature was dead wrong. With conscious, determined effort, people were to fight nature, fight to keep the lean body of youth.[24]

The fat-to-lean ratio standard had an even more arbitrary history than the ideal-weight standard. When insurance companies had first established that overweight was unhealthy, they explicitly stated this adverse effect occurred whether the overweight was caused by muscle and bone or fat. Even though no long-term studies correlating overfatness, or fat-to-lean ratios and mortality had yet been conducted, this belief now changed. The idea was merely a presumption and a very persuasive one, since it endorsed entrenched preju- dices. It was fat that people found disgusting, not muscularity.

The official campaign against overweight became much more potent and pervasive in the seventies because it was embedded in a larger philosophical and social change—the development of the health ethic. By the end of the decade, popular and professional health controversies were adjudicated and drawn into an entire government perspective and policy, what Joseph Califano, Jr., Secretary of the Department of Health, Education, and Welfare, described as an effort to start the "second public-health revolution in the history of the United States." The first Surgeon General's Report on Health Promotion and Disease Prevention, *Healthy People,* was published in 1979, and it announced a new medical philosophy and a new medical program for the nation. Its goal was disease prevention, its premise that people could and should control their own health through their personal habits. This emerging health ethic put the war against fat into a broader and ever more compelling context.[25]

The first public-health revolution had been the successful struggle against infectious disease. By the 1970s only 1 percent of Americans under the age of seventy-five died from them—a remarkable achievement. Now authorities felt it was time to get control of the new killers, which were accidents, substance abuse, and, above all, cardiovascular diseases and cancer. Just as knowledge about sanitation, sterilization, and antibiotics had helped control infection, so experts now urged an attack on the "new" root cause of mortality: an affluent society with bad habits. "We are killing ourselves by our own careless habits," wrote the Secretary of HEW in his introduction to *Healthy People.* These habits included "smoking and drinking . . . habits of diet, sleep and exercise, whether one obeys the speed laws and wears seat belts." In revealing language, the Surgeon General estimated that almost half the mortality in 1976 was caused by "unhealthy behavior or life-style."[26]

And of course, that most venerable of bad habits, overeating, was promi- nently discussed. First on the list of ways to avoid heart disease, according to the report, was maintenance of "lean body weight," followed by "regular vigorous exercise, smoking avoidance, consumption of small amounts of al- cohol, and a diet with relatively more vegetables, fish and white meats than red meats." The same recommendation applied to cancer (with avoidance of smoking first), and again a reductive approach to eating was iterated: "Only sufficient calories to meet body needs and maintain desirable weight (fewer calories if overweight)." A lean body was at the very center of the health ethic.[27]

This new "health revolution" encapsulated two shifts in medical philosophy and goals. Because causes for mortality were perceived to be the result of personal habits, people were told they were responsible for their own health, and because health care had advanced so far, scientists sought not merely treatment and avoidance of disease, but optimal health, an improved quality of life. The government had compelling economic reasons to urge optimal health among older Americans. Medicare and Medicaid had begun in 1965, and the government was footing a hefty portion of Americans' medical bills: In 1979, eleven cents of every federal dollar went for health. But younger Americans wanted to be more than disease-free. They also wanted to feel good and vigorous. They expected it as a right and also saw it as an obligation, so that to fail to be healthy was to fail.[28]

The health ethic became immensely potent because its roots were popular, not official. The radical youth of the sixties' counterculture re-entered the mainstream and brought many of their attitudes and values with them— including their distrust of America's institutions, from its food systems to its life-styles—and these became firmly embedded in the national psyche. There was one Establishment concern that particularly meshed with their values, one that they could embrace wholeheartedly: how the modern, "fatogenic" society endangered individual health. For the ex-protesters and ex-flower children, health was a question of physical well-being as well as a matter of higher consciousness and political righteousness; for the Establishment it was a crucial policy concern. Their ideas dovetailed, and the counterculture generation slowly joined with the Establishment in a new, evolving national consensus that healed much of the divisiveness of the sixties. They agreed everyone should strive to get healthy, stay youthful, live longer.

The radical generation turned to health in part because the political activism of the sixties had dissipated, as much because of its successes as because of its failures. After the cataclysmic events of 1968—the murders of Martin Luther King, Jr., and Robert Kennedy, the violence at the Democratic Convention, the failure of the Children's Crusade in the presidential elections of 1970, and finally Altamont, where the "Woodstock generation" had to acknowledge its own loss of innocence—a sobering cynicism began to spread, and it intensified in the seventies with the recession and the debacle of Watergate. The radical generation shifted its emphasis from saving the world to saving the self, from liberating the oppressed to personal liberation. Through the human-potential movement, they sought "higher consciousness" and self-actualization. The creation of the self came to be seen as the highest form of creativity. Initially, this process of self-creation focused on the mental and emotional, but these were also seen as inextricably linked to the physical and spiritual, and gradually, emphasis shifted to the physical, to creating bodily health and strength as the avenue for self-perfection.

The radical generation embraced the new ethic for other reasons as well. Times were changing. Inflation and recession dried up funds, and the collegiate rebels were no longer college-aged. They had to accept poverty as a way of life, not just as a moral gesture, unless they joined the money-making world. Even worse, many of them were approaching or had passed the dread age of thirty, and they sought a way of being over thirty without becoming middle-aged. When they returned to the mainstream, they brought these conflicts with them. They found one cause that resolved some of these paradoxes, preserved some of their anti-Establishment values, and also bridged their gap with the Establishment: health.

Youthfulness was still their ideal. Their goal was to age without suffering the ills of aging, either mentally or physically. They infused in the mainstream a reverence for youth and for perpetual "personal growth" and an abhorrence of middle-class, middle-aged stability, which they equated with personal stagnation. Hugh Hefner distilled the essence of this attitude in 1974 when he commented, "After their thirties, too many people 'settle down' into a kind of dull, gray tedium that's rationalized as maturity. It's an ongoing process that might more rightly be called hardening of the emotional arteries." In her best-selling book, *Passages,* Gail Sheehy contended that "creative solutions" to the crises of middle age and beyond could involve discarding loyal spouses of thirty years or abandoning old careers for new ones. It was never too late to retrieve the opportunities of youth, and a vital person should not let repressive, middle-class notions of responsibility and duty interfere with the quest for personal growth. Articles about fitness often specifically articulated this creed, as in a 1977 interview with one expert in *Vogue.* The ages between thirty-five and forty-five, he warned, were "a very dangerous time of life. You have unfortunately become complacent, professionally and physically. You've achieved a particular goal, and if you're not careful, you can be satisfied with that." Complacency was anathema.[29]

The health ethic also resonated with other counterculture values. Implicit in it were radical criticisms of the Establishment, of modernization, and of capitalism. In their greed, and with the aid of scientific advances, capitalists brutalized nature and threatened its very survival. They even threatened the physical well-being of Americans, who docilely went wherever modernization led them, never stopping to analyze the consequences. Americans showed the same lack of consciousness in their personal habits, willy-nilly eating the abundant and highly refined foods prosperity and modernization offered them, happily falling into physical lethargy as technology relieved them of the need to exert themselves. To many of the radical generation, these developments even seemed an insidious government/capitalist plot: "Blitzed out" by television, junk food, and beer, Americans would remain politically apathetic and spiritually numbed. To a generation busy reconciling two sets of values, the health ethic seemed an ideal philosophic principle. It was a way to stem the tide of these modern developments, a way to return awareness and higher consciousness to the conduct of daily life, and a way to preserve political and personal purity.[30]

This flavor of righteousness soared in the seventies when suddenly, seemingly from nowhere, American abundance was threatened. Oil and food shortages and escalating inflation made many believe that less, not more, was the wave of the future. Comforts could no longer be taken for granted. We were told to save on energy—keep our houses less warm in winter, less cool in summer; walk instead of drive, or just stay home to save gas; turn off lights. Worldwide crop failures meant our surpluses were needed elsewhere, and we felt even guiltier about having so much when so much of the world had so little. In the fifties mothers had told their children to clean their plates with gratitude: "Think of the starving people . . . " But as the world shrunk into a global village, just the opposite was said. To clean your plate while others starved seemed the acme of selfishness, of capitalist America's greed. The anticipated collapse of "fatogenic" luxuries strengthened rather than diluted the thin/fit imperative. "Less is more" became the new slogan for the age—and less food and less weight were prominent goals. We had to use fewer energy resources, but we could develop our own energy through exercise. In a balance between selflessness and selfishness, the body was hit from both sides. Fitness was for yourself; starving was for the world.

The health ethic also resonated with the counterculture's distrust of Establishment professions, especially medical science. The secretary of HEW's claim that "you, the individual, can do more for your health and well-being than any doctor, any hospital, any drug, any exotic medical advice . . . . " was a counterculture conviction. The most thoroughgoing of the critiques leveled against medicine came from Ivan Illich in his 1977 book, *Medical Nemesis,* in which he thundered that doctors had "expropriated" people's health. The golden age of medicine, when doctors and medical science were revered, was crashing to a close, and the new health ethic confirmed that people could and should take control of their own bodies and their own health.[31]

Finally, the health ethic meshed with the ex-counterculture's ambivalence toward materialism and the work ethic. Younger Americans did not want to be like the fifties corporate man in the gray flannel suit. After extensively interviewing young men in 1979, Gail Sheehy observed that they dreaded the idea of "waking up at the age of fifty-five from the money-power-fame success grind they watched their fathers pursue to find they have only a few years left to enjoy life between the first and final heart attacks." This ambivalence was part of their rejection of conventional middle-class notions of adulthood. But it was also part of their refusal to let professional success be the only focus and only aspiration in their lives. Sheehy was stunned to find they rated personal growth and fulfillment as more important than success in work. Quality of life was an overriding concern, and they didn't place much faith in the rewards of professional work. One successful young man underlined the new cynicism and disaffection as follows: "The principle difference between my contemporaries and our parents' generation is that they believed what they were doing was full of purpose and virtue. I don't think we kid ourselves. We have more sense of how limited and almost purposeless what we do is." Sheehy astutely observed that these young men were trying to forge a "hip capitalism" whose most salient feature was maintaining the "appearance of being laid back." They spoke of "unstructured time and unlimited space, of loosely arranged but loving relationships, of the body as temple and the mind as instrument for the most personal expressions." Beneath this appearance, Sheehy noticed the rigid success ethic of their fathers. The health ethic served their needs well. It meshed with their goal of cultivating more than just their careers, and it gave them a larger, more meaningful goal: perfecting themselves. Despite the rise of feminism, which did not endorse such cynicism about careers, women, too, shared these attitudes.[32]

The health ethic also meshed with another major preoccupation of the era—sex and the growing search for other sensual pleasures. The "new hedonism," as some called it, did not extend to the pleasures of a full stomach, which was deemed unhealthy as well as unerotic, and a variety of diet books recommended that you "reach for your mate instead of your plate," that appetite and hunger were better served through sex than food—a popularized extension of the psychoanalytic notion that repressed erotic drives made people eat. It was considered axiomatic that only the well-tended, healthy body was sexually appealing and sexually vital.

The health ethic escalated the mania for thinness and helped transform myth into obsession. Maintaining lean body weight was its principle rule and, in addition, weight loss came to be vaunted as more than just insurance against disease or an aging appearance. It was also seen as a way to prolong the biological stage of youth and possibly, to postpone aging itself. But most powerful were the new associations thinness had gathered, of political and moral righteousness, of a "hip" with-it life-style, and of higher consciousness. For, central to the self-creation and self-realization so fervently sought by the radical generation was the pursuit of youthfulness, beauty, and health—and, above all, of their public badge, slenderness.

The ethic escalated diet-mania also because, like the behavior modification theory, it reconfirmed the notion that people could and should control their body size through self-discipline. No medical miracles had been discovered for weight loss. Even amphetamines were discredited because studies repeatedly showed they were not effective and were both dangerous and potentially addictive. In an era reeling with the effects of increasing drug abuse, such aids were regarded with suspicion. One implicit purpose of the official health ethic was to restore clean living to a nation that had seemed increasingly drug dependent. The ex-radicals were on a parallel quest, looking for a "natural high" to replace the now-defunct glamor of drugs. In both viewpoints, an individual's mental and physical state were seen as matters of individual choice and action. Although new research intimated that individuals might not have absolute control over their body weight, the health ethic absolutely reconfirmed the venerable scientific and popular notion that fatness was caused by gluttonous habits. The overweight had no excuses for their shameful fat.

Of all the bad habits condemned by the health ethic, fatness alone remained a result of moral failure. Other habits and behaviors that had once also been deemed moral failings were recategorized. Drug and alcohol addiction began to be viewed as physiologic dependencies that the addict could not combat even with the sternest will. The addict was an invalid, not a criminal. Homosexuality ceased to be regarded as a form of psychopathology or even of social deviance. Gay liberationists insisted it was a legitimate, even desirable, sexual alternative, a viewpoint society began to accept. This reshuffling of moral and legal categories was occurring on all levels of American society. Impoverished ethnic minorities were no longer held solely responsible for their poverty or for their crime rates: Oppressive, racist conditions were seen as the primary cause. Fatness alone remained a "crime" and a sin for which the individual had to take total responsibility. Indeed, it was one of the few bona fide sins left in America.

The health ethic also introduced a new feature in American life: a passion for exercise. Moderate medical advice was carried to extremes, often by scientists themselves, and a new quasi-scientific orthodoxy developed. We came to believe that vigorous exercise made us lose weight, reduced our risks for cardiovascular disease, and was the pathway for self-transformation and spiritual transcendence.

In the sixties exercise had been regarded as an important adjunct to diet, but by the end of the seventies it was vaunted as an absolute necessity for weight loss and for the kind of body people wanted to have once the weight was gone. Jean Mayer's studies contributed to this shift in emphasis, as did an increasing number of studies that corroborated his findings. In addition, the relationship between low calorie intake and weight loss became more puzzling. Americans weren't eating more, but they continued to get heavier. The government's large-scale nutrition studies revealed that between 1965 and 1977, Americans ate 10 percent fewer calories but had nonetheless gained an average of 2 to 6 pounds. By the mathematical rules applied to weight gain and loss, they should have been losing, not gaining, weight. Many experts concluded that the reason for this discrepancy was self-evident: Modernization kept accelerating, and Americans were becoming less active. They pointed to the increasing use of the automobile, increasingly passive entertainments such as television watching and spectator sports, and to the phenomenal rise of automation in the home and in industry. For example, while in the 1950s, 40 percent of longshoremen were doing heavy physical labor, by 1972, only 5 percent were. In 1982 the authors of *The Dieter's Dilemma* expressed a widespread conviction: "Americans had reached activity levels that were approaching an all-time minimum for the human species. Only women in purdah, and a few other exceptional classes of people could have maintained such a low output."[33]

Another reason for the increasing popularity of exercise was the emergence of new scientific theories—many of them refurbished older theories—which suggested that exercise did more than just burn calories. The mechanical model of body weight, with its mathematical equation of weight gain and loss was beginning to seem suspect. To many researchers, it began to appear that the body "defended" a certain weight. Studies from the sixties and seventies showed that people's metabolic rates, the speed at which calories are burned to perform the body's maintenance functions, changed with changing caloric intakes. Most conscientious dieters know the despair of "the plateau," when the same monotonous diet suddenly ceases to produce the miracle of weight loss. The body simply reduces its own expenditure of energy to conserve fat stores. Overfeeding, on the other hand, accelerates metabolic rates, and after initial weights gains, the body stabilizes at another, higher plateau. The most vivid and startling evidence of this phenomenon came in the late sixties and early seventies, when Ethan Allen Sims's experiments indicated that it could be as difficult to make people gain weight as it was to make them lose it. These findings were corroborated by other studies and caused the old theory of *luxuskonsumption* to be revived and reformulated as *homeostasis* or, in the late seventies, as the *setpoint theory.* Though these theories differed, they argued essentially the same principle: The body was programmed to weigh a certain amount. Deviating from this amount by more than 20 pounds up or down required considerable effort and usually resulted in dismal failures. Overweight people who dieted but could not lose weight may not have been suffering from a failure of will but rather, like those who could not gain, from a biologically determined body weight.[34]

Physical anthropologists even developed a theory of adaptation to explain this phenomenon. Many observed that in prehistoric times—both during the hunting-gathering stage and in the agricultural stage—famines and dearth were common. They speculated that the survivors were those who "overate" during times of plenty and so stored ample reserves of fat to sustain them during food shortages. The human predilection for fat and sweets could be explained by this model—nature simply insured that these good-tasting, caloric foods would be consumed in large quantities during the brief periods they were available—as could the reason women are fatter than men. Women had to be able to store and conserve fat more efficiently than men because of their reproductive functions. In this construct, the fat person was a primitive vestige, burdened with a biology developed for a more primitive food environment. This explanation did not account for those who seemed to have trouble *gaining* weight, and it too presumed that fat had no modern biological function, but it did become widely accepted as a legitimate hypothesis.[35]

These theories took a prominent place in the chaos of theories about over-weight, but they did not cause a truce in the war on fat. Instead, many proponents argued that the secret to weight loss was to lower one's setpoint or to change the body's metabolic rate. For reasons that were not entirely clear, exercise seemed to do just that. It wasn't the calories a particular activity burned that mattered most—though this was still of great importance—but rather, that with exercise, the metabolic rate improved or the setpoint was lowered. A person might actually eat the same amount as in pre-exercise days and still lose weight. Many extrapolated from this fact that the more you exercised, the higher your metabolic rate would become, and the more weight you would lose. By the late seventies the exhortation to exercise moderately exploded into an urge to exercise more often and more vigorously.

Exercise also became central to weight-loss efforts because the new defini-tion of slenderness as a lean, fat-free body required it. Fat, not just high body weight, was unhealthy and ugly. Dieting alone clearly could not solve this problem. Without exercise, how could even the slender get rid of extra flab and fat? Many exercise advocates also began to argue that exercise was *better* than dieting because dieting burned both fat and lean tissue like muscle, while exercise burned only fat. The popular fitness "guru," Covert Bailey, observed that "all of us can think of friends who have gone on diets only to end up looking gaunt and haggard . . . . But it isn't the loss of fat that gives them a wasted appearance. It's the muscle loss!" Muscles made a body look good and shapely while fat made it look bad and lumpy. More appealing still was the argument that even if you didn't lose weight by exercising, you did exchange fat for muscle, and this was just as good. As a San Francisco exercise physiolo-gist explained, "I've lost 20 pounds of fat since I've started running and put on 20 pounds of muscle." She had also lost inches and dropped two dress sizes. What else did a woman need to hear to get on the running track?[36]

Other advantages to exercise were explored by scientists and popularized in the seventies. Many experts pursued earlier research about a link between heart disease and exercise, and a host of studies appeared suggesting that exercise reduced risk factors such as high blood pressure, high cholesterol levels and, of course, overweight. As knowledge about cholesterol became more sophisticated, it appeared there was a difference between HDL (high-density lipoprotein), the "good" cholesterol that helped prevent fat deposits from forming in the arteries and LDL (low-density lipoprotein), the "bad" cholesterol that tended to be deposited. Many researchers suggested that exer-cise raised the ratio of HDL to LDL while others argued that exercise could lower high blood pressure. While no one questioned whether moderate exercise improved general well-being, these other claims proved highly controversial. As the decade progressed, there was a massive proliferation of scientific articles on the ways exercise did or did not improve specific health problems. In the popular press, we usually heard only about the studies that confirmed its value.

Exercise advocates didn't just argue that exercise was healthy. In the early seventies health officials also made glowing promises about its other rewards. In 1971 the U. S. Surgeon General, Dr. Jesse Steinfeld, claimed that overall well-being improved with it: "We will sleep better, eat better, digest our food better." We were also told it would improve our working capacity. In 1973 the head of the Presidential Commission on Physical Fitness claimed that with regular exercise, productivity would improve 15 to 29 percent, a promise not lost on corporations and businesses whose efforts to provide exercise programs increased dramatically in the seventies. As another example of how the former counterculture had been absorbed into the mainstream, still others promised that it could alleviate tension and create a sense of emotional well-being more effectively than the drugs that were being so widely used. Paul Dudley White, dean of American cardiologists, wrote that "vigorous leg exercise is the best antidote for stress and emotional nervousness that we possess, far better than tranquilizers and sedatives to which, unhappily, so many are addicted today." In 1971 the Surgeon General stated that being in shape would even improve sex. In a decade reeling with the sexual revolution, this was an important claim. And finally, health officials promised that exercise brought a joy of living, and renewed vigor and energy. The Public Health Service wrote in 1970 that "people on exercise programs have more pep, vigor, and enthusiasm. . . . "[37]

All these claims came to seem comparatively modest, for by the mid-seventies belief in the purported health and emotional benefits of exercise escalated markedly. So did the amount of exercise deemed desirable. Running or jogging moderate distances had become popular during the late sixties and early seventies, but by the late seventies, ordinary people were running marathons. In 1972, for the first time in sixty-four years, Americans watched one of their own, Frank Shorter, win the Olympic marathon. The same year, a California pathologist and a devoted marathoner, Thomas J. Bassler, wrote a letter to the prestigious medical journal, *Lancet,* in which he presented what is popularly known as the marathon hypothesis. Bassler argued that marathon running provided immunity from heart disease. (The argument eerily echoed those of physical culture advocates a century earlier, who believed a strong body could resist all infectious disease, the killers of that era. It was tantamount to a "microbe killer," exclaimed an 1873 ad for Whitley exercise equipment. The strong, healthy person "could walk unharmed amid all contagious disease . . . may with impunity eat the tubercule bacilli, drink them, breathe them, sleep among them, and escape tuberculosis.") Popular interest in running longer and longer distances mounted, and when James Fixx's *The Complete Book of Running* came out in 1977, it brought the marathon hypothesis to millions of readers. Marathon running ceased to be the passion of only a fringe group. It became wildly popular, the goal of many a modest jogger. The number of entrants in the New York Marathon alone zoomed from a few hundred in 1976 to 16,005 in 1980.[38]

The radical generation embraced running because it seemed an ideal alternative to the commercialized spectator sports and the team sports they so violently castigated. Everyone could run. No one had to be banished to the passivity of the bleachers. And unlike team sports, which required organization and planning, running could be done anytime, anyplace, with a minimum of equipment. It was the sport for a free, impulsive spirit. More important, the radical generation criticized American athletics for encouraging militarism and cutthroat competition. Running was quite different. It was a competition only against the self. It was the height of romantic individualism.

Another reason for the popularity of running was that it tied into the whole mystique of the fitness ethic. Its adherents promised not only health but a kind of metaphysical euphoria known as *runner's high.* It was described in ecstatic tones and words that bore an eerie resemblence to those used by religious devotees in earlier centuries when they described their conversions and their faith. It was regenerating. By the late seventies scientists speculated that there was a physiological explanation for these sensations. Endorphins, opiatelike substances released by the body, reach high levels during vigorous exercise, and some people, though not all, apparently experience this rush of endorphins as a "high." To the generation that had tripped out on psychedelics, meditated to a Zen state, and enthused about nature and the natural, this all made sense. Nature simply provided a "natural" high, one that we had rediscovered.

Behind the public's enthusiasm for exercise was the continuing weight obsession and diluted counterculture values. Behind the medical community's excitement appeared to be a strange paradox, a confusion between fitness, which is the ability of the body to do work, and health, which is the absence of disease. With very few exceptions, more and more doctors and fitness gurus held out the promise of immunity through fitness.

For the vast majority of people, the lofty goals of health, self-creation, and self-realization were inextricably bound up with the desire to look good. Looking good was an outward symbol that one had the will and energy to transcend one's limitations, the higher consciousness to see through the ills and traps of modern capitalist society, and the courage to defy conventional notions about how adults should behave. Above all, looking good meant having a fat-free, streamlined, efficient body. The exercise ethic gave renewed and almost mystical support to the notion that people should slim down, erasing every ounce of fat from their bodies. The lean and hungry look—and often wraithlike emaciation—of the long-distance runner became an ideal. The exercise ethic did not free people from rigid dietary regimens. It just locked them into a concentric, equally rigid routine. And it reinforced the notion that people could and should control their body size and their health.

I am not suggesting that people who exercise moderately don't feel better. I am arguing that the standard for exercise became extreme in the seventies and that its purported benefits soared beyond the reasonable. This escalation was evident to only a few, but their voices could not be heard in the din of scientific and popular enthusiasm about exercise and the health ethic of which it was a part. And, at the heart of both was the decades-old phobia about fat. It had not been displaced but rather buttressed, dignified, and magnified. The quest for a fat-free body had become an American obsession.[39]

9

The Rise of Food Fetishism

Although exercise became central to weight-loss efforts in the seventies, diet did not decrease in importance. Rather, the health ethic expanded and escalated concerns about food. In the fifties and sixties Americans had both rejoiced and worried about their culinary abundance, and their primary concern had been how to enjoy this bounty and yet keep the calorie count down. But the criticisms leveled against the standard American diet in the sixties—by scientists concerned about cholesterol and by a young, life-style-conscious generation—exploded into a nutrition upheaval in the seventies. Americans were deluged with confusing and often conflicting advice which underscored that America's food supply and eating habits were fattening and also hazardous in and of themselves. In 1972 *Time* ran an article unnervingly entitled, "The Perils of Eating American Style." Like exercise, "eating right" came to be valued as more than an aid to weight control. Nutrition, once regarded as a rather dry and bleak subject, now inspired passionate public interest. Since the most fattening foods were also deemed the most unhealthy, the taboos associated with them were powerfully reinforced.[1]

These emerging food attitudes were another pivotal aspect of the health ethic. Like the exercise craze, they were also created by the health and medical community's sincere though biased research into disease, by the diffusion of counterculture values, and by our long history of weight obsession.

Nutrition consciousness grew out of the same wariness about modernization that had sparked fat-phobia. Food is so integral to cultural values and habits that it is usually consumed in an unconscious way. But when these are disrupted, or when there is rapid cultural change, conventional food habits and traditions may become dysfunctional and conspicuous. Both occurred in the seventies, as changes in America's food culture accelerated. From hoping for a chicken in every pot, Americans had come to find a McDonald's or some other fast-food chain at every crossroads. In the late sixties and early seventies these chains were multiplying by 26 percent a year. New convenience and prepared foods and mixes, and imitation and snack foods, which often were made or mixed with a new array of preservatives and additives, soared in popularity. By 1981 it was estimated that more than 50 percent of the foods Americans ate were processed and packaged, and that 50 percent of them had been introduced only during the seventies. One food critic observed that the mainstream American diet in the seventies consisted of "Oreos, peanut butter, Crisco, TV dinners, cake mix, macaroni and cheese, Pepsi, Coke, pizzas, jello, hamburgers, Rice-a-Roni, Spaghetti-o's, pork and beans, Heinz catsup, and instant coffee." Americans were moving toward an industrialized, mass-produced, and mass-marketed food supply. Food production itself kept shifting away from small, family-based farms to enormous agribusiness corporations that used modern and, to many, suspect techniques to improve their yields.[2]

Personal control over food was being relinquished to these giant concerns. American food patterns moved toward uniformity and standardization, diluting ethnic and regional traditions. In 1974 food and beverage ads accounted for 20 percent of all television commercials, and the vast majority of them promoted new products. Youngsters began taking their food cues from the colorful ads on the Saturday-morning cartoon shows instead of from their elders. Other changes in our eating habits were taking place as well. The traditional, home-cooked meal, once a focus of family life and daily rhythms, began to seem like a ghost from the past. Restaurant eating soared. By 1977 the average family spent as much as 25 percent of its annual food budget on restaurant and preprepared meals, with the fast-food chains getting larger and larger shares of the market: In 1971 they claimed 22 percent of the restaurant market, in 1978, 35 percent. Many in this generation were delaying marriage, which meant that many adults no longer even lived in a setting that revolved around family meals. Between 1970 and 1980 the proportion of single-person households jumped by 31.6 percent, two-person nonfamily households by 107.1 percent, and three-person or more nonfamily households by 133.3 percent. Even within the traditional household, mother wasn't home much anymore to do the cooking: 54.3 percent of married women with one or more children under eighteen were now working outside the home. They simply didn't have the time to prepare those meals their mothers or grandmothers used to make. Researchers found that mothers who did stay home didn't necessarily want to be "liberated," but they also didn't want to be "a slave in the kitchen like my mother was." Feminism was playing its own role in separating women and the kitchen. Antitraditional values of many sorts were altering our food attitudes.[3]

As the ritual of family meals was diluted, so were the rules constraining eating. Many observed that American eating patterns had become irregular and unstructured, and resembled "grazing." People snacked a lot. Researchers found that the average American had about twenty food contacts a day instead of the three square meals common in earlier generations. Many worried that these changes would be for the worse nutritionally, tending toward prepackaged, refined, calorie-laden foods. Beneath these concerns, another could be detected, one similar to that voiced by Sylvester Graham in the 1830s. The emotional associations between home, mother, and food were being disrupted. Modernization not only expropriated control of food from people; it also depersonalized food and eating. A *Washington Star* editorial fretted over this decline of intimacy between people and their food, and warned that Americans, especially children, needed "on-site food preparation" and "an awareness of real people preparing and serving the food." Stripped of traditional culinary rituals and associations, eating could indeed become—or be viewed as—merely a form of "pleasurable entertainment," a bad habit that had to be broken.[4]

A rising tide of health, political, moral, and aesthetic indictments were brought against the new, prefab American diet. They came from a wide range of groups—from scientists, government authorites, amateur nutritionists, the growing ranks of gourmets, and from the radical generation, whose political activism gave way to nutrition activism and who joined consumer protection groups and/or the growing ranks of health-food adherents who would eat only "natural" or organic foods. Despite the diversity of their critiques, their general point was always the same: The American diet was changing for the worse. Industrialization and abundance had corrupted the quality and healthiness of Americans' food supply and caused the rising incidence of degenerative diseases. The continuing agricultural revolution was not a leap forward but a leap toward the grave.

These critics began looking at primitive tribes and Third World groups and even at history to relearn food knowledge that had been lost. Journalists John and Karen Hess, for example, contended that "the rule of tongue is that the older, that is, the more primitive the society, the tastier its foods." Lay people and scientists flocked to study these groups, not to help them modernize as in the past, but rather to learn from them how people should eat. They idealized preindustrial, regional, and ethnic foodways and vehemently condemned those associated with modernity and prosperity. This was the crux of America's growing food fetishism. It was a counter-revolution against the "industrial" revolution in America's food culture, and it had broad political and social implications.[5]

Medical research in the sixties and seventies paved the way for these escalating concerns about the national diet. It broadened its focus from how much to what Americans ate. Comparisons revealed that they were eating larger proportions of certain foods—especially meat and saturated fats, sugar, salt, and refined foods—than their forebears and than most other cultural groups with low incidences of the diseases typical of advanced industrial nations. Different experts linked each dietary change to a different disease, arguing that they explained the high rates of heart disease, hypertension, diabetes, and cancers of the breast, stomach, and colon. Although scientists were in considerable disagreement, they all were placing remarkable emphasis on the role of diet in disease, and they thus laid the groundwork for a health ethic in which specific foods could be regarded as having preventive, curative, or pathogenic powers.[6]

As we have observed, the nutrition-consciousness of the 1960s had political overtones. As one Berkeley health-food store owner explained, "I see [natural food] as a way of understanding oppressed people and the political implications of food. Eating is a way of subverting Safeway. The food industry is a heavy political thing." Newly awakened advocates also objected to the inhumane treatment of animals under mass industrial production methods and to the quality of meat obtained from animals raised, they charged, on chemicals and antibiotics, and kept unnaturally cooped up for most of their lives. They fretted that the nutrients had been processed out of all American foods. And many complained that their mothers, who had conscientiously fed them a standard American diet, had been poisoning them.[7]

They did not trust modern medicine and were convinced that scientists knew little about nutrition. Instead they turned to homeopathic medicine and its holistic approach. They sought cures for emotional problems and disease through foods and herbs rather than through physicians and pharmaceuticals. They avidly popped vitamin pills and other supplements, convinced that if recommended dosages were beneficial, high dosages would be better. The health-food faddists, one health-food store owner marveled, "come in here like people going to Lourdes, wanting a cure for some real or imagined disease. Or they secretly think that there is some mystical something in ginseng, bee pollen, or royal jelly, like the wafer in the Mass, that will transubstantiate them and keep them young and beautiful forever." The faddists were no longer unique in this expectation. Ordinary Americans, too, came to think that what they ate was a matter of life and death, that there was magic in some foods which could transform them.[8]

The most potent fear unleashed by these groups was that the chemicals used in animal and agricultural production and as additives were contaminants that caused cancer. This conviction was as much a reaction to the increased use of food additives—up 60 percent between 1960 and 1980—as it was a profound distrust of the Establishment. Ralph Nader, crusading consumer advocate of the era, thundered that the FDA and other agencies responsible for the safety of our food were tools of the very food interests they were supposed to police. American food producers and sellers were viewed as profit-hungry capitalists who would poison the public cheerfully to make a buck, a viewpoint that finally led some to warn of a new McCarthyism: There weren't communists everywhere, but rather, unscrupulous capitalists who were poisoning our food supply. In essence, nutrition activists were advocating a return to small-scale, preindustrial farming techniques.[9]

The nutrition activists had an impact on mainstream America. Partially because of its sheer bulk, the radical generation was reshaping fashions in food. But their influence would never have been so widespread had it not been for the 1969 FDA ruling that cyclamates be banned because they caused cancer. A shudder of disbelief ran through the middle classes. By 1969 an estimated 75 percent of Americans were using the sugar substitute. Many had used it for eighteen years, never dreaming that the FDA would revoke an earlier ruling that it was safe. Diet-drink sales dropped precipitously, and Americans panicked about their food supply. If the nutrition activists were right in this case, chances were that their other indictments were also valid.[10]

For the next several years, the public reeled with other food scares, from DES to DDT, mercury nitrites and nitrates, MSG, BHT, BHA, and other "poisons" camouflaged by innocent sounding letters. Artificial flavors and colors were also attacked. *Chemical* became a loaded term, signifying all the dangerous, usually synthetic substances concocted in laboratories, then put in our food to make it irresistible—and poisonous. Consumers began avidly reading food labels, which were required by 1938 legislation, but while federal agencies debated about requiring more detailed labeling, manufacturers began complying to popular demands for it. Conscientious shoppers were assaulted with lists of terrifyingly unfamiliar and sinister-sounding chemicals—many of them merely scientific names for everyday substances—which added to their growing panic. Nothing in the supermarket seemed safe. The American shopping basket seemed a veritable pile of poisons. It was easy to believe the advocates of fasting: Fasting seemed healthier than eating.

Americans were caught in a cross fire of conflicting nutritional advice. Even scientists could not agree about whether dietary change might protect against degenerative diseases. Their disagreements, combined with nutrition activists' attacks on the average diet and on the scientific establishment itself, caused a crisis of authority about food. This vacuum in authority allowed food faddism to surge into the mainstream. The circulation of Robert Rodale's magazines, *Prevention* and *Organic Gardening,* leapt from 1½ million to 3 million between 1971 and 1977; more and more people began to regard Adelle Davis as a nutrition guru: by 1973 more than 10 million of her books had been sold, and she was introduced on television talk shows and in popular magazines as a respected nutritionist—despite repeated criticisms of her by scientists and even by federal agencies for her misinformation, her misquotation of scientific articles, her distortion of scientific facts, and for the infant deaths caused by overly zealous parents who followed her advice; and natural and organic foods became a billion-dollar-a-year industry.[11]

As the welter of nutritional advice became more confusing, and as nutrition activists became more strident, Senator George McGovern's Select Subcommittee on Nutrition and Human Needs shifted its focus from undernutrition in the United States to resolving some of these controversies. After listening to extensive expert testimony in a wide variety of areas, the committee published its conclusions in the 1977 *Dietary Goals.* Its five main recommendations for all Americans (with some exceptions for children and premenopausal women) were: Increase complex-carbohydrate consumption by eating more fruits, vegetables, and whole grains; eat more fish, poultry, legumes, and less red meat; lower saturated fat and cholesterol consumption and decrease the ratio of saturated to unsaturated fats; reduce sugar consumption and salt intake. In effect, Americans were to move away from processed, refined foods and toward a semivegetarian diet.

Yet the McGovern committee report didn't resolve the controversies. It escalated them. It gave government sanction to the notions that the American diet was unhealthy and that dietary change could significantly affect health and longevity. The committee estimated that if all Americans followed its guidelines, the number of deaths from heart disease would drop by 25 percent, from diabetes by 50 percent, and there would be a 1 percent annual increase in longevity. It provoked scientific controversy, for many official scientific bodies did not agree with its premises or recommendations, most notably the AMA and the most respected nutrition authority in the country, the Food and Nutrition Board (FNB) of the National Academy of Sciences, which had been setting American nutrition guidelines since 1941. And because it criticized so many staples—the eggs and bacon, cheeseburgers and fries, steak and potatoes, and snack and prepared foods that were the nation's staples and culinary pride—it attacked an enormous network of behavioral and economic structures.[12]

It also helped turn food, with its emotional and economic components, into a highly charged political issue. Within the government, the U. S. Department of Agriculture (USDA), the FDA, HEW, and other agencies fiercely competed to see who would set national nutrition policy. Journalist Margaret Eastman wrote in 1977 that nutrition had become "Washington's newest kickball." Larger political issues also emerged. Although many nutrition activists felt it did not go far enough, the McGovern recommendation aligned the government with their emerging position and with their critique of the Establishment. Proponents charged that agricultural and industrial interest groups were blocking reforms, and that health was being sacrificed to capitalistic greed, adding force to the charges of consumer advocates like Ralph Nader. If scientists didn't agree with the recommendations, and many did not they were accused of being the patsies of corporate interest groups. Proponents saw McGovern as a lone hero who dared battle against a powerful and reactionary Establishment. Scientific questions had become political issues.[13]

Other developments gave added political force to McGovern's recommendations and even influenced those recommendations. Worldwide crop failures in 1973 caused worldwide food shortages, and although Americans didn't suffer personally, they watched food prices skyrocket with inflation, shortages, and world demand for their surplus. "Food may never again be cheap," experts warned McGovern's Subcommittee. The Malthusian pincers seemed to be closing: World population kept soaring while food productivity seemed to be stabilizing and even declining. Along with the spectre of permanent energy shortages came the spectre of permanent food shortages. Americans' habits of overeating and of eating large quantities of luxury foods like meat, sugar, and fats seemed more than just unhealthy. They were wasteful of land and labor resources which, many argued, could be more economically and more humanely used by growing the basics needed to feed a hungry world. A host of books appeared to prepare Americans for a culinary future that would be less luxurious but equally healthy, such as Frances Moore Lappé's *Diet for a Small Planet.* "Eating right" now had as much to do with health as with the world's need for resources. The counter-revolution appeared progressive and politically righteous.[14]

In the unstable food atmosphere of the seventies the relatively radical and highly controversial recommendations of the McGovern report began to seem moderate. Scientists and popularizers of every persuasion transformed the indictments of the standard diet into often fantastic beliefs about its dangers. Those foods generally limited in weight-loss diets—fats, sugar, and salt—got the brunt of the attack.

As we have seen, saturated fats and cholesterol—found in dairy products, eggs, and meat—were the first foods specifically condemned as unhealthy. Warnings about them had become strident in the sixties, despite continuing controversy. By the seventies various scientific and government groups lined up for or against the recommendation to eat less of them. In 1973 the AHA took an even stronger stand on the issue and urged at-risk Americans to reduce their total fat intake from the average 40 percent of daily calories down to 35 percent or even 30 percent. By the late seventies scattered epidemiological studies suggested that the high meat/saturated fat content of modern diets might be associated with breast and colon cancer as well as with cardiovascular disease. The McGovern committee recommended that Americans reduce their red meat/saturated fat and cholesterol consumption.

Although this recommendation resembled that of the AHA, in fact it was radically different. It advised *all* Americans to make this dietary change, while the AMA and even the AHA had advised it *only* for Americans who had known risk factors for heart disease and who also had elevated cholesterol levels. In effect, the Committee was advocating a radical life-style change— meat had long been a staple of the American diet, its protein-rich properties acclaimed for creating American health and strength—originally directed only at a specific high-risk group. The Committee further argued that this dietary change should be national policy and that private industry should be pressured to help Americans meet it. In 1979 the Surgeon General's *Healthy People,* which articulated the new health ethic, endorsed it, and the following year, HEW and USDA did the same.[15]

New data were interpreted as confirming the benefits of the recommended dietary shift, which added urgency to the command. Between 1968 and 1976 deaths from—though not the incidence of—strokes and heart diseases began to drop significantly, by about 13 and 20 percent respectively. The Director of HEW's Heart, Lung and Blood Institute pointed to healthier habits as the reason: "fewer smokers, more people exercising, a 50 percent drop in the consumption of animal fat, and greater attention to the danger of high blood pressure." *Psychology Today* published the news in an article entitled, "The American Diet Shifts and Pays Off." Americans had hearkened to the dietary advice of the era. Between 1965 and 1977 egg and butter consumption had dropped and margarine consumption had increased. The only glitch in the data was that beef consumption had risen, not dropped, from 74 to 93 pounds a year, so dietary shift could not really explain the changed mortality rates. Nonetheless, the statistics were widely publicized as proof of the diet-heart disease link.[16]

It seemed that a consensus had been reached, and many authorities began to advocate even lower consumption of saturated fats and meat. As usual, the mass media turned medical recommendation into popular gospel. In 1979 *Vogue* interviewed Dr. Mark Hegsted, administrator of the Human Nutrition Center for the USDA. He told *Vogue* that the current American diet was bad, and worst of all was its high fat content. "Fat is the most serious problem," he reported. He went beyond the AHA guidelines, urging people to reduce their fat to "25 percent—or even 20 percent if you like" of total calories. He defended this low percentage on the grounds that "in other parts of the world where there is very little atherosclerosis and where heart attacks are almost unheard of, the people eat less fat than that." Dr. Hegsted was doing what other health reformers were doing—extrapolating from a nonadvanced nation's dietary habits and concluding that if followed, they would bring a similar reduction in cardiovascular disease,and he was repeating what Americans had heard for decades: Fat, in our food or on our bodies, served no purpose.[17]

Some scientists and popularizers went even further, insisting that people really did not need all the protein once deemed essential for good growth and health and promising that low-fat, semivegetarian diets could wipe out cardiovascular disease and possibly even cancer. Dr. Alex Comfort proclaimed in an article that "about 50 percent of adult male deaths in the United States are probably precipitated in whole or in part by animal fats, a fatal number, second only to those precipitated by cigarette smoking." Nathan Pritikin, coauthor of the 1974 book, *Live Longer Now,* had no training in medicine or nutrition, but his books and his longevity institutes became wildly popular, as did his recommended diet, which was almost devoid of fat—only 10 percent of calories. He promised that his diet not only protected against heart disease but could even cure it, and in later books he promised that it would also protect against gout, diabetes, hypertension, and a host of other diseases. A few years later Patricia Hausman and Richard Marek argued in their book, *Jack Sprat's Legacy,* that "very low-fat diets can actually unclog arteries that were coated thickly with cholesterol plaque"—a claim not made by reputable scientists. Popularizers had escalated into a cure and a panacea a diet recommendation originally made only for at-risk people who *might* thereby be able to reduce their risks.[18]

These tenets became quickly and permanently embedded in the American consciousness: A 1977 Harris poll reported that three out of four Americans were concerned about the cholesterol in their diets. Advertisers exploited the new data for all it was worth, filling the media with advertisements about the advantages of their low-fat products and quoting the authorities who endorsed such diets. The popular press also widely disseminated the prescriptions of nonscientists like Pritikin, who could easily become gurus because they seemed merely to carry to logical conclusions the admonitions of health authorities and because the public had been led to believe that there was some secret nutritional pattern that would bring them better health and longer life. In addition, many began to claim that the FNB's Recommended Daily Allowance for protein was much too high, so there was no defensible reason for keeping up our high-meat diets. And finally, the public was credulous because the new dicta fed and bolstered persistent prejudices about fat and overweight.[19]

World food concerns especially bolstered the attack on eating red meat. Stock raising seemed a deplorably wasteful way to feed a shrinking planet. Lands that cattle grazed on, many charged, could be used instead to grow grains, and the idea that cattle were fattened on grains that hungry people could eat struck many as too high a price to pay for Americans to indulge their taste for tender, fatty meats. *Diet for a Small Planet* outlined a virtually vegetarian regimen, one in which vital protein needs would be met through the increased consumption of legumes like dried beans. In the United States, as in other advanced industrial nations, these larger policy concerns were inextricably mixed with domestic health prescriptions.[20]

As with the exercise ethic, with which it was linked, dietary fat-phobia was not just imposed from above. It became a central feature of the new, fashionable life-style. Succulent, juicy roast beefs and T-bones no longer graced the tables of the sophisticated diner, who eschewed such hackneyed and unhealthy American fare. Adherence to a low-fat diet marked those with a higher consciousness about politics, health, and life—and those who had taste and style. Adherence to it also became something to boast about, clear evidence of admirable self-control.

The fate of sugar in the health-diet consciousness of the seventies was similar to that of fats, though it earned an even worse reputation. Scientific fact and fantasy melded, and sugar—primarily white, refined sugar—became another nemesis of the decade.

Sugar first got its bad name, as fat did, because of its links with a degenerative disease, diabetes, with dental cavities, and above all, with overweight. Sugary treats were full of the "empty calories" all dieters had to eliminate. In the seventies attacks against sugar escalated; foods high in sugar were dubbed "junk foods"—an unappetizing designation for energy-rich but nutrient-thin products. At the heart of these terms was, it appeared, the curious assumption that a food that did nothing but feed you and provided no other nutrients was a bad food, a corollary to the increasingly prevalent notion that eating merely to eat was also "bad."

Health-food faddists such as Rodale and Davis had long condemned the evils of table sugar, and concerns about it became widespread as industrialization of the food supply accelerated. It seemed Americans were eating more and more of the growing supply of "junk foods" like soft drinks, candy, cookies, and ice cream. Sugar was also used increasingly in refined and processed foods not ordinarily thought of as sweet: Sugars of all kinds accounted for 84 percent of food additives, white sugar (sucrose) for 62 percent of them. Various authorities, including the McGovern committee, worried that these developments would entail the replacement of well-balanced meals with sugar-rich prepared foods that provided insufficient RDAs (Recommended Daily Allowances) of necessary nutrients and that this shift would both increase the obesity problem and spread malnutrition.[21]

McGovern's committee recommended that Americans reduce their sugar intake from the average 24 percent of total calories down to 15 percent (though the amount Americans actually consumed was hotly disputed) and government agencies, such as the USDA, began to call for policies that would prohibit sugary snack foods from school campuses. Again, there were powerful political issues involved. The committee kept expressing its concern that profit-hungry manufacturers would stand in the way of such reforms. And again, the McGovern committee was urging *all* Americans to adopt a dietary change once targeted only for specific groups—diabetics and overweights. In doing so, it seemed to endorse the idea that there was something inherently bad about sugar and thus set the climate in which indictments against it could escalate.[22]

The indictments were directed almost exclusively at white, refined sugar. Many nutrition activists suggested that unprocessed sugars like honey and molasses were acceptable and even beneficial. In part, this belief stemmed from their antimodernization sentiments. Since the turn of the century, when technological advances had turned refined sugar into an affordable and widely available commodity, health faddists had warned against it, just as they warned against refined rice and flour because the nutrients had been processed out of them. The new generation of diet reformers took up this banner and praised unprocessed sugars like honey, which still had multiple nutrients, as one faddist explained, such as "copper, iron, calcium and potassium—in addition to other important minerals—and all nine essential amino acids." Honey was also touted as having beneficial side effects, which ranged, depending on the proponent, from acting as a mild laxative and sedative to being a safe sweetening for diabetics, to being a cure for arthritis. While the mainstream tended not to go to these lengths, the idea that sugar was an empty and absolutely useless foodstuff became widely accepted. In June, 1973, *Harper's Bazaar* told its readers that Americans "consume large amounts of empty calories daily," that there "is no physical need for sugar . . . only a psychological craving."[23]

The claims against refined sugar escalated beyond its "empty calories." The idea that it was also bad for us became axiomatic in the seventies. In 1973 the highly respected British physician and nutritionist, John Yudkin, in his book, *Sweet and Dangerous,* introduced many of the themes that would dog its trail. He argued that soaring consumption of refined sugar was responsible for the illnesses in advanced nations. Like so many of the nutritional dicta of the era, his was based on the presumed dietary differences between advanced and less advanced nations. The mass media publicized his theory widely even though the scientific community rejected it because the data did not support it and because his hypothesis was based on a study of only twenty people. The notion nonetheless remained popular. Even more durable was his claim that refined sugar was addictive, not merely "bad," but a drug.[24]

This idea that sugar could be an addictive and a mood-altering substance gained ground among isolated members of the medical profession and among nutrition activists and then spread to the general population. "Anti-sugarites" argued that when sugar hit the body in its pure form (refined and white), it caused a rush of blood sugar or glucose, producing a "sugar high" or energy surge. Of course, as with most drugs, a corresponding "low" followed, brought on, it was said, by an overstimulated pancreas that pumped excessive levels of insulin into the bloodstream, causing a precipitous drop of glucose levels and feelings of irritability and fatigue. These lows—in glucose levels and mood—stimulated a desire for more sugar, locking the sugar-eater in a vicious cycle that resembled addiction. This idea, originally suggested in 1924 by internist and medical nutritionist Seale Harris, survived among health-food faddists and then was resuscitated in the early seventies by psychiatrist R. H. Hoffman and diabetes specialist E. M. Abrahamson whose book, *Body, Mind and Sugar* argued that sugar and caffeine had become the "drugs" of choice for many normal people. Once again, the indictment was brought only against refined sugar: "Natural" sugars like honey presumably did not have the same metabolic effects.[25]

These ideas rapidly made their way into the mainstream via radio commentators like Carlton Fredericks, the new nutrition gurus, and the popular press. In 1976 William Duffy published *Sugar Blues* in which he spelled out sugar's frightening effects. Duffy proved to be a vital link between a fringe view and popular culture. The publication of his book was followed by his marriage to Gloria Swanson, which made both highly visible and strident proponents of these views. Dr. David Reuben, switching, as Alex Comfort had, from telling us everything we wanted to know about sex to telling us *Everything You Always Wanted to Know About Nutrition but Were Afraid to Ask,* was another vital link. In this book, he warned about the cocainelike effects of sugar. This was quite a leap beyond the older notion that psychological problems could lead to a psychological addiction to food. Now blame was put on the food itself. It was inherently addictive, like the illegal drugs that were becoming so widely used in this permissive era. Appetite was being thoroughly discredited. The yen for something sweet had been transformed into an unsavory compulsion that was beyond our control. If we felt like having a sugary food, we feared we had an unnatural craving, even an addiction.[26]

This view became so pervasive that parents began trying to keep their infants from ever tasting the refined stuff so they would never develop a taste for or an addiction to it. In playgroups, there was an unwritten rule that no sweets be given; only unsweetened fruit juice was acceptable. Unenlightened grandmothers got the evil eye when they tried to fulfill one of their traditional roles—giving candy to baby. And some began warning pregnant women to avoid the stuff as well, for it presumably entered the amniotic fluid, producing infants who would crave it throughout their lives.[27]

Sugar eating was even identified with a spreading but unrecognized disease—*hypoglycemia*, a disorder that causes low blood-sugar levels. Nutrition activists, among others, argued that excessive sugar consumption caused, *The Disease Your Doctor Won't Treat*, as one popular book was titled. Hypoglycemia was associated with a wide range of symptoms from anxiety to depression, fatigue, shakiness, confusion, allergies, and behavioral problems, and popular magazines advised us that many of our vague emotional and physical ills might really be a result of this disorder. By 1973 these beliefs had become so widespread that the American Diabetic Association, the Endocrine Society, and the AMA felt compelled to intervene. They reported that the disease is extremely rare, is not caused by sugar consumption but by an unusual pancreatic disorder, and could not be associated with the psychological and behavior problems popularly attributed to it. " . . . [T]here is not good evidence that hypoglycemia causes depression, chronic fatigue, allergies, nervous breakdowns . . . . " If even hypoglycemia didn't cause these reactions, it seemed ridiculous to presume sugar eating would do so in a normally functioning body. But the hypoglycemia idea proved hardy, and, in modified form, even entered respectable nutrition books: *Jane Brody's Nutrition Book,* published in 1981, acknowledged that true hypoglycemia is a rare disorder but nonetheless warned that "the body was not designed to handle sugar in concentrated forms, such as in a piece of cake or candy bar," because they cause "overproduction of insulin."[28]

Even without the hypoglycemia idea, sugar was still regarded as a bad drug, one that powerfully affected behavior. In the seventies it was blamed for learning disabilities and for hyperactivity in children. In a more dramatic variation of this idea, it was also blamed for adult criminal behavior. In the sixties Adelle Davis had argued that the infamous Manson "family" had committed the Sharon Tate murder because for days prior to the murder, they had been eating only candy bars. In 1978 this fringe idea had become sufficiently mainstream to be used as a defense in a court of law. San Francisco Councilman Dan White, who shot mayor Harvey Milk, was defended in an argument that became known as the Twinkie Defense. White's lawyer claimed the defendant had been subsisting on a diet of junk food that interfered with his reasoning and moral judgment. The public was surprised, but not unduly shaken, by this line of thought. It merely reconfirmed their convictions about the evils of sugar and about the powerful impact of nutrition on mood and behavior.[29]

By the end of the decade, it seemed axiomatic that sugar was bad, even if the exact reasons for this remained vague and confusing. The McGovern committee, by advising all Americans to cut back on sugar, seemed to endorse the spiraling fears about it. It seemed sinister, as dangerous as the other drugs that caused addiction and deranged morals. Although overeating was still viewed as subject to conscious self-control, sugar itself was caught in that reshuffling of moral categories so prevalent in the seventies. Sugar "addicts," at least, could claim their overeating was caused by a physiological dependency that left them powerless, and some researchers began to investigate whether these popular claims had some scientific basis. Sugar was no longer condemned just for being fattening. It now seemed dangerous in and of itself. And like fats and meats, its absence—or at least its restriction—became a feature of the new fashionable life-style.

Salt was the third foodstuff that came under direct attack in the seventies. Its fate was similar to that of fats and sugars. Hypertension had long been recognized as one of the risk factors for cardiovascular disease and, in the forties, researchers discovered that reduced sodium intake, particularly in the form of salt, helped control hypertension. Again, as with sugar, increasing industrialization of the American food supply caused mounting concerns about salt. It was the second leading additive after sugar, accounting for 15 of the 153 pounds of additives consumed each year by the average adult. And the idea emerged that this increased salt intake not only aggravated hypertension but also might cause it. McGovern's committee urged *all* Americans to cut their daily salt consumption down to 5 grams a day.

At the popular level, as with prohibitions about fat and sugar, the recommendations of health officials were transformed into panicked warnings and implacable taboos. As with so many of the food dicta, differentiations between cause, effect, and treatment of diseases got muddled, and from a variety of sources we began to hear that high sodium intake *caused* high blood pressure, kidney disease, and other illnesses. Author Marietta Whittlesay demonstrated the escalation of fears about salt in just the title of her book, *Killer Salt,* in which she wrote of the "shocking evidence linking depression, bloating, weight gain, migraine . . . and kidney disease to the salt we crave and consume—with fatal ignorance." While salt escaped being categorized as a drug, it was identified as an acquired taste, one that millions scrambled to divest themselves of and that conscientious parents tried to prevent in their children. Food manufacturers, always closely attuned to the fears and desires of the American public, rapidly began to reduce the sodium content of their products and to vaunt them as health-promoting.[30]

These emerging food convictions helped spawn a new culinary aesthetic. In the fifties and sixties weight-loss diet philosophy reflected the eating habits of the better-off classes. Complex carbohydrates like bread, pasta, potatoes, rice, and grains, the staples of the lower class diet, were deemed the most fattening foods and so bore the double onus of being fattening and unrefined. Weight-loss authorities recommended instead the more expensive meat, fresh fruit, and vegetable diets typical of those at the higher end of the social scale. Meat usually meant beef, for pork was not only considered more fatty but was also associated with lower-class diets. In a sense, this dietary advice encouraged the lower classes to adopt the habits of the better-off classes.

The effort primarily succeeded, in part, because modernized techniques helped make these once luxury items increasingly available. But as this occurred, food reformers began to idealize the eating habits of preindustrial, peasant societies and of the American past, and many scientists came to share their views. Complex carbohydrates were central to these diets, and gradually, they lost their onus as fattening—we learned that the sauces and fats they usually were served or cooked with made them fattening—and as unfashionable. Instead, rich, fat-marbled roasts and heavy, epicurean sauces came to be viewed as unfashionable, unhealthy, and fattening. Simultaneously, the modern, preprepared, and refined foods, once bought proudly by the affluent classes, became cheaper and more common—and lost their former status. In the forging of this new culinary style, one of the more durable fashion dynamics seemed to be at work: competition for status. The middle and lower-middle classes had no sooner begun to adopt the foodways of the elite then the elite food rules began to change.[31]

It was not just class competition that created the new food rules. Critics of modernization genuinely feared where it was leading, and their fear mingled with nostalgia for a culinary world that was disappearing. As so often happens in periods of change, critics idealized what was disappearing and sought to preserve it. Their reactionary sentimentalism also proved to be progressive. Again, as so often happens in such circumstances, these idealizations of the past provided a vision of how to direct the present. It enabled food critics to forge a new culinary aesthetic, one that did not reject modern innovations but that did allow them to integrate the best of the past into the present.

A new gourmet cuisine was born, one that followed the new precepts about healthy diet and natural foods and that also turned "undereating" into an art: nouvelle cuisine. The French, past masters of the culinary arts and subject to these modernizing trends, came through again. Nouvelle cuisine developed in the sixties among a new generation of chefs, including Paul Bocuse, Paul Guérard, and Jean and Pierre Troisgros. Despite variations, their cuisines shared common principles, which bore startling resemblances to the food rules articulated by nutrition activists and later, by the *Dietary Goals,* and which were in direct contrast to the emerging industrial food culture and its depersonalization. They favored a *cuisine du marché*—meals composed of the freshest ingredients available in the market every day rather than of the products "bastardized and polluted by food technology and overproduction." They incorporated peasant traditions and yet found ways to use new technology, such as the microwave, to create high-quality fare. They sought the "least transformation" in their food; that is, keeping it as close to its original state as possible to bring out its distinctive and forgotten flavors, which entailed significantly reduced cooking times for meat, fish, poultry, and vegetables, and avoidance of rich or complicated sauces that would mask natural flavors. The new chefs simplified gourmet traditions and pared food down to its simplest and purest form. And there was no danger of overeating. Nouvelle cuisine presentation called for small, beautifully arranged, highly decorative portions. In a sense, it was the art of minimalism translated to food.[32]

Nouvelle cuisine provided an epicurean solution for Americans caught between their desire for healthier nutrition and for refinement. By the late seventies affluent Americans, inspired by their travels to Europe (which had increased dramatically in the sixties), by Oriental influences, and by the "natural" foods movement, had found a new, sophisticated, and dietetically acceptable way to improve the quality of life—and of the table. "The sexual revolution is passé," announced *Time* in December, 1977. "We have gone from Pan to pots. The Great American Love Affair is taking place in the kitchen." And it marveled over the 20 percent rise in specialty-food spending between 1972 and 1977, the increasing popularity of restaurants with gourmet chefs and of the chefs themselves, who were becoming celebrities, the exploding popularity of home vegetable and herb gardening and of old-style farmers' markets, and over the vast amounts spent on cooking utensils and on elaborate kitchens for the home gourmet. Affluent Americans embraced the principles of nouvelle cuisine, which gave them a way to pleasure the palate without lots of cholesterol, fat, sugar, salt, additives, or calories.[33]

It appeared that a new system of foodways was being established, one that now had the endorsement of many governmental agencies, scientists, epicureans, and popular nutritionists. And the spiraling panic about the American diet seemed to be justified. But, in fact, although many authorities endorsed the comparatively moderate McGovern Report, no consensus had been reached. Experts who testified before the committee had not been in agreement, a fact not widely publicized and one obfuscated by political accusations. Many were outraged and dismayed when the AMA and many other scientists objected to the *Dietary Goals,* and a furor erupted when the FNB issued its 1980 report, *Toward Healthful Diets,* which disputed the recommendations. Yet the FNB, after meticulously reviewing the evidence, tried to demonstrate how many misconceptions had spread, how little scientific evidence supported the recommended changes, and how unnecessary the mounting food panic was.

The FNB objected to the upsurge in "magical" thinking about food, particularly the idea that it could prevent or cure illness, and to the notions that the typical American diet was inherently unhealthy and had caused an increase of degenerative diseases: Americans' life expectancy continued to increase; mortality from cardiovascular disease had dropped 20 percent in the previous twenty years and was continuing to decline by 2 percent a year; cancer rates had remained stable or declined since 1930—except for those associated with smoking. In short, American health had improved, not deteriorated, with the modernization of the food supply, and nutritional-deficiency diseases had been virtually eradicated.

The FNB acknowledged the legitimacy of asking whether dietary changes might also reduce the incidence of degenerative diseases. But it cautioned that epidemiological studies, which had implicated the diet of advanced industrial nations in these diseases, established coincidence, not cause and effect. They provide hypotheses that can then be tested, and when a sufficient number of studies from different scientific fields confirm the hypotheses, then there are legitimate grounds for recommending change. After meticulously reviewing the evidence linking diet to disease, the FNB concluded that this evidence was inconclusive and contradictory, which explains in part why Americans were so confused. For these reasons, the FNB disagreed with the specific presumptions and recommendations of the *Dietary Goals*, most of which, as we have seen, were carried to extremes by nutrition activists and food faddists. The advice, the FNB claimed, was not warranted by the scientific evidence and might adversely affect the century-long improvements in national health.[34]

In a variety of publications, those who agreed with the FNB explained why they were opposed to the advice that *all* Americans cut back on meat, saturated fat, and cholesterol consumption. The AMA and the FNB cautioned that the diet-heart disease link and even the cholesterol-heart disease link were inconclusive and controversial: Only 50 percent of the incidence of cardiovascular disease in the United States could be explained by some or all of the suspected risk factors—cigarette smoking, hypertension, overweight, stress, inactivity, family history, and high cholesterol levels—and even in these cases, it was not clear whether they were just associated or causative factors. The connection between high serum cholesterol levels and cardiovascular disease was especially unclear: Many epidemiological studies had shown no connection, and Dr. Michael DeBakey, world-famous heart surgeon, had reported that his own experience had shown "[no] definite correlation between serum cholesterol levels and extent of atherosclerotic disease." In short, the fundamental causes for cardiovascular disease were still not known. More importantly, they pointed out that trials to alter the incidence and mortality rates of coronary artery disease through diet had generally been negative.[35]

Even the relationship between diet and serum cholesterol levels was not clear-cut. The human liver produces its own cholesterol, anywhere from 800 to 1,500 milligrams a day. In the seventies Americans consumed an average of 450 milligrams of cholesterol a day, down from the range of 509–576 mgs common between 1900 and 1970. Human beings do not absorb much dietary cholesterol—only about 10 to 15 percent of that consumed. The FNB concluded that "no significant correlation between cholesterol intake and serum cholesterol concentration has been shown in free-living persons in this country." While saturated fat consumption was associated with elevated cholesterol levels, the evidence again was not clear-cut. What the body does with this consumption is variable. At one extreme are those who seem to have internal regulatory controls, so that their livers alter production of cholesterol to balance it with the amount consumed. No matter what these people eat, their cholesterol levels remain low. At the other extreme are people lacking such controls, whose livers do not alter production with consumption. Most people fall within these two extremes, and there are even others who have excessively high cholesterol levels because of metabolic abnormalities, which no dietary modification can control. Considering this evidence, the FNB underlined the fact that for individuals without other risks for heart disease and certainly for those without high serum cholesterol levels, no purpose would be served by dietary modifications. And they objected to the spread of false hopes that such changes might make a difference.[36]

The FNB also felt it was premature to make specific food recommendations. Many earlier presumptions about which foods raised cholesterol had been wrong, which explained some of the mounting confusion. Milk, once a nemesis, had been found to have two substances that make the liver reduce cholesterol production, so that it appeared this dairy product might lower, not raise, serum cholesterol levels. How many other valuable foods were also being condemned unjustly? The Board was also uneasy about the advice to increase the proportion of polyunsaturated fats: An unsettling though inconclusive association had been made between polyunsaturated fats and cancer. And finally, the FNB did not believe that the recommended dietary changes were entirely benign. There was concern that the trend away from meat eating might compromise protein intake and the intake of trace nutrients found primarily in meat.[37]

Finally, the FNB stressed that the fatty diet-cancer link was even weaker than the fatty diet-heart disease link. Both the FNB and the National Cancer Institute concluded that "no direct cause-effect relationship has been observed for nutrition and cancer in humans." The most consistent evidence of such a link had been between large consumption of polyunsaturated fats and *increased* risks of cancer.[38]

In addition, many experts were concerned about the growing belief that dietary fat and cholesterol were inherently bad. Frederick Stare, professor emeritus and founder of Harvard's Department of Nutrition, and Elizabeth Whelan, Ph. D., of Harvard's School of Public Health and executive director of the American Council on Science and Health, stressed that both had been unfairly condemned, and elementary biological facts had been lost in the public hysteria. Both serum cholesterol and dietary fat are essential for human life. Serum cholesterol is vital for many complex body functions: It is an important component in the cell walls; the body relies on it to make male and female hormones; the human brain itself is rich in the substance. The body also needs dietary fat. Public-health researchers in the the early fifties found that when dietary fat was reduced below 30 percent of calories, protein metabolism was impaired. Stare and Whelan explained that dietary fats "contribute to a feeling of satiety after a meal" and are essential as a transport system for the four fat-soluble vitamins.[39]

In essence, the FNB and these other authorities were trying to stem the rising tide of hysteria about dietary fat and cholesterol and of unfounded hopes about what eliminating them might do. Whelan, Stare, and others particularly objected to the accusation that the dissenters were patsies of interest groups, and pointed out that the industries that supported reform, such as vegetable oil and health food producers were interest groups that were themselves becoming almost as powerful. The FNB certainly did not recommend that we gluttonously consume fats and cholesterol. It argued that a varied, balanced diet—the kind recommended for decades—was still the best, and that if we did not have elevated cholesterol levels, there was no need to fear cholesterol or fat in our food.

The rising panic about sugar appeared to involve more fantasy than that about fat and cholesterol. No scientific evidence linked it to degenerative diseases or to mood and behavioral disorders, or even to diabetes. Experts concluded that sugar consumption did not *cause* diabetes, and in 1971 the Committee on Food and Nutrition for the American Diabetes Association officially reversed the old dictum that diabetics avoid eating carbohydrates. Research had shown that this dietetic restriction did not alter the course of the disease. There was certainly no evidence that refined sugar had cocainelike or other pharmacological effects, and Stare and Whelan went into painstaking detail in their books to explain elementary metabolic facts about sugar consumption. Blood sugar (glucose) levels become low after a period of not eating, and they climb after we eat, regardless of the type of food. In fact, it is generally believed that the low glucose levels trigger the sensation of hunger, while their rise produces sensations of satiety and well-being (not hyperactivity). In a normally functioning body, sugar does not make glucose levels fluctuate beyond normal ranges. Only when people have hypoglycemia or diabetes do blood sugar levels deviate significantly enough to produce abnormal symptoms. But hypoglycemia is an extremely rare disorder, one that is not *caused* by eating sugar, and it is generally considered a *symptom* of disease rather than a disease in and of itself.

Similar scientific distortions fed the belief that unrefined sugars were good, refined sugar bad. The human body breaks all sugars down into glucose, whether they come in the form of sucrose (refined sugar), glucose (the sugar in our blood and in many plants), fructose (the sugar in fruit), or lactose (the sugar in milk), or in the form of unrefined honey (made of glucose, fructose, and sucrose). The body doesn't seem to care what form the sugar comes in;

it metabolizes them all in similar ways. Furthermore, few scientists could endorse the precept that unrefined sugars like honey were better because they had other nutrients. The extra nutrients occur in such minute amounts that people would have to eat huge quantities to have them figure into their nutritional picture. Consumers' Union estimated it would take about 200 tablespoons of honey to approach the daily requirement for potassium and 267 for phosphorous, depending on which type and batch of honey were used. This was another popular shibboleth based on considerable misinformation.[40]

Even the claim that Americans were beginning to eat unprecedented quantities of refined sugar was based as much on fantasy as on fact. Though there was some basis to the belief that Americans were eating more sugar than they had a century earlier (between 1870 and 1879 average per-capita consumption was approximately 39.7 pounds a year, while in 1970 it was about 101.9 pounds) the statistics were misleading since traditional home-produced sweeteners such as sorghum, maple sugar and maple syrup, corn syrup, and molasses were not measured. Furthermore, between 1925 and 1980 refined-sugar consumption had remained fairly constant, dipping and rising in response to price fluctuations—and to rising fears about its effects. In 1925 average consumption was 104.3 pounds a year, an amount that dropped gradually to 97.6 pounds in 1960 and then rose again to 101.9 pounds in 1970, only to be followed by another drop in 1981, when it was 79.5 pounds. There was also dispute about the McGovern committee claim that refined sugar consumption amounted to 24 percent of total calories. The USDA, the FDA Select Committee on GRAS (*Generally Recognized as Safe Substances*), and the National Research Council estimated that in 1974 it was closer to 14.1 percent of total calorie intake, somewhat less than what the Committee recommended. Finally, and even more surprisingly, the advanced industrial nations were not consuming more refined sugar than other nations. In 1980 Costa Rica, Cuba, Guyana, Jamaica, Iraq, Malta, and Mexico, among others, were all consuming far more of it per capita than Americans were, at least according to United Nations statistics, and presumably they did not suffer all the debilitating effects described by the antisugarites.[41]

The most durable shibboleth was the notion of an "empty calorie," an indictment brought against sugar and against junk foods. There is no such thing as an empty calorie. A calorie is a measurement of food energy, and sugar is a useful source of energy, providing four calories per gram, just as other carbohydrates do. Furthermore, few people eat pure sugar—candy bars, cakes, and cookies are also full of eggs, milk, flour, and fats. As nutritionist Frederick Stare explained, "Just because sugar tastes good doesn't mean it's not good for you. Sugar is a first-rate source of energy. Relax and enjoy moderate amounts if that is your desire." Nutritionists also pointed out that even the infamous fast-food chain meals and snack foods provided energy, and some met many of our other nutritional RDAs. They are not addictive or unhealthy.[42]

The advice to reduce salt consumption was one of the few dietary guidelines the FNB supported. But it still tried to clear up the misguided hopes associated with this dietary change. It stressed that salt intake did not *cause* hypertension. Rather, high sodium intake seemed to exacerbate the condition for those who had it and possibly brought out its symptoms in people who were genetically predisposed to it. According to its estimates, only 15 to 20 percent of the American population fit this category. Nonetheless, because there seemed to be no evident *need* for more sodium than occurred naturally in foods, and out of prudence, the FNB recommended this reduction. But it stressed that this dietary change could not be considered a guarantee against developing hypertension. Certainly, for the 80 to 85 percent of the population without a family history of or predisposition to hypertension, this dietary change would serve no purpose.[43]

Similarly, the reasonable demand for caution about new food-production techniques had spiraled into unjustified hysteria. Americans were convinced that their foods were riddled with a plethora of dangerous synthetic substances. In an effort to clear up the confusion, many nutritionists hastened to explain that additives and preservatives had made the American food supply one of the safest in the world. Nor were the additives dangerous. Ninety-three percent of the additives used are sugars and salt—which may not assuage the worries of those concerned about these substances—but they are hardly unnatural or synthetic. They have a venerable history: For centuries, salt and sugar preserved essential foods that otherwise would have been unavailable to a hungry population. Of the other 7 percent, three additives comprise 90 percent of them; the remaining 10 percent is made up of 2,600 additives. They are used to enhance flavor and color, as preservatives, texture agents, leavenings, and nutrients—such as the Vitamin D added to milk and the enrichments mandated for white bread. Which of these additives were natural instead of synthetic also wasn't always clear. For example, calcium propionate, used to inhibit mold in bread, is also produced in the human body and occurs naturally in many foods, such as Swiss cheese. Was its use in bread, then, artificial and so unsafe?[44]

Many of the indictments the FDA brought against various additives— cyclamates, BHT and BHA, nitrites and nitrates, among others—proved to have been premature, based on individual studies whose results could not be duplicated or whose results, when re-examined, proved to have been misinterpreted. The lifting of FDA bans on these additives never received much publicity. Political pressure from nutrition activists may have been responsible for the premature bans, as well as a highly controversial aspect of the Delaney Amendment of 1958, which regulated them. It stipulated that any substance known to cause cancer, regardless of the amount administered, be banned. But amount was crucial. The most harmless, even healthy, substances and foods can have toxic effects if taken in large amounts. Vitamin A, for example, is necessary for good health, but too much of it can cause irreversible damage to the central nervous system and even death. Some seafoods have traces of arsenic, as do many fruits, vegetables, cereal products, meat, and dairy products; carrots contain carotoxin, a dangerous nerve poison when ingested in large amounts; beets, spinach, and some other vegetables are far higher in nitrates than the allowable amounts of nitrate artificially added to foods such as bacon; oranges contain a chemical toxic to human embryos—but we don't become ill when we eat them because we don't eat sufficient quantities. Many scientists felt that the Delaney Amendment's dismissal of this fact distorted policies. They insisted that a benefit/harm ratio be established, for many of these products had benefits that far outweighed their potential harm.

Similar misconceptions dogged the terms *chemical-free, organic,* and *health food.* The FDA tried valiantly to come up with acceptable definitions of these terms to regulate the advertising pitches of food manufacturers. They could not do so because the terms were so unscientific. Even the buzzword *chemical* was a problem. All foods are made of chemicals. The list of scientific names for the ingredients of a cantaloupe could stop the heart of a conscientious food shopper as readily as the list of ingredients in a Twinkie. If eaten as part of a well-balanced diet, all foods are also "organic" and "health foods," because they promote health. Even the term *natural foods* caused perplexity. All foods are "natural" or made from "natural" ingredients. The FDA simply could not come up with scientifically acceptable definitions to justify these terms.[45]

I am not trying to suggest that we don't need to be watchful about the effects of modern industrial techniques, including the use of additives. There are dangers inherent in many modern methods. But a legitimate wariness about new industrial techniques had boomeranged into a hysteria that had little scientific foundation, and Americans had been terrified, unnecessarily, about their food supply. The food revolution had not caused a cancer epidemic. Experts worried that people were paying higher prices for "organic" foods, which offered them no better nutritional quality nor any other benefits than the cheaper supermarket versions, and they worried about the long-forgotten dangers that might be revived when modern techniques and preservatives were *not* used. Experts were also alarmed about the fantastic claims made about megadoses of vitamins and certain foods. They explained that people eating well-balanced meals shouldn't need supplements. And more was not better. More vitamins and nutrients did not bring added protection or benefits, and in excessive dosages some could be harmful, even lethal.

The FNB concluded that cancer and cardiovascular diseases had "multiple and poorly understood etiologies," which were "not primarily nutritional, although they have nutritional determinants that vary in importance from individual to individual." Many scientists also expressed a deep and valid concern that the emphasis on diet and on dietary programs might divert research and research moneys away from investigation of the other underlying and perhaps more significant causes of these diseases. High—and unfounded—hopes had been raised by the new dietary recommendations and by the soaring popularity of food faddists. Food, many nutritionists tried to explain, was not a medicine or magic talisman. It was needed to ensure good health and was supposed to taste good and be enjoyed.[46]

Despite these admonitions, Americans embraced the new dietary dicta, in part because the etiology of cancer and cardiovascular diseases did remain obscure, and a disease of unknown causes is terrifying. Throughout history, people have adopted a variety of rituals to protect themselves from such dangers. Prudence dictated that if there were even a chance dietary modification would provide this protection, then it was a ritual worth adopting. Many scientists embraced the dicta for similar reasons. In addition, they were following a venerable historical pattern. When the cause of a disease is unknown, personal behavior and habits—particularly diet and bowel patterns—become the prime suspects, for food is the one thing we bring from the external world into the internal environment of our bodies.

But Americans were credulous mostly because the restricted foods were also those that caused weight gain. Food could be enjoyed—as long as we were not fat. This was key, for at the core of all the new food rules was an enduring—and constantly mounting—fat-phobia. It was a paramount feature of nouvelle cuisine: Michel Guérard's 1976 *La Grande Cuisine Minceur*—the "cooking of slimness"—had been enormously popular in both its French and English versions, and cultural historian Stephen Mennell underlined that all the new chefs had "the dietetic implications of their work constantly in mind." Fat-phobia was also central to the McGovern committee's *Dietary Guidelines* and a primary reason they were so widely accepted. The committee's original goal was to address America's number-one health problem—obesity—to find what nutritional patterns had made it epidemic and how they could be changed. It estimated that if its guidelines were followed, obesity in America would be reduced by 80 percent. The committee admirably and sincerely tried to squelch the soaring popularity of fad diets by presenting healthy and sensible nutrition guidelines, which indeed resembled diets the medical profession had been recommending for decades—for weight loss.[47]

Despite many scientists' efforts to quell the mounting food fetishism, even they were not loudly telling Americans to eat the foods condemned by the McGovern committee, precisely because these foods contributed to weight gain. After explaining that saturated fats could not be causally related to cardiovascular disease and cancer, the FNB and authors Whelan and Stare nonetheless admonished us to remember that "all fats and oils, from whatever source, are high in calories . . . . If weight control is a problem, as it is for many, you will need to avoid excessive amounts . . . . " The same was true for sugar. Those who advised Americans to reduce their sugar consumption had at heart a perfectly reasonable concern about the replacement of well-balanced meals with treats that provided insufficient quantities of the Recommended Daily Allowances of nutrients. Nonetheless, it is hard to avoid the conclusion that sugar's relation to weight gain, and its suspect deliciousness, caused its identity as a bogey. Even Stare and Whelan, after reassuring us about the innocence of the substance, observed that "as long as the RDA is being met for all nutrients, there is no harm whatever in using snack foods to fulfill additional calorie requirements. If you have a weight problem, you won't have room for many of these "extras"; if you are on a reducing diet, chances are you will temporarily have to do without any at all . . . . " Though the "fattening" properties of salt—which caused apparent weight gain because of water reten- tion—were not stressed by officials, they strongly influenced the public's fear of it. Popular diets had often warned against these "fattening" properties, and many would-be dieters abused diuretics to keep their weight low, their bodies lean and unpuffy. *Weight gain* and *bloating* were the key words in the porten- tious catalog described by Whittlesay in her book, *Killer Salt.* [48]

Several studies, including those of British physician Dennis Burkitt, had stressed the fattening properties of "fiber-depleted starchy carbohydrate foods" and had attributed the better health and leanness of Africans to their high-fiber diets. These ideas were immediately popularized by Dr. David Reuben, osteopath Sanford Siegal, and Barbara Kraus, author of the *Barbara Kraus Guide to Fiber in Foods,* all of whom assured us that fiber fills our stomachs, so we eat less, and decreases the transit time of food through the intestinal tract, "thus lowering the number of calories your body receives from the food you eat." The high-fiber diet was fundamentally a way to lose weight. Even health foods were touted for their ability to keep us slim.

Summing up the chaos of opinions, journalist Chris Chase aptly concluded: "Salt *may* give you high blood pressure and heart disease and strokes, sugar *may* leave you toothless and hopped up and less able to combat bacterial infections, meat *may* set your heart to attacking you, *and all of it will make you fat.* " Fat-phobia had powerfully influenced the new health-food precepts, and they, in turn, powerfully reinforced America's endemic calorie-conscious- ness. Diet-mania had simply moved to higher ground. [49]

As the seventies moved into the eighties all the concerns about fat, sugar, salt, additives, and processed foods ceased to be a confusing jumble, and they ceased to be radical. They merged together, creating a new food philosophy in America. The political thrust behind them dissipated, and the health thrust became overwhelmingly important. Few bothered to explore more closely the scientific accuracy of the new precepts. And no one could tell where the experts' cautions ended and the faddists' claims began. They were part of a long and, by now, believable continuum. And they were nourished by those romantic images of preindustrial foodways. It was no accident that in the eighties Jane Fonda's health and nutrition ideas became wildly popular and mainstream. Her background made her uniquely representative of the era. She had become a highly visible symbol of the counterculture and of its indictments of modernization and capitalism, she had a history of fierce diet-mania (and had verged on bulimia and anorexia), and she had the Hollywood glamor and beauty everybody wanted—though she went to great pains to separate herself from commercial standards of beauty. It was the welding of these concerns that raised diet-mania to yet a higher pitch of intensity in the eighties, when even the term *diet* came to be castigated. The low-calorie, low-sodium, low-fat, cholesterol- and sugar-free, fiber-rich, natural-foods regimen was the way we were to eat throughout our lives, the way we could "eat to win."

10

Her Body Must Be Thin, Firm, and Beautiful

Behind the growing dominance of the exercise regime and health (and health-food) consciousness were new standards of beauty, far more exacting and more body aware than ever before. A woman now had to be thin *and* boast a firm body with all adipose tissue taut and shaped. Paradoxically, in this decade of change—of permissiveness and personal liberation, of reverence for the natural, of resistance to superficiality and conformism, and especially, of Women's Liberation, when all traditional notions about women were challenged—a compelling standard of female beauty emerged, one that locked women into a war with their own bodies. The health and exercise ethic sanctified and intensified their preoccupation with fat, food, and fitness—and with physical perfection.

Though Twiggy had disappeared from the fashion scene, her successors—Lauren Hutton, Roseanne Vela, Cheryl Tiegs, Farrah Fawcett and, at the end of the decade, Brooke Shields—still represented impossible standards. Their bodies, honed and taut, were even more compelling models for the female population. Many a woman knew that even if she dieted to disaster, she couldn't meet Twiggy's little-girl, little-boned look. But she did think she might be able to tame her flesh until it became as lean and taut as that of Cheryl Tiegs. She thought so also because, in the sobering environment of the seventies, fashion magazines like *Vogue* abandoned the carnivalesque fantasy of the sixties and presented models in realistic settings and clothes, which made them seem far more imitable than their predecessors. The new look didn't end the war on fat but rather escalated it.

The ideal shapes of models in the seventies were taller and leaner than ever before—5'7" or 5'8", sometimes even as tall as 5'10"—with weights often as low as 105 pounds. And yet again, fashionable standards were in collusion with medical ones. With the medical community urging a low fat-to-lean ratio, with fat both on and in the body a sin against health, no authorities, medical or otherwise, protested or set limits on the heightened urge for thinness.

A vivid example of how extreme fashion standards had become is documented in Aimee Liu's autobiographical book, *Solitaire,* in which she described her sufferings from anorexia nervosa. She noted that she began a modeling career, and continued to get modeling jobs, during her illness. A true anorexic was not regarded as too thin to be a paragon of beauty. While waiting for one photographic session to begin, she became faint from hunger and felt like she might "pass out." Another model, laboring under the same deprivation, passed out first. While agencies denied that their models dieted and fainted frequently—insisting they were naturally thin—other sources suggested this was not a rarity at all. But even if the models were "naturally" thin, their thinness was extreme. The woman modeling a "tiny bikini" in a 1975 *Vogue* was to resemble Botticelli's *Venus Rising from the Sea,* but she more nearly resembled a skeleton rising from the sea. The models showing bathing suits in the 1977 fashion shows were all bones. They looked more like concentration camp victims than like normal, healthy women.[1]

Other women in the public eye, who formerly had subscribed to somewhat different beauty standards than those for models, were also striving to get slimmer. L. M. Vincent, a physician who specialized in the health care of dancers, harrowingly chronicled the emaciation they sought in *Competing with the Sylph,* published in 1979. Though he did not question the aesthetic value of slenderness for classical ballet, he argued that the standard of thinness had become dangerously low. He found professional dance students and dancers depriving themselves of almost all nourishment or following bizarre, inadequate diets even though they danced strenuously six to eight hours a day, and he found disturbed body-image perception, vomiting to control weight, and frank cases of anorexia nervosa. He described twenty young women associated with the New York City Ballet, where George Balanchine's emphasis on line had produced extremes of elongation, whose frighteningly low weights had brought on amenorrhea. A 5'4.5" sixteen-year-old weighed 97 pounds; a 5'5" eighteen-year-old weighed 95 pounds; a 5'6" teenager weighed 90 pounds; a 5'6.5" twenty-year-old weighed 95. Between 1978 and 1980 other researchers reported similar findings among professional dance students, with close to 38 percent of some samples exhibiting attitudes and behaviors akin to those found in anorexia nervosa.[2]

When Vincent asked a physician why he had given a diet to an already sylphlike dancer, the physician shrugged and responded that the ballet subculture demanded these low weights. When Vincent told a ballet company official that many of his dancers were not menstruating, he, too, shrugged and said, "They're not menstruating. So what?" These young women had no authorities putting a brake on their compulsion for thinning. And they were no longer an idiosyncratic enclave, subject to aesthetic norms that did not apply to ordinary women. As fitness—and leg warmers—surged into fashion, ballerinas were seen as the aristocrats of body strength and bodily beauty, the ideal all women strove to emulate.

Those other beacons for the normal eye, beauty queens and *Playboy* center-folds, also slimmed dramatically. The radicalism associated with skinniness dissipated, and the Miss Americas joined the trend. Already, in 1970, the average contestant's weight had dropped to 117—the lowest it had been since 1937 and 1938, but she had also gained an inch in height. By 1979 the average contestant dropped 2 more pounds, down to 115, but she had inched up yet again, to a shade under 5'7". This downward trend became even more marked in the eighties.[3]

Playboy, the bastion of female voluptuousness, had up to this time sustained the view that erotic and haute couture figures were different, and it had celebrated fuller-bodied, amply breasted girls. But in the seventies the *Playboy* centerfold's shape began to resemble the new ideal. The typical Playmate's figure, once an hourglass, was elongating into the boyish, athletic form. Her hips became slimmer, her waist thicker, even her famous bust got smaller. Her legs were longer and leaner, coltish, not kittenish. The Playmates' average weights dropped from 11 percent below the national average in 1970 to 17 percent below it in 1978. Only the sexy girls in the cartoon illustrations still had the ample curves preferred in earlier decades. The voluptuously endowed woman had long been banished from fashion; now she was also being banished from erotica. She remained as a faintly comic figure; serious romantic passion was identified only with a lean, taut silhouette.[4]

In making this transition, *Playboy* was responding to new social currents and tastes. But as it responded, it helped mold tastes as well. Men who reached puberty in the fifties and early sixties may still have had sexual fantasies about soft, voluptuous women, but those whose sexual awakening was later had been exposed to a different erotic ideal. To them, leanness was sexy; the small-breasted woman began to appeal as much as if not more than the full-breasted one. Ironically, it is possible that this development had a more powerful impact on women than men. Men may have sought lovers who approximated this ideal, but women literally wanted to embody it, to have the kind of figure no man could resist. They, far more than men, sought this standard in real life.

This trend toward a singular body ideal was caused, in part, by the break-down of barriers between "high" culture and popular culture. International café society, the young, the restless, the Studio 54 crowd, and media celebrities became elite Society, producing a new intermingling between beauty subcul-tures. Verushka, a *Vogue* supermodel, appeared in *Playboy* in 1974—not, to be sure, as a Playmate, but as a seductive woman of multiple moods. Nonethe-less, she posed provocatively in all her long, scrawny, flat-chested nakedness. Actress Farrah Fawcett went from TV's "Charlie's Angels" to a poster that became wildly popular and revived the pinup tradition, to *Vogue,* which in April, 1977, gushed over "Far-ra-out Farrah" and described her as the "Sex

Goddess of the 70's." Diane Keaton, with her Annie Hall look, bridged the film world and the fashion world, and Brooke Shields went from the provocative movie, *Pretty Baby,* in 1978 to a "naughty" advertisement for Calvin Klein jeans, to the covers of *Vogue.* This fluidity produced an unprecedented standardization and rigidification in American images of female beauty.[5]

From the professional beauties, the lean, long, taut body standard made its way into the lives of ordinary women. Excursions to fashionable boutiques could be exercises in despair. Writer Kennedy Fraser remarked in *The New Yorker* that a visit to the chic New York department store Bendel's—where "skeletal salesgirls" and "ethereal customers" seemed to weigh no more than 90 pounds and where anything above a size 4 was an "unmentionable"—could send a shopper "empty-handed onto Fifty-seventh Street, feeling dazed and overweight." And women were assailed by the media images and the women's magazines, which all pushed the look and insistently and incessantly gave advice about how to get it. The magazines carried yet more diet articles, and exercise advice began to dominate their pages, eventually moving to magazine covers as a come-on for buyers. By the end of the seventies the leading women's magazines carried a minimum of two or more exercise articles per month. Exercise books designed especially for women surged in popularity, such as Kenneth Cooper's 1972 *Aerobics for Women.* The goal was lean, taut fitness and, always, the promise was the same. As *Vogue* put it in May, 1974: "Make your bid for fitess now to have the happiest summer of your life."[6]

The seventies produced a kaleidoscope of styles that varied at a dizzying rate: Hems rose and fell and rose again until even *Vogue* told women they could choose any length they wanted. The "new classicism" and the soft disheveled styles of the early seventies gave way to the disco-minded and exercise-chic fashions of the late seventies, yet throughout this period styles also careened from peasant to exotic to space age to primly corporate to New Wave, and to the most dominant style of all, blue jeans. But always, despite these shifts, the focus on the body continued and even mounted. When minis were replaced by longer dresses and skirts, demands on the female body did not relax. When it introduced the midi, *Mademoiselle* explained that the longer hems should not be interpreted as a relaxation of the thin imperative. "Some creampuffs . . . hypothesized a midi would cover a multitude of sins— slump, dump, or just plain flab—bared by a mini. We caught them before they had put in an order for their bonbons and explained what makes a midi work . . . beneath it, a body in fabulous condition. If you don't have it, your svelte 1970 midi is going to look like a frumpy 1935 housedress . . . . So, creampuffs, there's no escape. Whip yourself into super shape and stay that way." In any case, minis remained popular and, in 1971, hot pants hit the fashion scene. So did bared midriffs, which now could be worn in the city as well as at the beach resort.[7]

As the decade wore on, fashion traveled the gamut from the revealing to the classic, but the imperative to think of the body first remained. *Mademoiselle* was prophetic when it warned that the midi would not give a reprieve to the flawed body: The apparent concealment afforded by longer dresses and layering was deceptive, for these clothes were increasingly made of loose, soft, clingy fabrics such as cotton jersey and Indian cottons, which satisfied the urge for comfort and fell in aesthetic folds. But such dresses took their shape, not from the stiffness of their material or from their cut, but from the body on which they hung. This unconstructed style—a boon for manufacturers since it lent itself so well to mass-production techniques—put added demands on women's figures.

By 1977 designers from Ungaro, Givenchy, and Dior to those designing for the mass market, were using light, semiopaque, or sheer fabrics that revealed the contours beneath them and that were hung loosely over the body in what some called the "freed body fashion." The same year, Studio 54 opened, *Saturday Night Fever* reached its peak of popularity, and disco-mania swept the country in full force, bringing the slinky, stretchy, electrifyingly colored disco-dress that was, above all, exhibitionistic and body-conscious. As Carrie Donovan wrote in the *New York Times Magazine* in November of that year, all the new styles were "designed to celebrate the body" and to expose it. The body literally had become the core of fashion.[8]

Once the body became the focus of fashion, it was subject to the same scrutiny and strictures as clothing styles. Never before had women's magazines discussed so thoroughly every detail of female anatomy or set such specific standards for it. In 1970 *Vogue* detailed these specifics in a feature about "the new young body . . . " In the accompanying picture, a nubile young girl sits astride a barebacked horse in the forest. She wears nothing but tight jeans, and her long, straight blonde hair flows over her naked shoulders and breasts.[9]

The message was clear. The physically ideal woman was young, her slim-hipped body just barely swelling into adolescence. She was lithe and lean, without a trace of cellulite, flab, or jiggly adipose tissue. She was innocent but erotic in a "wholesome" way. Above all, she was natural. She had the freshness of the forest around her, and her body was not unlike that of the magnificent horse she rode—sleek, athletic, and infinitely well-bred. It seemed as if no artificial aids or adornments produced her. This was natural beauty, and there was only one way to get it. The following year *Vogue* heralded the "1971 Figure" and subtitled the article, "Exercise: Everybody Wants It." Without it, how could anyone look like that model? This pubescent body ideal proved to be an enduring trend and culminated at the end of the decade with Brooke Shields and other "baby models."[10]

Throughout the decade, the fashion magazines earnestly spelled out how we could make this body and alerted us to flaws we might never have noticed before. "The New Young Bosom," *Vogue* proclaimed in 1970, and in subsequent years, articles discussed how exercise and diet helped produce such a firm, upright, delicately swelling bosom—and, if these failed, the advantages and disadvantages of plastic surgery on the breasts. And, by the mid-seventies, we learned from the French of another beauty blight, cellulite. In 1973 *Vogue* advertised *The Cellulite Book* and explained that there was "a general lack of awareness concerning cellulite in this country." Within a year, *Mademoiselle* was explaining that "cellulite is thin woman's fat," composed of unsightly lumps, bumps and bulges, and offered the "Cellulite Shape-up Plan." Another bodily "flaw," presumed to be abnormal and unnatural, had been called to our attention. It certainly was no longer enough to be slender. We had to hone every inch of our once-private flesh to silky-smooth perfection.[11]

These new standards helped to redefine modesty. It was now perfectly acceptable to display publicly a near-naked body, but only if it met the new standards. As *Vogue* warned, the body-baring styles required that new care be taken of the body, for it would now be exposed to elements and to public scrutiny that in the past had been "faced only by the face." Feelings of shame and modesty no longer had to do with exposure but rather with the quality of what was being exposed. To avoid such shame, women had to diet and exercise.

Pressure to diet and exercise mounted also because undergarments, not just outergarments, had ceased to perform their venerable role as aids, even molders, of the stylish figure. Throughout the seventies sales of brassieres, and especially of girdles, plummeted, cast off by a (theoretically) liberated generation of women as unhealthy and sexist symbols of constraint. Women had lost one of the handmaidens of public beauty: the secret foundation wear that made the dressed body approximate the fashionable form. Dupont marketing researchers noted that this trend had grown steadily from 1970 on, particularly among the "young, the working woman and the higher-income-bracket women who were the mainstay of the apparel industry"—the most fashion-conscious groups. The body-revealing styles, the soft fabrics, and the abandonment of body-shaping underwear caused a revolutionary turnabout in fashion ideology. Women were now told that they had to be beautiful if they wanted their clothes to look good, and the responsibility was entirely theirs. They had to make the clothes work; the clothes no longer worked for them.[12]

In fact, of course, with the "freed body" styles and the abandonment of girdles, women had simply exchanged an external constraint for a more powerful, internal one: diet and exercise. The Dupont researchers found that women felt they no longer needed girdles because they "kept their weights down with diet and exercise." Pressure on women mounted as responsibility for achieving this figure dropped squarely in their laps. They couldn't even rely much anymore on diet pills or on the diet doctors who prescribed them. In 1972 the FDA cracked down on the manufacture and dispensing of these pills which, in any case, had accumulated a sinister reputation as word about their addictive, unhealthy qualities spread and as they came to be associated with the "speed freaks" of the drug subculture. Women believed their own efforts, not nature or beauty aids, would bring them the ideal body.

Fashion magazines never again told women they could go out and buy beauty. They still promised that everyone could have it, but now it was a question of self-discipline, not of money. In 1972 *Vogue* explained that "exercise is making the most of yourself. A graceful body with good weight distribution depends as much on good muscle tone as on diet. There's nothing mystical about it." In March, 1974, *Mademoiselle* assured readers that cellulite was caused by "poor eating habits, lack of exercise, insufficient water intake, poor breathing and circulation, stress and fatigue." By 1979 *Vogue* summed up the new pathway to beauty: "Living—What It Takes Now: The New Discipline." Beauty had become a matter of character.[13]

As always, these developments in the world of fashion were stimulated by larger cultural changes which, in turn, also intensified women's lust for physical perfection. The radical generation's rejection of tradition and its quest for individualism and personal expressiveness, and women's liberation all undermined fashion traditions and their presumptions. As we saw, this process began in the late sixties, but in the seventies the discombobulation became widespread and deeply entrenched. Women in the seventies rejected classical high fashion and all the rules associated with it. They rejected clothing that smacked of elitism and privilege. They opted instead for blue jeans, once the uniform of the manual laborer, and Paris designers were putting out the equivalent of T-shirt dresses. Clothing manufacturers were distraught to find that women weren't even spending much money on clothing anymore.

This rejection of conventional fashion was spurred by more than the democratic impulses of the decade. The radical generation rebelled against the commercialization of American culture and against the commercialization of beauty in particular. Their quest for inner meaning and higher consciousness, for what was real and natural, made them violently hostile to the artifice of traditional fashion and to its concentration on superficial appearance. It was vanity, an "ego trip" that had little to do with the inner self. The Women's Liberation movement expanded this attack with its own thoroughgoing repudiation of women's pursuit of fashionable beauty, which was perceived to be the result of sexist oppression. These critiques spawned a new fashion demand: Clothing was either to demonstrate one's lack of interest in fashion or it was to be boldly individualistic, a creative expression of an inner self freed from the dictates of fashion moguls. An antifashion fashion had emerged.

With this assault, and with the general chaos in social mores, the old dress code disintegrated. With the yen for natural, comfortable styles, city wear and sportswear intermingled, and dress once appropriate for the beach was worn in the city. Sexual differentiation gave way to new unisex styles. Women wore jeans and corporate suits, and they also fought ferociously for the right to wear pants and pantsuits in formal settings. Evening wear became relaxed and casual. Hats, gloves, matching purses and shoes, and other ladylike, matching accessories disappeared. Age distinctions in dress relaxed and then virtually disappeared. In essence, the old formality of dress was replaced by a new informality.

Along with this informality came one of the most radical changes of all: a redefinition of what constituted modesty, of private as opposed to public exposure. The rise of the psychotherapeutic mentality and the craving for openness and honesty led to a new informality in manners and to a new frankness in public conversation about what once had been deemed personal matters. Nothing was to be hidden, secret, or private. The same frankness applied to the body. Body exposure was no longer regarded as shameful or immoral but rather as a signal that one was liberated, "out front," and in tune with the new values. This attitude undermined yet another linchpin in the traditional dress code and helped launch the body-baring styles.

Throughout the seventies fashion seemed to be in search of a new language and standards, new dress codes, and new definitions of beauty that meshed with the new values. It, too, began to express scorn for slaves to fashion. By the end of the seventies *Women's Wear Daily,* whose existence depended on the notion of fashionable dress, coined the term *fashion victims* to describe women who looked *too* fashionable. Another result was that fashion leaders acknowledged that the "woman of today" had "more than fashion on her mind," as *Vogue* put it in 1972, and the magazines began to resemble self-help manuals, loaded with articles about how to handle bosses and subordinates, how to get to the top, how to manage money, and even how to repair cars. Another, more profound, result was that fashion increasingly came to advertise its wares by flattering the consumer: celebrating her independence, assuring her the products would promote her self-expression, and that she used them, not to impress or please others, but to please herself: "Because you'd rather be yourself than anyone else," intoned Charles of the Ritz cosmetic ads; "This I Do for Me," Miss Clairol ads read.[14]

In the prevailing atmosphere, fashion leaders could not promote even a beautiful figure just for beauty's sake. They groped for a new definition of beauty and found one: Beauty came to be equated with physical health, the kind celebrated by the health ethic—lean and energetic. In 1971 *Vogue* began to run a regular column entitled "Health and Beauty." By 1975 it had moved even further away from the old definitions of fashionable beauty. With obvious contempt, it claimed, "We are well past the days when beauty was an ideal way of passing the time . . . . " Now, attention to looks wasn't just "icing on the cake." It was "one of the responsibilities of everyday life." Why? Because it was inseparable from health. Beauty was to be achieved not through work on the outside of the body but by working from the inside out. *Vogue* advised five beauty basics that sounded like a litany of the health ethic: proper nutrition, exercise to improve circulation, proper sleep and proper breathing—and of course, a lean body weight.[15]

By 1978 *Vogue* was calling on the AMA to justify its claim that preoccupation with beauty was the same as preoccupation with health. "Fashion is not an ego trip," the magazine declared. "It's healthy to want to be as attractive as we can—the better we look, the better we feel and vice-versa. Call it vanity if you like. We'd call it wholesome—and so would the AMA." The following month, the magazine elaborated on the new American woman. Suddenly, she had the "look women all over the world want to emulate." That look was one of inner qualities such as "self-knowledge," and above all, "self-confidence." How did it show? Through her "waving, burnished and healthy hair, and through her body, which gave all her clothes "a superb plus." "Fashion," this premiere clothes magazine acknowledged, "is only as good as you look and feel." Pursuit of fashionable beauty, then, was neither superficial nor intended to impress others.[16]

The wildly bouncing bodies and desperately exuberant smiles of the seventies' models were a far cry from what fashion magazines had idealized in the past. These models didn't have the refinement, or cool hauteur of their predecessors. They certainly lacked glamor as it had traditionally been defined. They were without mystery and, therefore, the body, too, was exposed without mystery. In fact, the very idea of "natural" beauty was contradictory to fashion. Historically, fashion has always been a plastic art, based on artifice and on the use of beauty aids to achieve a certain look. But in the seventies this changed—at least in principle, for "natural" cosmetics became the rage.

The growing liberalization of American society also contributed to the new body emphasis. Other racial groups began to infiltrate the fashion world and its magazines. In the seventies black and Asian models appeared on the runway, in advertisements and catalogs, and even on the covers of fashion magazines. Although windblown, girl-next-door blondes still dominated, they no longer represented a single standard of beauty. In this heterogeneous environment, only one standard could be applied to all: the ideal body. It seemed the penultimate beauty value for a democratic society, for it was theoretically accessible to anyone.

At the core of this growing equation between beauty, health, and energy was a new, feminist conception of women. In a 1975 issue of *Vogue* Susan Sontag argued that, traditionally, woman's beauty had been based on her "power to attract," not on her "power to do." Beauty was passive, not active. In an age of feminism, this was unacceptable. Passivity was rejected. *Lady, Mademoiselle* informed its readers, had become a four-letter word. The new, liberated woman had to be active, self-confident, assertive. She had to be strong. When fashion searched for a visual rendition of this new beauty, it landed on the most natural and most energetic thing we possessed—our own bodies. It was one acceptable measure of beauty because, presumably, how they looked reflected how we felt, and the beauty we thus achieved was not for show, nor to attract a man, but for ourselves.[17]

This was one reason feminists did not condemn the slender, fit ideal even while they rebelled against the Miss America Pageants and the sexist commercialism that produced the tyranny of fashion and turned women into sex objects. In addition, they were seduced by the ideal's naturalism and by its

association with healthiness, which gave its frankly cosmetic purposes a dignified and righteous veneer.

The new, somewhat androgynous beauty standard also meshed with other
feminist goals and values. Liberated women, seeking acceptance as equals
among men, eschewed the full-bodied voluptuousness traditionally assoicated
with a sex-pot or an Earth Mother. They did not want to project conventional
femininity, particularly when they entered male occupations. They wanted to
de-emphasize female sexual characteristics in order to project serious-minded-
ness, not flirtatiousness; businesslike competence, not seductiveness.

The look appealed also because it was so decidedly unmaternal. Marriage,
let alone motherhood, was not a high priority for the liberated women who
wanted to prove themselves in traditionally male occupations. Between the
mid-sixties and 1980, the age of first marriage for females rose, and the birthrate plummeted to a historic low of 1.7 children per married females as women
postponed the encumbrances of husbands and children so they could make
their mark in the world. The liberated woman had little respect for the matron
whose life revolved around family and whose head was filled with domestic
concerns, the woman who had never managed to get out there and achieve.
She did not want to be a nurturer, a passive dependent. She did not want the
matronly body associated with such traditional roles. The slender body seemed
to symbolize her ideal of independence and self-sufficiency. Just as she did not
need a man or the security of a stable male relationship, just as she did not
need pregnancy and children to be fulfilled, so she did not need food. Her lean
form was proof of her self-reliance.

The slender, taut body also meshed with deeper feminist convictions. In
their proclamations for equality between the sexes, feminists insisted that
biology was not destiny, that there were no inborn differences between males
and females, other than reproductive functions. They argued that traditionally
accepted differences had been caused by cultural conditioning, which itself had
been shaped by centuries of sexist oppression. Men and women, beneath this
conditioning, were the same. The new ideal body was virtually androgynous,
a visual rendition of the faith—or hope—that there were no differences between the sexes. Women, they charged, did not have to be weak and passive,
unable to do physically demanding jobs usually reserved for males, and vulnerable to physical aggression, especially rape. Feminists did not regard exercise
as a cosmetic device. It served a more important purpose: empowering women.

The slender ideal's explicit presumption that people could mold their own
shapes also echoed feminist ideals. One of their earliest and most vehement
demands had been for women's right to control their own bodies. Feminists
challenged husbands', lovers', doctors', fashion's, and society's presumption of
such rights. They wanted to be independent, masters of their physical experiences and physical destinies. These attitudes meshed perfectly with the cultural
demand to be thin and fit. Women did not have to be fat. They could mold
their bodies as well as their destinies.

Feminism also contributed to the thin/diet obsession by denigrating women's traditional associations with food and nurturing. In the feminist perspective, concern with food and eating was trivial, the food for minds trapped in the mental universe of home. Paradoxically, in trying to liberate women and bring them the respect and opportunities they deserved, feminists radically devalued women's traditional roles. The homemaker was trapped in a menial service job for which she didn't even get paid. Many feminists made these points not to undermine women's contributions in the home but rather to underline that they should have the right to other, more high-minded challenges as well. This fine distinction wasn't grasped by many and, in any case, it didn't alter the gist of the attack. Traditional woman's work was virtually meaningless, and woman's traditional association with food was de-meaning. Women now had a triple indemnity to contend with when they got fat. They were doing something very unhealthy, they were destroying their chances of being beautiful, and they were exposing the fact that they hadn't gotten their minds out of the kitchen.[18]

The health-food and gourmet trends were not at odds with this develop-ment. In the former case, the concern was health, not pleasure or indulgence of the palate. And gourmet cooking was not the same as what used to be thought of as home cooking. Cultural historian Stephen Mennell trenchantly observed that there is a world of difference between the chef of haute cuisine and the domestic cook. From its inception, haute cuisine was practiced by men rather than women precisely because it could be elevated to the status of an art only if it were not associated with humble domesticity—that is, with women—and only if it were set apart from the monotonous routines of every-day life. The liberated female and the rising number of male home gourmets of the seventies generally met these criteria. They usually did not prepare such meals for the family's daily fare but rather for special occasions and weekends when they had time and when dining could be an event out of the humdrum of ordinary life. In addition, the new-style dining involved more art than appetite. Nouvelle cusine, as we have seen, was meant to satisfy the eye without affecting the figure. As food became more cosmetic, it became less nutritive and more decorative, and the home gourmets more artists than traditional cooks. They were emphatically different from the frumpy, overweight housewives who overfed their families.[19]

Sexual liberation, which the radical generation brought into the mainstream, played a far more vital role than feminism in escalating women's quest for a slender, perfect body. The sixties and seventies were truly a golden age for sex. With the pill and the IUD, pregnancy could be avoided easily without any interruption of a passionate moment. Abortion was legalized, which meant that if contraception didn't work, a woman still had the option to terminate, safely, an unwanted pregnancy. All known venereal diseases could be treated simply and effectively. In these days before herpes and AIDS, Americans had found in sex what they sought in food: a pleasurable activity without any permanent consequences.

These technical advances were less important than other new perceptions of sex. Women had declared they had erotic appetites as early as the 1920s, but up through the fifties and sixties, they were circumscribed by social, moral, and religious rules that discouraged premarital and extramarital sex. The youth culture and feminists attacked these rules, particularly the "double standard," which gave less sexual liberty to females than to males. In the sixties and seventies women demanded the right to the same freedom, and declared that, contrary to the popular ideology that underlay the double standard, women were no more emotional about sex than men. This attitude had been spawned by the radical generation's romanticization of everything natural. They overturned age-old convictions by arguing that sex was innocent and wholesome, that no rules should govern this pleasuring of the body: Any sexual behavior or experimentation was acceptable—even encouraged—as long as the people involved did not hurt or coerce one another. Swinging singles and swinging couples, homosexuals and lesbians, liberated women and erotically gyrating disco dancers all proclaimed their right to sexual freedom and their sexual availability. This development was partially responsible for the amalgamation of the erotic and haute couture ideals: All women, whatever their backgrounds, now wanted to signal their sexuality explicitly. Some called it hedonism; others called it liberation. Regardless of what it was called, this new preoccupation with sex had a powerful impact on women's attitudes toward their bodies.

Sexual permissiveness led to the relaxation of censorship laws in 1969. Suddenly, everywhere in the media, in the arts, and even in academic circles, the sexual act was portrayed, described, or investigated in explicit and thorough detail. So was the ideal body. The average woman, eyeing the television or film screen, the magazine photo or the billboard, or reading the latest literature, became acutely aware of how she was supposed to look when undressed. She now had explicit images with which to compare herself. And, with the new bent on realism in these images, the average woman believed these models represented a norm she could resemble.

The nature of female sexuality became an overriding interest. A rising spate of articles and advice books encouraged women to explore their own sexuality, to scrutinize their bodies without shame, to learn to love and talk about them, to masturbate—both to give themselves this pleasure once granted only to men and to find what gave them the greatest orgasmic experience so they could instruct their lovers—and to admit to and act out their sexual fantasies. Women were being encouraged to focus on their bodies, to expect transports of joy from them, to develop and perfect them. These formerly intimate, private matters had suddenly become public and, as a result, so had the female body.

Sexual liberation contributed to women's growing obsessions about their bodies in other, subtler ways as well. Americans had begun to regard sex as life's ultimate experience. They began to pursue sexual fulfillment with the zeal of religious converts and to expect from it the ecstasy and fulfillment once associated with religion. And they no longer linked it to love, marriage, or procreation. They didn't even demand a pretense of romance or sentiment from their lovers, and in this decade, they certainly didn't demand commitments. The liberated woman was supposed to be independent, needing stable relationships with men no more than she needed food. Men and women pursued sexual pleasure as an end in and of itself.

Sex became curiously impersonal, almost masturbatory. Its technical aspects became more important than its emotional aspects, and books like Masters and Johnson's *Human Sexual Response* and the proliferating sexual therapy programs invariably emphasized the mechanics, not the emotions, necessary to give and get good sex. Lovers were judged on the basis of their technical prowess. Sex was becoming a matter of performance, subject to the standards ordinarily associated with competitive sports. Men and women were seeking the sexual ecstasies that "high performance" brought.

Having an ideal body became crucial. It was the tool with which a woman gave and received the joy of sex. Where once voluptuousness was the implicit guarantee of this capacity, in an explicit world, the voluptuous body was a failed body, incapable of high sexual performance. After twenty years of the antifat campaign, women didn't even question this assumption. A fat body submerged sexual desire, buried sensuality beneath layers of numbing tissue, slowed responses, and made the gymnastics sex now demanded difficult. Fat people ate away their sexual cravings. Even more, every woman knew fat women were loathsome. No one desired them. A fat woman couldn't choose her sexual partners. She had to wait to be chosen, and then chances were that he was someone no one else wanted, a leftover. A nice body was imperative for a proper affair. Already in 1970 *Vogue* ran an article on the "Cost of an Affair." One of the biggest expenses—$800 worth—was for the "21 Days of Shaping Up With Miss Craig" in New York. After all, like for any other competition a woman had to get her tools in top form.[20]

The new sexual mores made women frantic about every flaw in their anatomies also because promiscuous social encounters and one-night stands were increasingly common. In the sixties, with the "love generation," sex had still been associated with love—even if it hadn't been the conventional love that led to marriage—but in the seventies such sentiments became passé. From popular novels like Erica Jong's *Fear of Flying* to magazines like *Cosmopolitan*, and even more conventional ones like *Mademoiselle*, such encounters were glowingly described. In the throbbing atmosphere of the discos, strangers were to connect as lovers through "body language" and suggestive dancing instead of through the far more banal—and in the noisy setting, impossible—convention of conversation. This promiscuity, akin to anonymous sex, meant that nakedness, once revealed only to an established lover or husband, had suddenly become rather public, as strangers became bedfellows. Women were infected with insecurity, fearing their transient lovers would judge their flesh with the cold eye of an objective observer instead of with the forgiving, accepting eye of a sweetheart. They feared they would be compared with the flawless forms pervading the media and believed males expected such a form—certainly they expected it of themselves.

A perfect body could serve as armor against any possibility of criticism, rejection, or shame. Modesty indeed had become the embarrassment connected with a flawed body. Even the staunchest feminist, able to stand up for herself against any sexist attack, could wither at the slightest hint that she was fat or flabby. Her shame that she hadn't dieted or exercised enough was her Achilles heel. Somehow the idea had emerged that men had the right to expect, and to search for, lovers with ideal figures. Even women in theoretically secure and stable relationships succumbed to such panic and insecurity. After all, the obligations of the superwoman included successful, vital marriages sealed by sexual attraction.

If sixties' "free love" had invaded mainstream culture and matured into a kind of sexual Olympics, this was not the only legacy of the period that endured and further contributed to American women's obsessions with their weights. Although in the seventies many of the counterculture had passed the dread age of thirty, they still revered youth. As we have seen, everyone wanted to look, feel, and prove they were still youthful. The rising numbers of books that appeared about the "crisis of middle age," from Eda LeShan's *The Wonderful Crisis of Middle Age* to Fred McMorrow's *Midolescence: The Dangerous Years,* to Gail Sheehy's *Passages,* all urged the middle-aged to forget the "shoulds" that bogged them down and to embark on a "voyage of personal discovery and self-actualization," to avoid stagnation through continual personal growth. Little value was placed on wisdom or knowledge of the past or on the "pillars of society" who upheld cultural traditions. Many have argued that the seventies and eighties brought the demise of childhood. On the contrary, they brought the demise of middle age as a valuable and distinct life stage. The "generation gap" had been closed by encouraging everyone to behave as though their young adulthood had just begun.

One reflection of this attitude was that clothing ceased to vary for different age groups. The styles that evolved were cruel to any but a young and lean figure, but they were meant to be worn by everyone. If a woman wanted to dress stylishly, she had no choice but to exercise and diet herself into shape. Fashion magazines once had insisted that true beauty never dies. Now they also insisted that a beautiful body could last forever—with diet and exercise. Medical experts, too, insisted that the mature woman should keep her svelte shape, that there was no reason for her to add fat with the years, and that it was even unhealthy if she did so. *Vogue* had warned women that at thirty a decision had to be made about whether "to let your body go" or "to fight it all the way." Clearly, the fight was better than abdication. There was no need to ask why.[21]

In the seventies middle-aged women did have special reasons to panic about creeping middle age and creeping overweight. Sexual liberation, the new permissiveness, and feminism had put them in a vulnerable position. With the insistent identification of youth and sexiness thrown at them by the media, they knew they could never compete in the romance game. Mrs. Exeter's column in *Vogue,* addressed to the society matron, had disappeared from its pages in the sixties, foreshadowing the demise of a mature female ideal. In the same period, these women had seen all their own rules about love, sex, marriage, femininity, and childrearing overturned. They could hardly act as wise guides for their offspring or for the younger generation as a whole—the "generation gap" was too wide. And feminists, many of them their own daughters, were in a fury of rebellion against them and their values, charging that they had been victims of sexist oppression, that their lives had been wasted as menial servants for their families. The homemaker was devalued, and the middle-aged women who had been—either happily or unhappily—housewives, now found that few regarded their life's work as worthwhile.

Worst of all, many could no longer feel secure that their mates would defend them, nor could they feel secure about their marriages. The new permissiveness had eroded even this citadel of society. With the divorce rate doubling, with books encouraging divorce as one solution for midlife stagnation, and with "open marriage" widely propagated, even women who had achieved marriage could not feel secure. In this environment, middle-aged and even younger wives felt doubly pressed to retain youthfulness and the youthful, sexy shape that signified it. It was one way to shake the nagging fear that their men would search for a liberated woman with longer, slimmer legs, fuller breasts, and firmer thighs and buttocks. Even more important, the many women who suddenly faced divorce now found themselves back in the courting game long after their youth had ended. They had to retain the coquetry and sexual allure once appropriate only for courting girls—though only thirty years before, *Vogue* had ridiculed women who tried to preserve girlish beauty. For women of all ages, sexual competition had become intense, but it was especially so for the married woman and the divorcée, who had to vie with the lithe bodies of the young.

The thinness lust now infected more age groups and, because of larger social changes, more social groups. The democratization of physical ideals through the influx of black and Asian fashion models suddenly extended the culture of beauty—and its body demands—to women who had considered themselves hopelessly outside its boundaries and who had tended to subscribe to different standards. Though weight loss had been a consistent theme in magazines for blacks since the fifties, in the seventies there was a crescendo of features about black personalities who had shed their excess poundage. Even Puerto Rican matrons had begun to watch their weights, though in the past American Puerto Ricans would accuse "a married woman too concerned with her weight and shape . . . of selfishness and coquetry." A Gallup Poll found 41 percent of nonwhites considered themselves overweight.[22]

A similar trend occurred among white ethnic minorities, particularly southern and eastern European women. In the sixties and seventies liberalization and increasing affluence allowed more and more of these women to attend college and begin their climb up the social ladder. Many of them had nose jobs and straightened their hair to meet the prevailing standard of American beauty. Most of all, they tried to shed their excess poundage. Sociologist Marcia Millman observed that for many families, especially Jewish and Italian Americans, slimness was "associated with upward mobility, and fatness with one's ethnic orgins." She also observed that children from these backgrounds tended to populate the diet summer camps. Sadly, many of these youngsters were not even significantly overweight. They were sent by parents who considered themselves fat and who feared if they didn't take prompt action, their children would also be fat.[23]

These groups frantically pursued slimness not just to be beautiful but also because slenderness indeed had become the crucial insignia of social status and of Americanization. The identification between richness and body weight was embedded in the national psyche. A well-bred person had to be slender, for a fat body was an uncivilized body. And, as long as the faith prevailed that people could control their body size, slenderness seemed a pre-eminently democratic value, consonant with America's cherished self-help ideology.

In fact, the new body emphasis seemed as much a reaction against the increasing democratization of fashion as an expression of it. Ironically, as high fashion—or imitations of it—became more affordable, it lost its status. The elite could no longer explicitly signal their status through their clothing. This was one reason fashion designers began to put labels on the outside, rather than the inside, of clothes. Labels were distastefully crude, and the competitive impulse behind fashion instead shifted to a more worthy object: the body. The jacuzzied, exercised, tanned, and ineffably taut form could only belong to the woman who had the leisure and the money to make it look that way.

Even more, the tall, lean form reflected and codified the social hierarchy. In 1973 the National Center for Health Statistics reconfirmed Stunkard's finding that obesity was most prevalent among the poor and racial minorities. Black women between the ages of twenty and forty-four formed the largest subgroup of overweight Americans: 29 percent of them were overweight as opposed to 18 percent of white women in that age bracket. People of northern European ancestry, the Public Health Service observed in a 1965 publication, tended to be taller and slimmer than the stockier and "relatively short-statured southern and eastern Europeans"—probably because of genetics. Other studies showed that these groups also tended to encourage hearty eating. In short, the new standard of status and beauty, slenderness, still militated against certain ethnic types and cultural habits.[24]

As the tyranny of slenderness spread and intensified, prejudice against the overweight also mounted. American society, at least in theory, had outlawed slurs against all minority racial, religious, ethnic, and sexual groups. Yet, it closed ranks against the overweight. And much like the attitude to poverty in the nineteenth century, there was a feeling that fat was a self-selected defeat, morally contemptible and indefensible. By March, 1975, *Newsweek* was writing: "Discrimination Weighty Problem: Bias Against Overweight Job Seekers." Researchers reported in the *Journal of Criminal Justice* that businessmen and scientists would hire an employee who had been in jail or in a mental ward over someone who was fat: Criminality and insanity seemed less intransigent and less deplorable failings than fatness—and possibly less criminal. A 315-pound woman appeared at a Miami court for a misdemeanor charge. Her sentence: three-years' probation—if she lost three pounds a week. If she went off her diet, she had to go to prison. The poundage didn't have to be so excessive to threaten one's job. National Airlines fired stewardess Ingrid Fee because she was "too fat"—she was four pounds "overweight."[25]

There had to be a reaction. There was. The National Association to Aid Fat Americans (NAAFA) was formed in 1969. Its purpose was to help fat people who, it contended, were "the victims of prejudice, stigma, exclusion, exploitation and psychological oppression." The group was radical in that it did not try to help its members lose weight nor suggest that they should lose weight. Instead, it argued that there was nothing wrong with being fat, and it supplied a supportive social context so fat people could shed their guilt and shame and accept themselves. But no matter how much happier members were, they could not convince the outside, thin world of this fact. When Mike Wallace did a "60 Minutes" segment on them in 1978, he concluded that their self-professed happiness was a mask: " . . . [B]ehind their mask of pride or joy or liberation, America's fat people, especially America's fat women, suffer. . . . " In 1972 radical feminists in Los Angeles organized a Fat Underground with a Fat Liberation Manifesto in which they attacked head-on the medical and cultural presumptions about fat: "Biology, not eating habits, is the main cause of fat. Health problems of fat people are not inherently due to fat, but are the result of stress, self-hatred and chronic dieting." The movement foundered, and its collected essays remained unpublished, rejected by both mainstream and leftist publishers who "could not believe that fat could be other than a sickening condition caused by bad eating habits." The essays were not published until 1983 in *Shadows on a Tightrope*. They are a testament to the anguish suffered by fat women and an exposé of the myths and misinformation that surround Americans' fat-phobia.[26]

Toward the end of the decade this resistance became less defensive. In 1978 *Ebony* magazine proclaimed to its black audience: "Big Can Be Beautiful," and it featured big women in glamorous clothing and poses. Interestingly, the magazine was responding to a new development. Some clothing manufacturers had realized that an estimated 28 percent of potential buyers were overweight, yet stylish clothes rarely came in any size larger than an 18. Manufacturers mobilized to tap this market, and *Ebony* was advertising clothes designed for the big woman. "So what if you wear a size 42, have a 36-inch waistline and weigh 230 pounds. The days are past when big was synonymous with ugly," *Ebony* enthusiastically announced.[27]

The following year Carol Shaw and her husband, Ray, launched *Big Beautiful Woman,* a magazine that also advertised attractive clothing for the big woman and attacked the prejudice that only thin could be fashionable. Shaw argued that big women seemed ugly, not because they were "naturally dull-eyed, bloated and pasty-faced," but because they were filled with shame and self-loathing and didn't groom themselves. She urged them to dress up. But Shaw didn't stay meekly on the defensive and just proclaim that big could be beautiful. She also charged that thin was ugly. She went on to stage Big Beautiful Miss America contests and told reporters and her audience: "Hey you fellows under thirty, this is what a woman is supposed to look like—nice round curves. You thought women were supposed to look like young boys?"[28]

Tragically, but not surprisingly, in the same period, cracks started appearing in the injunction to get thin and exercise. Some girls and women were taking it too far. In 1974 pathological eating disorders came to public attention. *Mademoiselle* ran a chilling piece in January, 1974, entitled "Dieting to Disaster," by a woman who had slipped into a deadly battle with anorexia nervosa for no apparent reason. The article, movingly written, was tucked at the front of the magazine as "An Opinion." It stood alone, with no further editorial comment, a stark contrast to the photos of leaping, happy, skinny models, and to the exuberant articles about how women could finally take control of their lives, their bodies, and their health. It was the treacherous, and perhaps inevitable, underside of these developments. The following April, *Seventeen* cautioned: "Thin Isn't Always So Beautiful." In 1975 six articles on anorexia nervosa appeared in popular magazines, and Hilde Bruch, who had referred to anorexia nervosa as a rare disease in 1973, noted in 1978 that it had ceased to be rare. Even "normal" women were suffering from emotional and behavior patterns similar to those of anorexics. The following year Susie Orbach came out with her powerful book, *Fat Is a Feminist Issue,* which underlined the fact that the thin imperative had particularly devastating effects on women.[29]

In March, 1977, Americans were alerted to yet another eating disorder. *Psychology Today* ran an article by Marlene Boskind-Lodahl and Joyce Sirlin, called "Gorging-Purging Syndrome: Bulimarexia." The binge-purge pattern had been known since antiquity, when the Romans institutionalized the "vomitorium," in the thirties the practice had been referred to with wry humor; Jane Fonda recalled that in her college days, she and her friends, after reading about the Romans, had adopted a similar practice. In the fifties and sixties psychiatrists and others had referred to both self-induced vomiting and laxative abuse as purge methods used by overeager dieters and some anorexics. Clearly, the binge-purge pattern was not a modern invention. But the Boskind-Lodahl/Sirlin team had discovered something new: Some of these binge-purgers went to dangerous, life-threatening extremes. For them, binging and purging were not occasional occurrences but rather, something they did several times a day. The facts were chilling. From the outside, these women seemed normal: attractive, of normal weight, well-adjusted socially and sexually, competent, and high-achieving. Yet, they had been possessed by a secret demon. They were dominated by their obsession with food and weight and by the binge-purge syndrome itself, which made them compulsively buy huge quantities of foods, down them quickly, and then purge them amid repeated—and hopeless—resolves never to do it again. Their excessive abuse of laxatives and vomiting, and the often wildly careening weights that resulted, were life-threatening. This indeed was a pathological disorder, one that had not yet even earned a name from the medical profession. What most alarmed researchers was how many women "came out of the closet," confessing they had been suffering from the syndrome for years. Many had been victims of earlier weight consciousness and had suffered from it for decades, though only now did they testify to their plight. Bulimarexia proved to be more common even than anorexia nervosa. It became one of the most common female psychological disorders of the era, and perceptions about even occasional laxative use and self-induced vomiting changed dramatically. They seemed sinister.[30]

While traditional psychoanalysts attributed these disorders to individual, often mythopoetic, psychosexual abnormalities, others began to attack the slender ideal. Feminist psychotherapist Susie Orbach charged that slenderness was one of the cruel and arbitrary demands put on women by the fashion industry and that women were susceptible to its blandishments because of their oppressed condition in society. Orbach thus gave overweight women a new digity. They were not failures but rebels who refused to bow to fashion's and men's dictates, who refused to be "sex objects." Oddly, despite her radicalism, Orbach's point of view was also rather traditional. Like Dr. Theodore Rubin, she suggested fat women were fat because, unconsciously, they didn't want to be thin. They were unconsciously protesting against their plight as women in a sexist society. "Fat," Orbach wrote, "is a response to many manifestations of sexist culture. Fat is a way of saying 'no' to powerlessness and self-denial, to a limiting sexual expression which demands that females look and act in a certain way, and to an image of womanhood that defines a specific role." In a sense, Orbach presumed women overate and got fat out of anger, frustration, and defiance, but psychotherapists and analysts had been saying something similar for decades. Orbach just presented a feminist explanation for the anger. Eating was still, in her view, a largely symbolic act. But if Orbach regarded eating and fatness as primarily symbolic, she nonetheless did demonstrate how much both obesity and chronic dieting were caused by societal pressures, and she uncovered one of the cruelest traps in the thin imperative: The very effort to diet creates obsessions about food that ultimately can lead to eating disorders.[31]

Others in the psychiatric community made a different and perhaps more persuasive connection between feminism and women's obsessions with their weight. They observed that feminism, by opening so many options to women, by encouraging them to "go for it," by promising they could "have it all," set up extraordinary personal expectations. Women and adolescent girls thought they should be high-achieving superwomen. Christopher Lasch made a similar observation about the "narcissistic generation" as a whole. The narcissist is terrified of being part of the "common herd" instead of one of the "great" people, a celebrity. Being normal or average was unacceptable. This attitude was part of the cultural romance with self-realization spawned by the human-potential movement. High achievement and success were still the American Dream, but they were not to be measured only in terms of professional accomplishment. They were also to be measured in terms of mastery of the self, of ability to transcend personal limitations.[32]

For young girls who grew up in affluent surroundings with every advantage and with doting parents, the compulsion to succeed, to stand out, became especially powerful. Failure could only be their own fault. They had few deprivations or obstacles they could blame for their inability to be among the best. They sought perfection. For all women, but for them especially, having a disciplined, exercised, infinitely civilized body, and living up to the health-fashion ideal, was central to that quest for perfection. In addition, with the confusion of values and gender roles, it was one value that stood out clearly. As these psychiatric experts pointed out, the proliferation of ideal bodies in the media, combined with the litany that Americans' main problem was their inability to control their lust for food, deeply affected these girls who strived so hard to be "good." For the high-achieving, liberated woman and for the girl bent on notable accomplishment, the contest for mastery over appetite and bodily flaws was irresistible. They could control their impulses toward food and laziness even if most Americans couldn't. This indeed could be regarded as a great achievement in and of itself.

Americans had been alerted to the treacherous underside of the thin imperative, but America's fat-phobia was not diluted. The very magazines that warned about "dieting to disaster" tucked their warnings between articles that kept reiterating the litany against overweight. In addition, the association between slenderness and the new ideal woman of the seventies was too powerful. Women seeking empowerment knew that food equals power, overeating equals powerlessness, had become one of the fundamental equations of the age.

By the end of the seventies the ideal woman was a high-achieving professional who strode into the boardroom and bedroom and onto the tennis court with self-assurance, or else she juggled with expert competence her roles of wife-lover, successful wage earner, and mother. This was a woman in control of her emotional needs and of every situation in which she found herself. She refused to be regarded as a subordinate by men or anyone else, including her family. The era was one of tremendous cultural chaos as old rules and roles were overturned by the various liberation movements. Sadly, the new liberalism in sex, fashion, and gender roles exacted a toll from women. With the new freedoms came a remarkably rigid body ideal, one that required women to exert incessant control over their bodies as well as over their needs for stable love relationships—and for food. Ironically, as the role of women was redefined, theoretically empowering them, these very freedoms trammeled them even more with one enduring traditional pressure—the pressure to be thin.

IV

THE OBSESSION AND
BEYOND

11

Obsession Becomes Religion:
The Fitness Epidemic

The health-fitness ethic escalated throughout the seventies. An expression of developments we have traced from the fifties, it grew from a trend into a national imperative. The national mood had changed. The political, moral, and aesthetic venturesomeness of the sixties and seventies was collapsing. The election of Ronald Reagan in 1980 inaugurated political moderation, and in many quarters, political apathy. He campaigned for a return—in both habit and polemic—to the social values the counterculture had overturned: family, business, success, social stability, and faith in America. Too many broken homes and hearts, loss of novelty, and herpes and AIDS dampened the fevers of sexual liberation. Yuppies—young, upwardly mobile, urban professionals bent on financial success and its material rewards—supplanted hippies as baby boomers discovered they might not be able to achieve the standard of living of their parents, let alone fulfill the American Dream and surpass it. The appearance of poverty ceased to be chic. Cocaine replaced marijuana as the drug of choice—the drug of a driven, high-powered generation. And right behind it were diet and exercise. Few wanted to be laid back now and few wanted to drop out anymore. This was especially true for women, who were fighting as hard, if not harder, than men for positions in the marketplace.

The quest for self-realization mutated into a drive for personal survival, and we believed the fittest survived best. We might be unable to control the external human and natural environment, but we certainly could control our internal environments and make ourselves into our personal best—strong and muscled enough to be winners. Jane Fonda, the female ideal of the eighties, now raised her clenched fist, not as a sign of protest, but to show her biceps. One's own body, its health and especially its strength, emerged as the new cause célèbre. We believed we could become as powerful and invulnerable as Superman—the mythic American hero who re-emerged in 1978—if only we followed the new precepts with an iron will. Americans had transformed an obsession into a religion.

We saw its manifestations in the first two chapters of this book. The diet-related industries burst far beyond the levels reached in the seventies as Americans' passion to shed fat intensified. The number of articles on diet in the popular press soared from sixty in 1979–80 to sixty-six in the *month* of January, 1980, in just twenty-two contemporary magazines. Between 1983 and 1984, the diet articles listed in the *Reader's Guide* alone had hit 103, and in 1984, 300 diet books were on bookstore shelves. While intestinal bypass surgery for weight loss declined in popularity, liposuction rose as a new panacea. It was a new surgical procedure that vacuumed out local adipose deposits, not to make a fat, aging body healthier but to perfect a well-kept body whose bulges wouldn't budge despite devoted exercise and diet. The technique was imported from France in 1982, and by 1984 approximately 55,000 liposuctions had been performed in the United States; by 1986 the number had risen to 100,000, and it became a common form of cosmetic surgery, despite the cost ($2,000–4,000), discomfort, occasional skin disfigurements, and its rare but potentially deadly complications.[1]

Exercise, too, soared in popularity. Between 1981 and 1985 an estimated 25 million Americans had joined the latest activity, aerobic dance classes, which proved to be primarily a female form of burning fat and building muscles: 90 percent of the "aerobicizers" attending the 50,000–100,000 studios in the country were women. When Reebok first put aerobic shoes on the market in 1982, sales amounted to $3.5 million; three years later they had reached $65 million, and in 1986, Americans spent $3 billion on all kinds of athletic footwear. The same year they spent over $1 billion on exercise equipment for the home and for the gym, all in an effort to put on those muscles modeled by Sylvester Stallone and Jane Fonda.[2]

The American public clearly had been smitten with health and fitness. Popular fitness magazines suddenly appeared and succeeded, such as *New Body, Shape, Fit, Spring,* and *Self. American Health* was hailed in 1985 as a success legend by *Newsweek* and the *New York Times.* More established magazines made sure they included at least one or two, if not more, articles on some aspect of health, fitness, or diet in each issue. By 1986 even *Ms.,* historically concerned with vital feminist issues, reported that "you our readers identified health coverage as the number-one reason you read *Ms.*"[3]

Jane Fonda became the female ideal of the era. She was uniquely suited for this role. She was a political activist who had found a way to be a "good capitalist"; a staunch and successful feminist—wife, mother, actress, and entrepreneur—and above all, a celebrated Hollywood beauty. Her marriage was, in some sense, symbolic of the times: This child of Hollywood wealth, whose actor-father had become an icon of American virtues, and who herself was a Vassar graduate and an international sex symbol, wed Tom Hayden, the scruffy, radical leader who came from stolid Midwestern virtues. It was the marriage of two distinct American subcultures, just as the election of a film star to the presidency was. This melding, with Southern California taking new leadership in the national culture, forged the new mainstream.

Fonda also became one of the most visible, outspoken, and successful priestesses of the new religion. She catapulted aerobics into a national craze when her *Workout Book* came out in 1981, and her subsequent books, exercise videos, records, studios, and clothing line were wildly popular, turning her into a flourishing cottage industry. Fonda pushed the new health ethic and its food rules—though her dietary advice contained much of the nonsense of food faddists like Adelle Davis, who powerfully influenced her, and many of the fringe ideas endemic to Southern California's cult of beauty.[4]

As we have seen, the health ethic swept into the mainstream in part because it mirrored so many counterculture values and because it came to be accepted and was then pushed by government and health authorities. HEW, the Department of Agriculture, the AHA, the American Cancer Society, and the Surgeon General himself called for Americans to reform personal habits, to exercise and eat right—that is, according to the McGovern committee's *Dietary Goals*. It seemed a consensus had been reached. From issuing edicts, these authorities went on to urge practice, and the movement developed a momentum of its own.

There were efforts to influence and even legislate private health habits in campaigns that bore an eerie resemblance to the Prohibition movement. Officials pressured American food industries to comply with the new dietary standards: Fast-food chains were urged to offer healthier fare, the meat industry to produce beef with lower fat content, and many schools began to ban vending machines of soft drinks and candy from their campuses. Cities began to pass antismoking ordinances. Ex-radicals never managed to get marijuana legalized, but in a remarkable about-face that was a sign of the times, they eagerly worked at a local level to get public cigarette smoking banned and felt victorious when they succeeded. They were exchanging their liberalism for a new conservatism. Now they believed government *should* regulate private habits, not only to protect consumers from corporations whose lust for profits led to carelessly made and unhealthy products but also to protect consumers from themselves.

The 1970s had seen a slow absorption into mainstream popular culture of both formerly radical and formerly specialized medical opinions, but it was in the eighties that faith in exercise and fitness swelled. Scientists began to research the value of exercise for good health and wrote reams of articles on the subject. Despite some doubts and cautions expressed in this literature, the public only learned about the scientists who vaunted exercise as a prevention for everything from aging, to osteoporosis, to depression, to personality problems. Most of all, they kept hearing echoes of the "Marathon Hypothesis": that daily, strenuous aerobic activity would prevent cardiovascular disease because it strengthened the heart muscle, vastly improved circulation, and countered many of the known risks for heart disease.

Belief in the value of exercise had been mounting since the sixties, but what characterized the eighties was the paramount preoccupation with it, the shift from moderate exercise to strenuous exercise—the passionate pursuit of the strength and endurance levels of professional athletes and an almost masochistic pleasure in the aches and pains that accompanied such efforts. By 1983 more than 400 marathon races were held yearly in the United States, with 157,000 runners completing the grueling twenty-six-mile course. They were determined to "break through the wall" of their endurance, whatever the physical pain. Bicyclers didn't go out for a nice neighborhood ride: They went for hours, mindless of the scenery, intent only on getting their pulse rates up and covering longer distances in shorter hours. Bodybuilding edged into favor for men and then for women as well. When Fonda's *Workout Book* hit the stands, women left the track for the gym to make "going for the burn *your* way of life," as the book cover exulted.[5]

Medical science seemed to endorse the popular idea that if some exercise was good for us, more was better, that the fittest were the healthiest—despite the protests of many within the scientific community that this was a patent distortion of biologic realities. Americans became convinced that visible muscles meant they were invulnerable to attack from disease. They called it body power, and body power was what they wanted. In May, 1986, *Esquire* featured on its cover a flexed, well-muscled model with a headline emblazoned beside him: "Body Power! A Guide to Muscles, Training and the Sports That Pay Off." And the fitness fanatics now also promised that body power brought improved abilities, the kind we needed to survive, not just in the jungle, but also in the complex, modern, white-collar world. It brought success.

Eating right preoccupied Americans more than ever. It went with being fit and presumably served the same purposes. All of the seventies' confusion about which foods were "good" and which "bad" seemed resolved, and the *Dietary Goals* became gospel, especially its warnings about saturated fat and cholesterol intake. In 1984 *Time* reported the results of a massive ten-year research study by the National Heart, Lung and Blood Institute, which seemed to prove that reducing cholesterol levels *did* reduce the incidence of cardiovascular disease. Cholesterol was frightening. As *Time* explained: "You don't sense your cholesterol rising or feel plaque developing . . . . For up to one-third of victims, the first sign of this secret disease is sudden death." A similarly insidious process presumably occurred unless we ate the diet recommended in *Dietary Goals.* The Food Marketing Institute reported that between 1983 and 1987 shoppers' concerns about salt had risen 22 percent, about fat, 78 percent, and about cholesterol 180 percent. A virtual demonology of food was now accepted by mainstream culture, which is why Fonda's mesh of dietary sense and nonsense could be accepted so easily. Interest in nutrition soared as people came to believe not just that certain foods were bad but also that certain foods and diets were superfuel for the superathlete: They were "power diets." As a best-selling diet book put it, we wanted to *Eat to Win.*[6]

Although some diets did not directly address the issue of weight loss, most of them did, and all of them assumed that people wanted to achieve their ideal weights. They didn't have to state it explicitly. It had become axiomatic. The Food Marketing Institute reported that concern about calories had risen 133 percent just between 1983 and 1987. The most crucial change in attitude toward diet was that now we were told dieting wasn't dieting. Jane Brody explained the new attitude in her 1981 best-selling *Nutrition Book:* "A final requirement [for permanent weight loss] is that you *give up the notion of a 'diet.'* A diet is something you go on and off. Permanent weight control means that the diet you go on today is the same as the diet you'll be on a year from now is the same diet you'll be on for the rest of your life. This is not really a diet, but an *eating management plan.*" Dieting was supposed to be a way of life. Our appetites had to be controlled at all times so that we always ate the low-fat, low-calorie way—whether we were thin or fat, fit or flabby.[7]

The new food rules became almost as strict as Judaism's kosher laws. They even carried similar moral overtones. Eating "bad" foods wasn't just unhealthy; it was also a violation of the injunction to control appetite. Overeating was an even more serious violation. Just as many bodily functions were banished from the public to the private sphere with the civilizing process, so was overeating, or eating with festive abandon, banished from public life. It was a shameful, even sinful, thing to do—unless the eater was superthin. Overeating had to be done in private, away from the prying eyes and stern judgments of friends and family. Eating had become loaded with a moral significance well beyond any it had had in earlier decades.

When pediatricians reported in 1983 something they called "fear of obesity" among nine- to seventeen-year-olds, and when in 1986 we found that third and fourth graders were dieting to lose weight, the public was horrified and asked how this disturbing state of affairs had developed. It is more surprising that they were surprised. They didn't seem to realize how monolithic the imperative to eat right and control appetite had become. They forgot that many authorities had been warning that the snares of obesity began even in the womb and that all children should be on a diet similar to that outlined in the *Dietary Goals.* The values of the wellness epidemic had penetrated our culture, leaving no age group immune. Even the once round and rosy Campbell Soup kids were thinned down in 1984. These observers didn't see that controlling appetite and thus, body size had become America's most prized virtue. The dieting fourth and fifth graders were simply trying to be good.[8]

There were many reasons the health ethic was so widely accepted. One was demographics. More and more Americans were living to the ages when degenerative diseases commonly struck. By 1980, 11.3 percent of the nation's population was sixty-five or over—a larger percentage than ever before in any society's history. Our very success in improving the nation's health was spawning its own set of problems. Health-care costs kept soaring, and the federal government and health agencies realized that something had to be done to sustain an increasingly elderly population. If there were even a chance that better diets, exercise, and weight loss could help control the soaring costs, then it was worthwhile to ask Americans to revise their habits. The new philosophy also shifted responsibility for poor health away from the government and medical establishment on to the individual.

The government and society as a whole also had to address other problems caused by a large population of elderly people. What kind of life could elderly Americans lead once they retired? This was a distinctly new social problem, and it was occurring in an environment where family and community ties were breaking down. Too often, older people were lonely and isolated, cut off from any sense of belonging or any sense of purpose. Society had to find a blueprint for those who could expect to live five to twenty years after retirement. The blurring of age distinctions brought on by the counterculture, by the human-potential books for the middle-aged, and by fashion provided a useful solution. Throughout the seventies and eighties older people were told what middle-aged people had traditionally been told: They could retrieve the opportunities and even the energy and health of their younger years if they kept active, did exercises once deemed appropriate for young people, ate right, and watched their weight.

Other demographic changes also helped the wellness epidemic take hold. The baby boomers who had brought in the counterculture and the human-potential movement still formed the bulk of the population. Their beliefs and concerns still set the tone for the culture at large. But the oldest of them were now becoming middle-aged, and it was vital for them to find a way to make this acceptable to themselves.

Here, too, Jane Fonda mirrored the concerns and beliefs of a generation. In her first book she emphasized how eating right and exercising had rejuvenated her: "Today at forty-three my body is stronger and more limber, and I look and feel better, than when I was twenty." Three years later, after her father's death and her forty-sixth birthday, she suddenly came face to face with the end of her youth. In her second book, *Women Coming of Age,* she examined the terrain of forty-five and over. She asked the following questions: "What, I wondered, can women in mid-life realistically expect of themselves physically? Is continued fitness, sexuality, and vitality possible? Do we have special nutritional needs now? Can we halt the aging process? Is there an equivalent of the childbirth technique to ease us through the transition into mid-life?"[9]

Her questions were oddly physical, as though aging were only a biological ordeal, not one that had to do with the mind and soul or with new responsibilities and values. Fonda was essentially asking whether the physical traits of youth could be preserved. She answered with an emphatic yes. The aging process was "negotiable." The technique that would "ease" us into middle age was resistance to aging through healthy diet and exercise. Throughout her book, Fonda kept repeating that all those dietary no-nos—fats, salt, sugar, processed foods, and too much meat—and lack of exercise caused aging. They also caused the even more deplorable middle-aged spread. She didn't present her ideas in moderate tones. With the zealousness of a convert, she assured us that "eating right" and strenuous exercise would keep us young.

Others in her generation seemed to share her feelings. *American Health* magazine noted that the baby boomers were in the vanguard of the fitness ranks: 57 percent of those between thirty and forty-nine were exercising regularly. And Fonda wasn't the only one concerned about being over forty. The women's magazines began to write more about how to take off five or ten years, about how to look and feel young at any age. Joan Collins, Barbi Benton, and Fonda herself were splayed across their glossy pages as proof incarnate that no one over thirty—even over fifty—had to bow out of the beauty-youth game. In 1982 *American Health* promised we might "break the age barrier" and headlined: "She looks 35. She acts 35. Could she really be 92?"[10]

In emphasizing how to look young at any age, the women's press was responding to an economic reality. Their major market was not twenty-year-old women who would have little interest in these issues. Rather, as had been the case since the sixties, it was the baby-boom generation, the group with the most people and the most dollars. In the sixties the women's press had addressed concerns of twenty-year-olds; in the seventies, of thirty-year olds; and now, in the eighties, it was forty-year-olds. This group's lust for exercise was part of its desire to remain youthful, and youth was being redefined just as thinness was.

At the heart of the health-exercise ethic was a desire on the part of Americans to control their own lives and deaths. For women, perhaps, to whom the issue of control was paramount, this was even more crucial. *Vogue,* echoing the Surgeon General's 1979 report, *Healthy People,* explained that "your health is your own doing. It depends overwhelmingly on what you did today and what you did yesterday. And what you do tomorrow." Even *Ms.* succumbed so much to what was, in essence, a holistic view of health, that it accepted advertisements from *Prevention* magazine, a publication that scientists repeatedly condemned as health quackery. But *Prevention*'s ad distilled the kind of thinking that was beginning to prevail in America. It read: "Illness isn't natural. It isn't even inevitable." Over the previous century, human mastery of nature and control of disease had succeeded so much that Americans now expected well-being as a birthright and regarded all illness as "unnatural," and preventable. They believed they could control nature, perhaps even death, through diet and exercise.[11]

The new ethic even held a promise of salvation. We began to hear that we might postpone, indefinitely, death itself. "Futurologists," many of them with professional degrees, had started promising in the seventies that scientists might soon unlock the secrets of aging and of mortality itself—and conquer them. By the eighties these ideas were becoming familiar and reinforced the ethic. In January, 1980, Diana Benzia wrote in *Harper's Bazaar* that "scientists forecast the ability to stop the clock on aging within fifty years, creating a society of immortals." She went on to quote Drs. Ivan Popov and Hans J. Kugler, both of whom argued that people could add thirty to forty years to their lives with "sound nutritional principles, exercise, and effective ways of coping with anxiety." It was almost too good—and too simple—to be true. The health-exercise ethic held out the promise that we just might cheat death itself.[12]

It wasn't just commitment to rejuvenation that turned the health ethic into a new religion, however. This ex-radical generation still cherished many of its earlier values, still had a penchant for panaceas, for grand solutions to old problems. Determined to reform the world, it embraced grandiose missions. This time, the crusade was not to bring world peace and justice, but rather to eradicate the worst injustices of all: aging, disease, and death. The ex-rebels had turned from outer to inner concerns, from other-orientation to self-orientation, from collective to personal destiny, from spiritualism to materialism.

It is easy to see in the passion for wellness a 180-degree turn from the youthful commitments of a radical generation. It seems a curious philosophy for a group that once rebelled against materialism and the superficiality of appearances. The generation that militantly sought world peace and mental and spiritual enlightenment, now sought physical perfection. This generation had come to merge the spiritual and the physical. And so the pendulum swung. Millenial quests had shifted from the external world of social man to the internal world of one's own body. And a television ad for Reebok shoes could show people exuberantly exercising to the strains of the Beatles, "You Say You Want a Revolution." Exercising was a continuation of their revolution.

But one could not achieve wellness without demonstrating it. Like Calvinist sinners, the elect—the fit—had to confirm visibly in this world their pretensions to salvation—that is, well-being. And like Calvinists, they could never be sure they had been "chosen", which leads to great anxiety. And, in a material world, the most fundamental demonstration of one's election and salvation was a thin, fat- and flab-free, taut, strong body—and it had to be achieved at any cost.

A thin body was the physical incarnation of such pretensions, for weight loss—achieving a fat-free body—was the linchpin of the health ethic. And the ethic, in turn, futher dignified and ennobled the weight-loss quest. It now basked in the glow of all the other pathways to good health—the newer virtues—such as not abusing drugs and alcohol and not smoking. Fat-phobia had expanded and intensified, moving to higher ground.

Americans did not work out zealously and deny themselves traditional food favorites just to be healthy or good. Mostly, they did these things because the new religion had become pre-eminently fashionable. The "with-it" people displayed in advertisements and commercials and on television and movie screens sipped light cola and light beer, mineral water and white wine, ate light, fat-free fare à la nouvelle cuisine, and dressed in casual sportswear like shorts and T-shirts, sweats, and spandex-type body-hugging pants and tops. By 1983 the marketing research firm, Frost and Sullivan, reported that "the generation that brought us radical chic in the late sixties and early seventies brings us fitness chic in the eighties." *Stores* magazine explained in 1984 that "this clothing line evokes a 'stay fit' ethic that has captured the imagination of the entire country."[13]

There was another reason for Americans' zealotry: They wanted to be beautiful. The new ethic had created a new physical aesthetic, for both men and women. The long, lean body cherished in the sixties and seventies gave way in the eighties to the muscled body. Sylvester Stallone and Arnold Schwarzenegger captured the essence of the male ideal. Schwarzenegger had helped popularize male bodybuilding; the film *Pumping Iron* spread it to the general public. By June, 1980, the *New York Times Magazine* announced that "a new 'ideal' body image is emerging: good healthy brawn." Men's exercise changed correspondingly. They went for "tougher, harder workouts" in order to re-sculpt their bodies. Many moved from the jogging track into the gym. And the decade's cinematic sex heroes, such as Nick Nolte, Harrison Ford, and William Hurt, now had to put on muscles before taking off their shirts. Such a body was a must for a hero. Only a man with evident musculature could fight corporations, criminals, and corruption—or have the strength to win an ardent feminist.[14]

While some kind of visible strength was a traditional masculine ideal, by 1980 women, too, wanted visible muscles, not just lean, taut flesh. Not since the days of ancient Sparta's female athletes had women wanted to wear muscles. Already, in the mid-seventies, the press had noted the fringe fad of female bodybuilding, which slowly moved to the edges of respectability. In 1979 Lisa Lyon won the first Woman's World Bodybuilding Championship, and the news hit the major magazines. *People* vividly entitled its article on the event: "Nobody Will Ever Kick Sand in Lisa Lyon's Face." Female bodybuilding gained more adherents: 5,000 women flexed competitively in 1984; by 1985 the number had jumped to 12,000. It also veered toward extremes and provoked confusion. Beverly May Francis, the star of *Pumping Iron II: The Women* was called "the next Arnold" because she had developed such extraordinary musculature. "She can make her biceps bulge and put her veins on view so vividly that observers frequently get grossed out. 'That can't be a woman,' is the typical response," *Newsweek* reported in 1985. Contests often ended in pandemonium as judges quarreled with one another over what criteria should be used to rate competitors. Should the women look like women or should they show off the musculature of men?[15]

Most women did not pursue the form of the bodybuilders. Instead, they pursued a more moderate version of it—the body build of a more established sex and beauty symbol: Jane Fonda. As though in some remarkable metamorphosis, Fonda had managed to be curvy and busty in *Barbarella,* skinny and straight in *Klute,* and so lean and muscled in *On Golden Pond,* that one journalist was moved to comment, "She has a body like wood . . . . You don't want to stroke her, you want to sand her down." Another complained that the film's climactic scene, with Fonda posed in a bikini, seemed like a "commercial for *Jane Fonda's Workout Book.*" In fact, Fonda's look was the new ideal for female beauty.[16]

In the spring of 1981 fashion magazines were abuzz with the development. "Muscle Chic," *Glamour* headlined, and *Mademoiselle* heralded, "Getting Strong: Developing Muscle Strength in Women." In July, 1981, *Glamour* underlined how new the new look was in an interview with Debbie Meyer-Reyes, winner of three Olympic gold medals in swimming. She recalled how embarrassed she had once been about her muscular arms, but now, she excitedly said, "firm muscles are great." Soon, Jane Fonda was joined by Raquel Welch, Linda Evans, Victoria Principal, and others, who were arrayed before us on the covers of their workout books and videos, flexing muscles, waving mini-barbells, and showing off perfectly sculpted, flabless bodies. In May, 1985, *Newsweek* marveled at the "New Flex Appeal" and reported that a full 50 percent of the 4.2 million users of Nautilus weight-training machines were female.[17]

Fashion magazines went full-steam ahead, redefining beauty to meet the changing standards. Beauty was no longer just equated with health: It *was* health. It was no longer just agility and energy and self-confidence: It was strength. The words *beauty, fitness, health,* and *strength* began to be used interchangeably. As Jane Fonda put it, "The glow and energy of the healthy woman is the ultimate beauty, the only beauty that will last." Beauty had become personal and individualistic. We were not to live up to an externally imposed physical standard but rather to develop our own best looks by developing our health and strength. The very qualities of the liberated woman and the standards of the health ethic had become beauty.[18]

But beauty, particularly fashionable beauty, cannot consist merely of inner qualities: It has to be translated into reality, embodied physically, visibly. In the seventies fashion's emphasis had shifted from the clothes that covered the body to the body itself. The new look was a culmination of this trend; now, the body *was* fashion—the object of plastic art—and clothes played an entirely subsidiary role. More than ever before, fashion and beauty took their cues from the (literally) raw material. Aesthetic standards had settled on the very surface of the skin, regardless of clothes, makeup, or hair styles.

If, in the past, we could associate a designer with a change in fashionable body shape, such as Poiret in 1907 or Dior in 1947, we are at somewhat of a loss to find an originator who could be credited with the muscled look of the eighties. It seemed a culmination of the trend toward democratization of fashion and beauty: Inspiration came less from specific designers than from women themselves. Also, no designer could be credited with a look that required minimal clothing and maximum exposure. The new look did not call for design in the traditional sense.

The new look was also a culmination of the body-baring trends in disco styles and exercise wear that had begun in the late seventies. Informality had reached a new peak, and women could be seen on the streets clad in the leotards, tights, and sweat clothes that once were appropriate only for the locker room. Their nonexercise clothes were now often made of exercise-wear materials, and they were ever more revealing. In May, 1985, *Harper's Bazaar* announced, "We're warming up to summer, and super body-baring clothes are the watchword of the new season's fashions." In the same issue, it described an even more surprising phenomenon: Crinolines were back, but as outerwear rather than underwear. Other clothes were designed to highlight, and show, lacy bras and camisoles. Calvin Klein came out with a more feminist variation of this idea: Men's thin, sleeveless undershirts, cut for women, were to be worn hugged to a braless torso. The female body had no more secrets or mysteries. Even the revival of lingerie was, in part, a comic parody: It was no longer to be accidently glimpsed, a hint of other, hidden delights. Now it was worn frankly and publicly, a wry reminder that nothing was hidden.[19]

At first, it seemed that the muscled standard would free women from their grueling battles with their weights. The rhetoric that went with the new look stressed qualities, not mere physical looks. And shape mattered more than weight. We even learned that the narrow, small-boned body was not the only beautiful body: Big-boned, mesomorphic forms could also be beautiful. *Mademoiselle* writer Annie Gottlieb reported that what her thighs and hips lacked "in voguish slenderness, [they] now make up for in firmness and line"—and that was acceptable. *Mademoiselle* even headlined some merciful, unheard of news in February, 1986: "Those Extra 5 Pounds—Use Them, Don't Lose Them."[20]

The new ideal also seemed more generous and accessible than earlier ones. Muscles are one of the more malleable parts of the human body. They can be developed with exercise. Manipulating the body into a facsimile of Twiggy— even a Twiggy with 10 or 15 extra pounds—had been a thankless task. Even if a woman managed to stay on a deprivatory diet long enough to get her weight down to prepubescent levels, certain unfortunate anatomic inheritances could not be dieted away such as big bone structure, a pot belly, "love handles," and cellulite. But with the muscle-exercise ideology, fashion seemed to have found a solution for such dogged flaws. A woman could indeed flatten a belly, tone up a thigh, a sagging arm, or jiggling buttocks—she could be big but shapely and taut. The new ideal seemed to give women the opportunity, and the power, to approximate its standards.

Best of all, the techniques for achieving this body—exercise—were vaunted as fun, even exhilarating, and as producing benefits far more important than fashionable beauty. Fashion magazines began to resemble health and sports manuals, and always, the underlying message was the same: Exercise meant getting healthy and strong, developing character and self-pride, rejuvenating the soul as well as the body.

This indeed was a beauty and a beauty technique to which liberated women could respond. Phyllis Theroux's 1982 article in *American Health*, entitled "The Size 7 Soul," signaled how feminists could accept both. In it, Theroux confessed: "There was a time when I thought vanity—rewriting the body— was the product of dishonesty. The woman who primped and exercised and watched her calories seemed silly." The women exercisers she now admired were different. They had character. They "squared up" to their mirrors, recognized their flaws, and did something about them. To Theroux, this concern was no longer a sign of traditional weakness, but rather, with these new premises, a sign of strength. It was "being honest—and to my way of thinking—almost virtuous." Women were not working out to improve their appearance or to attract a man. They did it to seek some physical perfection, and they did it for themselves.[21]

Even *Ms.*, which eschewed preoccupation with appearance, was conquered by this ideology. While it was one of the few magazines to defend the overweight and to argue that fat could be fit, it nonetheless endorsed the health ethic's precepts of proper diet and exercise—and its concept of natural beauty. The ideal of natural beauty, of course, was not new—from the mid-nineteenth century on, feminists and health reformers periodically had condemned the artifice of fashion and endorsed instead a natural ideal—but modern feminists generally had been hostile to concerns about beauty, and *Ms.* had focused almost exclusively on other political and economic issues. This changed. In 1983 *Ms.* initiated a policy of devoting every May issue to the "Beauty of Health." Its May, 1984 cover showed a bubble-bath clad model with as radiantly energetic a smile and pose as those that graced other women's magazines.

The new muscled ideal seemed too good to be true. It was. For it deepened, profoundly, women's battles with their flesh. It exacerbated their preoccupation with their bodies and their body shape. In 1984 eight articles on women's distorted body images appeared in the popular press. Eating orders continued to spread. America's fat-phobia had reached more virulent dimensions.

Superathleticism was simply a new fashion ideal, one connected almost exclusively with the corporeal self. As always, this brought increased scrutiny of the body and ever more exacting demands about how it should look. Under the guise of showing readers how to exercise and build up muscle strength, these magazines simply alerted them to more and more possible flaws, to details of their anatomies they probably had never before given a thought to and which they never dreamed should or could meet certain standards. A slightly loose upper arm, a slightly shapeless upper thigh, a small calf, who had worried about it? A jiggling inner thigh or a dimpled buttock—we might have been unhappy about them, but they were not a focus of concern. As long as we were thin, they weren't a terrible liability and, in any case, we didn't think we could do much about them.

Times had changed. No part of the body was immune from beauty's standards. It had no more "private parts." Every part was now public and had to match the prevailing standard. The exhortations of the exercise manuals were presented under the cheerful guise of health, fitness, and personal strength—though how a less flabby arm or tighter inner thigh or firmer buttocks were going to affect our "health" was never explained. It didn't need to be. Health and fitness had become synonymous with beauty.

Nor did the muscled body relieve us from our thirty-year-old war with fat. Fitness literally was defined as the absence of body fat, and that fat was now even more repugnant than it had been in the past. The new ideal woman was stripped of nearly every layer of adipose tissue: She was skin and muscle, and her body was, ideally, "close to the bone." Why did Fonda urge us to "go for the burn"—that painful sensation when a muscle is overworked? Because, she explained, "it means lactic acid, which burns fat away, is being released into the bloodstream." The new standard didn't give women a smidgen of room in which to stop worrying about their weight, either. Weight was useful only as something to convert into taut muscle, and excess weight would merely create grotesquerie. No one could possibly be consoled into thinking it had become acceptable.[22]

Paradoxically, although we were assured we could weigh minimally more, our standard of beauty had become even thinner. The marathon runners we admired were excruciatingly scrawny, with scarcely any fat to soften their harsh angles. When *Time* heralded the "New Ideal of Beauty," it remarked that it was "slimmer than before . . . . The frame, deprived of some adipose tissue, looks more sinuous." Our professional beauties, too, kept getting slimmer. The average Miss America contestant competing between 1980 and 1983 weighed 5 pounds less than she had in the period between 1972 and 1974. In the earlier period, 5'5" contestants averaged about 113 pounds; in the later period, they averaged about 108.5 pounds. Even more striking than these averages is the number of excessively thin women who won their state competitions. In 1983 Miss South Carolina, 5'4", weighed only 101 pounds. That same year, three of the 5'7" contestants weighed only 110. But state judges did not think they looked unhealthy or too thin, nor were they deterred from choosing these young women as paragons of American beauty.[23]

Our other beauty celebrities are exalted for, above all, their low weights. When popular magazines write about celebrities like Diane Dixon and Barbi Benton, or when fashion magazines describe the "best bodies" of models and beauty celebrities, we are supposed to read with awe and admiration about their spartan diets and strenuous exercise routines. We don't know how much stronger or healthier they are, but we always hear about how little they weigh. Weight—a low weight—is still the most fundamental measure of beauty.

At its heart, the exercise craze was simply another, more powerful weight-loss scheme. Much as exercise buffs argued that the goal was exchanging fat for muscle, and that scale weight was irrelevant, the bottom line was always the same: How much do you weigh? Certainly the most irresistible message of the exercise advocates was that with strenuous exercise, we burned calories. The plethora of charts detailing how many we burned per hour of exercise exposed the real root of the fitness fetish: We wanted to make sure we were burning off the calories we took in.

We even heard the irresistible: If we exercised enough, we could eat more and still not gain weight. Bodybuilder Christine Zane told *Newsweek* about the benefits of her sport. One, not lost on any woman, was, "Now I can eat all I want and stay thin." In fact, they could not. Most female bodybuilders stayed on spartan diets and even decreased their fluid intake before competitions so that no extra flesh or puffiness would mar the vision of their muscles. Nonetheless, exercise was vaunted as the magic answer for our war between our appetites and our wills. Perhaps this was why women so willingly went for "the burn." The avid exerciser was not just demonstrating a masochistic machisma; she was also willing to suffer in order to expiate the sins of appetite.[24]

A more fundamental reason this fashion ideal exacerbated weight and body obsessions was that women believed they could and should achieve it. The medical profession, fashion and exercise mongers, feminists, and many other cultural authorities assured them that with enough effort, they could shed those extra layers of fat and firm up those abdomens, thighs, and buttocks. They had learned there was something they could do—indeed *had* to do—about such flaws. The new look "represents an attainable ideal for all ages, races, walks of life," *Time* explained. "It requires little more than the will to work at them." The woman who did achieve the ideal body, *Time* went on, demonstrated that she "cared enough about herself to improve herself," that she had intelligence—"the brain that determined to shape [that body]," and above all, that she had self-respect. A 1987 ad for Reebok shoes captured the essence of this ideology in a full-page picture of a leotarded female shown only from her breasts to her ankles—her presumably Reebok-shod feet didn't even show. Next to her picture, where advertisers usually identify suppliers of the model's clothes and accessories, were the words: "Body developed by Kathryn Hamerski, aerobics instructor." Kathryn Hamerski was the model.[25]

Even more than in the seventies the observations of psychologist Erving Goffman are apropos. When a group believes a person is responsible for his or her own problems or imperfections, then that person becomes an object of ridicule, contempt, and prejudice. Compassion is replaced by scorn. As American society liberalized, it trapped the flawed body in an even tighter vice. It was the one failing still seen almost exclusively as an individual's fault. "You have no excuse for sporting anything less than your own best body," *Harper's Bazaar* told its readers. This attitude was vividly underscored by a woman who wrote a letter to *Ms.* to protest against an article which argued that fat could be fit and healthy. She argued that this "implies that obese women have no power to change; that they are victims of their fate. These are the ideas that have stifled women's progress for ages. It's time that these terribly overweight women realize that there is a healthier alternative: a choice. Isn't the opportunity to choose the essence of feminism?" A choice. As long as body size and shape were regarded as a result of personal choice, no woman could forgive herself—nor could others forgive her—for having a failed body. It was a sin, a crime, and a just reason for self-punishment and despair.[26]

Women could not easily rebel against this ideal as another form of oppression imposed by sexist society or by the fashion industry. If health, beauty, and fitness were all one look, there were no grounds on which to attack it. In any case, it was perceived as a fashion of exhilarating new freedom, not of oppression, in part because it resonated with feminist values that had gained currency as the women's movement became mainstream. Strength and physical autonomy were part of attractiveness, which now was a matter of stepping aggressively into the world, not waiting passively to be chosen.

The notion that women could take charge of their bodies also meshed with more fundamental beliefs of the women's movement. Even more than the fitness of the seventies, the muscled look seemed to be a logical development, and a more faithful visual incarnation, of the belief that biology is not destiny. The bodybuilders had defied all conventional notions about the female body and had proved that through hard work and determination, women indeed even could build the muscles of a strong young man. If most women sought the body of a Jane Fonda rather than that of a Beverly Francis, the presumption was the same: Biology—and genes—were not destiny.

The muscled look also seemed a further embodiment of women's quest for strength and independence. In her *Mademoiselle* piece, Annie Gottlieb waxed enthusiastic about the implications of the new look, arguing that feminism and a muscled body reinforced one another. Her "old body," she wrote, had looked "vague and wistful, as if it were made for waiting: waiting for me to lose 10 pounds, waiting for a man to say it was beautiful, waiting for a child to make it useful." It was, in short, associated with traditional female functions, and it was passive. But her newly muscled body, she enthused, was not made to wait but to act with strength and effectiveness. It symbolized the power to "carry your own weight financially," to carry heavy grocery bags up five flights of steps, if need be, and to fend off an attacker. Most gratifyingly, it produced emotional strength as well. This empowered woman no longer "desperately" needed a man.[27]

The rhetoric that accompanied all fitness/exercise articles repeated, in one form or another, the same underlying message and did so with the same rapture. Women were "getting strong," they were "going for it." They could have it all: homes, kids, careers, husbands. They were showing they could be as competent and as strong as males. And the media repeatedly echoed Gottlieb's point that the mind and body were one, that "the elusive strength of character women had been seeking for so long turns out to have one of its major roots in physical competence, something most men are expected to develop from earliest childhood."

The muscled look also reflected new social realities and ideals for women. They needed strength. More of them were entering the work force, either out of financial necessity or in pursuit of meaningful careers. Homemaking had been so devalued that few could stay home without damage to self-esteem. Colette Dowling's best-selling *Cinderella Complex* had argued what was becoming a common belief: Any homemaker who was not also working, or cultivating the skills to work, at a remunerative job, suffered from a debilitating "neurotic dependency." Fear, not commitment, kept her at home. And more women were struggling to compete on what formerly had been male terrain. Sometimes they literally needed physical strength to do so. In 1979 the federal government funded a fitness program for women so they could get strong enough to fill their allotted quota of jobs in the steel industry. More often, they needed the sense of independence and strength that would help them compete with men on male turf, or allow them to shoulder the combined burdens of their traditional and new roles: homemaker, mother, and worker. And they knew well that one out of two marriages ended in divorce: They had to be strong enough to cope with single parenting and self-support. Getting strong could be an exciting process of self-growth. It could also be a now-indispensable necessity. Women not only *wanted* to be strong and self-reliant—They *had* to be.[28]

At heart, the muscled look was androgynous. Traditionally, fashion has accentuated the differences between the sexes, except for brief periods when some male styles were incorporated into female clothing. In the seventies unisex styles and thin bodies had begun to erode sexual differentiation in dress and, to a lesser extent, in bodies themselves. Everyone was to look like a just-budding adolescent. The look of the eighties was more androgynous still. Women were not just dressing like men; they actually were trying to develop the musculature of men, and the physical strength it brought. Many fashion writers noted that in the past, only lesbians who assumed male roles and professional athletes—both outside the standards of traditional femininity—dared defy the injunction that women keep muscles discreetly small. Furthermore, the privilege of cultivating such softness had primarily belonged to women from the comfortable classes who did not have to engage in heavy physical labor. But, for the women of the eighties, the heavy physical labor once done only by men now had status. They wanted muscled arms and legs, abdomens as flat and hard as a sheet of steel, hips and buttocks taut as drums, and breasts reduced to small, firm, upright swellings—all without a hint of the jiggle that normally characterizes them. But this is not the body of a woman.

This androgynous body also reflected the ideal of equivalency between the sexes in all spheres of life. Men's and women's roles had become, at least prescriptively, almost indistinguishable. Women competed as equals in school, on the tennis court, and in the boardroom, and they were to enjoy sowing their wild oats as guiltlessly as any bachelor. They were also expected to bring home a good income. Men were to cultivate the sensitivity and emotional responsiveness of women, to share in the housework and in tending to baby and growing kids—if there were kids. Motherhood was still out of favor, and the woman with children was to behave no differently and look no different than her childless sister. The daily functions of men and women had ceased to be different. Among single men, one even began to hear what once had only been whispered by single women: "I'd like to find someone who's earning seventy grand a year. . . ." Men's and women's roles and responsibilities had become as similar as the bodies they idealized.

The muscled female ideal reflected some disturbing trends in American society. It seemed to symbolize hermaphroditism even more than androgyny. Betty Friedan, reviewing the Women's Movement in her book, *The Second Stage,* observed that "we must at least admit and begin openly to discuss feminist denial of the importance of family, of woman's own needs to give and get love and nurture, and tender, loving care." Friedan had summed up the distortions inherent in the new ideal. Women who struggled in the professional world, who didn't need anyone to help them lug bags of groceries up five flights of stairs, who postponed marriage and childbearing, who could opt for single parenthood if a mate did not appear (who could even have themselves impregnated at a sperm bank and so avoid intimate heterosexual contact altogether) clearly did not "need" anyone in a traditional sense. Women were to perform male and female functions all by themselves. A woman was to be thoroughly self-sufficient and, above all, to possess that traditional American virtue, self-reliance.[29]

The new body ideal also suggested a kind of mastery over heredity and nature. In the seventies, when the "natural" look was in, it was presumed that the beauties of the day got their fresh outdoorsy looks naturally and that they didn't devote much time to their appearance. The eighties are different. Every celebrity and every magazine assures us that exceptional beauty has been achieved through hard work. We might even speculate that readers would be dismayed had they found a much-praised beauty had done nothing to mold her looks. We want a beauty that has been forged by human will. We want to be self-sculptors so that we, like the model in the Reebok ad, can claim credit for the perfect machine our body has become, and demonstrate our mental strength and our exquisite control.

There are deep ironies in the muscled ideal. Presumably, it is a beauty for the active, not the passive, woman. Yet, bodybuilding traditionally has been a sport in which appearance, not prowess, is judged. Mr. Americas are not evaluated for their skill in performing difficult feats. They are judged by how their bodies look and by how well they have molded each muscle group. The competition is based on appearance as much as any Miss America contest is. Women have not escaped the trap of judging themselves—and expecting the world to judge them—on the basis of how they look.

Fashion has always been a plastic art, and beauty a measure of individual artistry and taste. It is still a plastic art, but its raw material is now our flesh, not our clothing. Beauty is no longer so much a measure of artistry as of self-discipline and character. Women have liberated themselves from one standard of beauty only to adopt a far more compelling one.

There is another irony in the body-sculpting craze. The body ideal entails tremendous concern with each detail of one's anatomy. In the rhetoric of the exercise craze, women are not shaping up to appeal to men but to appeal to themselves, to strive for physical perfection. The irony is that they end up, Narcissus-like, trying to fall in love with their own images. Gottlieb, in her *Mademoiselle* article, described her new appreciation of her muscled form: Her tummy was now "a vertical sheet, resilient as a drumskin, and faintly sectioned, like a clipper ship's sails in a light breeze." Her thighs, which had been going "doughy," now were firm and shapely. This kind of rapturous praise of one's own body was typical of the exercise-fitness literature and, in fact, was the ultimate goal of working out: pride in the female body one had forged. But in another time and place, such descriptions would apply to a lover, not to oneself. Hermaphroditism is thereby carried to its logical extreme: Women are urged to be autoerotic. It seems an appropriate ideal for an age that encourages us to liberate ourselves from our basic biological needs and destinies, and from social and emotional dependencies—to liberate ourselves from marriage, pregnancy, childrearing, and death.[30]

There is also irony in the larger cultural romance with muscle bulk and strength. There is no evident reason why urban, white-collar people, who compose the majority of these exercises, feel so pressured to be in the peak of physical condition, ready to act with huge energy reserves at any given moment. In primitive, medieval, or even early modern times, when physical strength often meant the difference between survival and death, or for modern soldiers or competitive athletes, it makes sense, but it is puzzling to see this concern among twentieth-century citizens who live in an advanced technological age. It is also puzzling that while Americans enjoy unprecedented health and longevity, they are so preoccupied with fighting disease and death. The fitness buffs believe fitness can bring physical and spiritual renewal, a belief also held by the physical culturists of the turn of the century. But a vast majority of the fitness buffs are well-educated people, including physicians, who must know that fitness is not the same as health, and that extra fitness and extra muscles cannot protect against cardiovascular or other diseases and who, one might think, would see self-improvement as more than just a physical proposition.

Our romance with strength and muscles clearly fills other, more important, needs. In a tight economy, upward mobility is no longer assured. Between 1973 and 1983 the median incomes for those aged twenty-five to thirty-four dropped slightly for the first time in forty years. At the same time, housing costs soared so much that many of the baby-boom generation began to wonder if they could ever afford what once had seemed to be an American birthright: ownership of their own homes. In May, 1987, *Time* reported a startling new trend: Many young adults were moving back in with their parents because they could not afford their own housing. And the baby boomers were facing an internal paradox: Their very numbers, which had made them so potent a cultural force, created fierce competition in the marketplace. Even would-be professionals—professors, doctors, lawyers, scientists—found themselves in the middle of a glut. No one was begging for their services. Professions that once promised instant access to the upper-middle classes no longer did so. This frustration was compounded by another persisting attitude. Many of those who had been part of the counterculture still refused to accept the Establishment professions' traditional mystique. Career success was once again vital, but it still was not to be the only purpose of life. The fitness ethic provided an outlet for career frustrations and a chance to excel at something other than careers.[31]

The fitness ethic also gave people a sense of mastery, at least over their private destinies. The rebellious generation had given up on trying to change or guide the destiny of the world, of their nation, and often even of their communities. The fitness ethic gave them a sense of molding change, at least in the private world of their own bodies. It also gave these highly charged, competitive people a new, worthy opponent: their own limitations. They could set fantastic goals for themselves—goals usually set only by professional athletes—and achieve them. They sought that peak moment of meeting a challenge and going beyond it, what runners call the "runners' high." This sense of surpassing one's own limitations gave the exercise ethic its peculiarly evangelical quality. It also provided a form of heroism in an unheroic age. Such heroism could appeal because, as historian Christopher Lasch observed, this cultural group had come to regard being average as equivalent to failure. People wanted to excel, to stand out, to be winners. Fitness—a perfect body—gave them a way to achieve their personal best.

But one gets the sense, too, that Americans indeed are working out to save themselves. On some profound level, they seem to feel they are in danger. Personal survival has become the buzzword of the decade, and its new imperative, perhaps partly because of social and economic realities. Americans may feel small and impotent in a world of giant corporations in which they are insignificant and dispensable cogs. They know that they are in a fiercely competitive environment with others standing by, ready to usurp their positions. Even more, they seem to sense no human interest, no personal loyalty from their employers. Harvard economist Robert B. Reich recently observed that in American-based Japanese firms, American workers use the pronoun "we" when referring to the company and its policies and projects. American workers in American corporations do not: the pronoun is "they." Americans have come to regard their companies—and all establishment institutions—as adversaries. They and society itself seem to be moving inexorably in accord with laws that the individual cannot comprehend and certainly cannot control.[32]

The sense of danger may also be connected to other changes. Just as companies' loyalties to the individual diminished in past decades, so did individual loyalties to anything or anyone outside the self. In part, this was a culmination of the romantic individualism spawned by the human-potential movement. Loyalties and commitments to a specific company, career, organized religion, hometown, and even family were subordinated to the need for personal realization and fulfillment. Harvard economist Robert B. Reich commented that American workers were ready to change their jobs at "the drop of a hat." They were ready to change cities, religious affiliations, and even mates and lovers with equal swiftness if any of them proved an obstacle to self-realization and success.

This philosophy informed the women's movement, too, and caused some profound changes in family life. The feminist injunction that women should have the choice to be something other than homemakers developed into the conviction that happiness and self-realization could not come from serving others. As the modern family was stripped of more functions, this argument gained credibility. Women had a right to personal, nonfamilial goals, and a right to expect to meet them. Several historians have underscored how much this new individualism affected the family and family ideology. In the nineteenth century and before, the family was seen as the basic unit of society. It was a harmonious unit in which members, prescriptively at least, subordinated private needs for the larger good of The Family. By the 1970s and 1980s the family was no longer the basic social unit. The individual was. And within the family, competition tended to replace harmony as mothers, fathers, and children vied for space and time to fill their own needs. The "good" of the family no longer took automatic priority. On some levels, the family had become a group of competing atoms, each trying to find meaning and fulfillment outside its confines—an attitude expressed most extremely, but also most succinctly, by radical feminists who charged that the family itself "oppressed" women. The personal had indeed become the political, and even these most intimate relationships, once a source of comfort and trust, had become battlegrounds between the sexes. Love itself had become unreliable. Single women complained about "hit-and-run lovers" and were terrorized by herpes and AIDS. And neither husband nor wife nor lover could rely on social institutions to ensure that their "significant other" would always be there.[33]

The only realistic commitment was to the self. It was also the only socially sanctioned commitment. No one was supposed to be dependent on another, nor need another. Dowling told us that homemakers stayed home, not out of commitment or a sense of responsibility, but out of neurotic fear. In the recent best-selling book, *Women Who Love Too Much,* we are even told that women who remain passionately committed to less than ideal lovers/mates are also suffering from destructive and hitherto unrecognized neuroses. Passionate romantic love, its agonies and ecstasies—the stuff of art—has been reduced to the equivalent of drug addiction or alcoholism. We are advised to deny or repress or lose our longings for love, trust, and security—just as we are to repress our biological need for food. On the most fundamental level, modern Americans are as alone as Rambo in the treacherous Asian forests. Only those with exquisite self-control—with body power and emotional self-sufficiency—can survive.[34]

Perhaps, too, the whole wellness ethic is a response to this social upheaval. All societies seem to need rituals for ensuring salvation and criteria for measuring goodness. The chaos of the sixties and seventies had overturned the traditional morality of the fifties, and few would condone a return to that system in which sexual freedom, divorce, single mothers, high-achieving women, and homosexuality were condemned. Nor could conventional religions easily reclaim adherents—though a notable number of ex-radicals, called the "new conservatives," were returning to them. But after the excesses of the sixties and seventies Americans seemed to need some sort of reaffirmation of values and rules for clean living. The fitness ethic, in part, fills that need. It restores some order, some hierarchy of values. It provides a code of conduct by which we can judge ourselves. It is, perhaps, the only suitable religion for a secular age, the only outlet for those seeking a clear moral system, or spiritual comfort, or salvation.

One can't help but wonder, too, whether much simpler motives drive the exerciser: loneliness and a sense of meaninglessness. Lipsyte described a man he had met at his gym. The man happened to remark that his kids were available only for "quality" time, his lawyer-wife had gone to jog after poring over briefs. He had no intentions of putting extra time into his firm, which was talking about merging into a mega-corporation. He simply had nothing else to do—and nothing else to strive for. The passion for exercise may be a way to assuage the loneliness of modern life, a way to put meaning back into lives that seem busy but strangely purposeless. The forced happiness that characterizes all the fitness ads and all the ads that use fitness to sell their products, speaks to a generation that has always expected happiness but is confused about how to achieve it. These ads lure us with expectations of the quick fix we once got from drugs, or of the religious rapture that has been lost in a secular age.[35]

All of these forces buttress the fitness ethic and give it its special power. The fit person is a fashionable and a romantic image. The vast majority of the fitness faithful want to capture this image as their own. Fashion's deepest persuasive power has always been on this level. People seek the qualities, the gestalt, symbolized by a particular style—even if they have to go to painful extremes to realize it in the flesh. Vanity and hope drive them. Fashion has great power, especially when its extremes are stridently reinforced by every authority in society and when no one stands up to mock or question their validity. People want to look fit for the same reason they have obeyed other fashion rules: They need to see that gleam of approval and respect in the eyes of those who behold them. Today, this need is especially pressing. We have little inner self-confidence because of the breakdown both of social institutions that once provided approval and security and of other values with which we judge ourselves—such as the church, family, and community. Women, like men, are not warring with death and disease as much as they are striving to *look* like they are conducting that war—or as much as they are trying to define themselves. And they have turned that war into a religion, in part to find meaning and structure in their lives.

The fitness ethic has affected women even more powerfully than men. It has escalated their war on fat and on their bodies. They struggle for fat-free bodies that surge with energy and strength, yet they try not to feed them; they strive for weightlessness yet weight-lifting abilities, for the celebration of female empowerment through masculinized bodies; for the strength to break any bonds that might chain them by chaining themselves to a ritual of self-control. The strong body symbolizes a Promethea Unbound, and yet it is still Promethea Bound. It is almost as though, in some cruel historical consistency, women's bodies remain the terrain on which cultural ambivalence is played out. They have won new physical and social freedoms, but with them came the imperative for a neverending ritual of self-control. Historian Norbert Elias observed that the civilizing process has entailed the exchange of external controls on behavior for internal controls. The new permissiveness in sexual conduct, body exposure, and gender roles certainly has eroded traditional external controls, but culture, as though following some primal law of balance, has exacted a price. They have been replaced by new, more potent internal constraints. The empowered woman is to have none of the traditional feminine, or human, needs for physical and emotional nourishment: food, protection, financial support, children, security, or love.[36]

It is a difficult standard for most of us poor mortals to meet, fettered as we are by all-too-human weaknesses. The new body standard has proved equally difficult to meet. The exhilaration of women's enfranchisement into body power has had a vicious underside. Women feel their bodies never quite measure up. Thin is never thin enough. Fit is never fit enough. Physical perfection remains elusive. The fitness craze has not freed them from concern about their physical appearance, nor from trying to live up to externally imposed standards, nor from their wars with their own bodies. It has done just the reverse.

12

Why Thin Is Never Thin Enough

Amidst wealth and success, Karen Carpenter dies from the long-term effects of starvation. Jane Fonda confesses to past anorexic and bulimic behavior—she used to gorge and purge. Statistics vary, but some estimate that as many as 5 to 10 percent of adolescent and young women may have anorexia nervosa and that perhaps 25 to 30 percent of college women are bulimic. These are not the only age groups affected. When *Seventeen* ran an article on bulimia, the UCLA Eating Disorder Clinic received thousands of letters from desperate fourteen- to sixteen-year-old girls, some of whom said they had been binging and gorging for six years. Similar publicity also brought letters from women in their late thirties and early forties who had been bulimic since adolescence. While some experts question these figures, none dispute that the incidence of eating disorders has risen dramatically in the past twenty years. And none deny that a vast majority of us will flirt with these extremes—or with weight-loss rituals only marginally less bizarre and drastic—if we have not already done so. We think we are too fat. Again, statistics vary, but at least 75 percent of us with normal or below-normal weights think we need to lose a few more pounds. Food, weight, diets, and exercise dominate our thoughts and conversations, as they dominate the magazines we read, the television programs we watch, and the beauty and health advice we hear.[1]

We are never thin enough to believe we are not fat. We are never taut enough to believe we are not flabby. We can never diet and exercise enough to believe we do not have to diet and exercise more. Our new religion has trapped us in a painful and futile quest. It offers no salvation, only a perpetually escalating cycle of sin and precarious redemption.

In the preceding chapters, we saw the multiple developments that made a preference for slenderness snowball, accumulating deeper resonances along the way, into a new religion. The imperative to be thin became monolithic as fashion's decrees were reinforced and pushed by all cultural authorities—the health industry, the federal government, employers, teachers, even religious leaders, and parents—until the concept became so self-sustaining, so internalized, that no reinforcement was necessary. Even Ancel Keys, one of the few experts who disputed the overweight-disease link, called the fat body "disgusting" and pointed to the fat in our food and in our blood, not that on our figures, as a pathogenic agent. These authorities had not fabricated a conspiracy of lies to hoodwink and oppress us. They were trying sincerely to find solutions to the most common modern illnesses. The fitness gurus were not trying to put something over on us, either. Jane Fonda, for example, comes across as very likeable, very open, and more than eager to help and reassure others.

But our judgments, and even those of scientists, are shaped by larger cultural values and concerns. The ideas that animal fat of any kind is repulsive and/or dangerous, a mortal threat to the body politic itself, and that we should eradicate it, developed in response to specific historical conditions. Many of these ideas date back to the nineteenth century, but were fully elaborated only in the twentieth century. They were an almost panicked reaction to modernization, affluence, and the democratization of American culture. More generally, they were an effort to exert control in a world where change seemed to race ahead with a momentum of its own, beyond human control. And finally, they supplied a new set of social truths. They resonated with American values—self-help, egalitarianism, perfectionism—and, at the same, filled the vacuum created by the collapse of other traditional values during the sixties and seventies.

And still, women were as affected—if not more affected—by the fact that slenderness was deemed beautiful as by the fact that it was deemed healthy, correct, or liberating. And because this beauty standard was endorsed so thoroughly by the culture—even by those institutions that traditionally had put restraints on the pursuit of beauty by condemning it as a sin of vanity and false values, and often, as unhealthy—it had special potence. But traps were hidden in the imperative to be slim, traps that at once seduced women and made failure inevitable.

Women were seduced by the new beauty standard in part because, as we saw, it was ideologically acceptable. It seemed egalitarian: The rich presumably had no unfair advantage in the competition for beauty, since it involved the body, not clothing, and so character, not money. It also resonated with feminist values, apparently liberating women from the traditional oppressions of fashion. The older generation went through a radical process of consciousness changing to arrive at this new definition of beauty; the younger, yuppie-age generation inherited it and, for them, its assumption is tacit.

But ideologically appealing as the fit/lean standard is, it has not liberated women from fashion. Instead, women have adopted a liberated fashion. It is full of inner contradictions that sabotage its ideological goals. As we saw in the foregoing pages, the new fashion has proved as elitist in its way as older fashions were. Few women have the time or money to work out for hours at the gym everyday, sun themselves long enough to get the perfect tan, get jacuzzi-bathed and massaged, or feed themselves those perfect, healthy, low-calorie meals when work, family pressures, and financial straits demand they do otherwise. And though American society and fashion itself have been liberalizing in the past decades, the ideal female body standard has become increasingly rigid and narrow. A more homogeneous, smaller society might have had better luck coming up with an anthropometric type that many tended to have, but in heterogeneous America, the historical melting-pot, this was well-nigh impossible. The ideal was biased against women not from northern European ethnic and racial backgrounds, whose genes tend to make living up to this lean, tall standard more difficult.

The perfect body is simply a new status symbol—one that was partially a reaction against the increasing democratization in fashion and in American society, where expectations of social mobility were heightened at the same time that they became more difficult to achieve. With the badges of upward ascent—expensive-looking clothing—suddenly available to even modest pocketbooks, how else could people distinguish themselves from those below them on the social ladder? The perfect, pampered body emerged as a vital outlet for one of fashion's most traditional functions: the game of competitive display.

There is another deception in the current standard. Whether we call it "natural" or "affirming your own uniqueness," we have simply established a new ideal women feel they must meet. The shift in emphasis from external adornments to the body underneath has produced a standard of beauty far more literally physical and physically exacting than any that preceded it.

The new fashion set standards in subtler ways as well. Women quickly, and probably unconsciously, began to imitate the strong, confident gait, gestures, posture, and movements glorified by film stars and the women's magazines—just as they imitated the slouch of the 1920s and the graceful droop of the 1830s. These, too, are fashion standards we try to meet. "Natural," by definition, seems antithetical to civilization which, as it molds the human animal into a social animal and so, into a human being, imposes constraints and codes of conduct and aesthetic values. It is especially antithetical to fashion, the plastic art that tries to help us humble, imperfect mortals meet prevailing standards of beauty. No matter how comfortable and casual our current dress practices are, we have not only been unable to dispense with the obligation to fulfill aesthetic standards—which may be impossible to do in any society—we have also failed to produce a more generous, relaxed standard. We have created an equally—if not more—rigid and compelling one. Why else would we need "natural makeup" to make us look natural?

In a rather cruelly literal twist, we have indeed developed a beauty standard based on the power to act rather than on the power to attract. It *is* based explicitly on performance: the ability to diet and exercise. These became direct tools—moral imperatives for what *Vogue* in 1980 heralded as "The New Discipline"—in the struggle for beauty. Living up to the new fashionable standard became a test of moral character, of a woman's ability to control her impulse to eat, or at least to compensate for it through exercise.[2]

As we have seen, the whole culture placed paramount value on the ability to control appetite and body size. Overindulgence with food was seen as the pathogenic agent of modern diseases and as a trait of the newly enriched classes who hadn't yet learned to act with restraint and refinement in the midst of plenty. The size of the body assumed overwhelming importance. So did the number of pounds we gained and lost. Paradoxically, while superficial appearance was increasingly scoffed at as unimportant, the appearance of the body was being tied indissolubly to moral character. We literally seemed to believe we could judge a person's character by his or her body shape. It became a measure of goodness. We had come to see our weight as the physical embodiment of our moral will.

This moral component has given the lean body ideal a special and rather destructive power. Fashion has always reflected, to some extent, the morals and preferred behavior of its era. The Steel Engraving Lady of the 1830s, for example, resonated with a sensitivity, demureness, and otherworldliness valued at the time. But today our beauty ideal does not merely echo these associated values. We have developed a specific, mathematical way to measure and to test them—one certainly cruder than any others in the annals of fashion: the clothing size we wear and the number of pounds we have lost or gained. Sadly, we do not just judge others by these criteria. We have internalized these standards and judge ourselves according to them even more harshly than we judge others. The slightest increments on the bathroom scale—amounts so small that they are physically invisible and would be unnoticed on someone else—become sources of shame and despair. We have adopted the crudest and most baldly physical standards to judge our beauty and our inner worth.

Although men generally are not aware of those minor flaws that strike women as tragic disfigurements, and although they tend to be much less stringent about desirable female weights, they, too, are caught up in this mystical numerology. In accord with the new social values, they believe that two statistics—height and weight—describe beauty or ugliness. At a ski resort recently, I overheard one male instructor trying to convince another to go on a blind date. His description of the woman in question was: "She's 5'4" and weighs 105." His friend, visibly impressed, replied, "She sounds beautiful."

Ironically and sadly, this "liberated" standard gives men as much, if not more, power over women as traditional ones did. The conviction that all women *can* make themselves slender and taut gives men the prerogative to ask them to do so. And women yield this prerogative because they also believe that their weights and shapes are a matter of choice and, perhaps more importantly, reflect their inner worth. The standard thus gives men the right to demand that women change their bodies in accord with their erotic fantasies: lose weight, firm up a sagging belly, behind, or inner thigh. It also creates expectations that can cause, or be blamed for, sexual tension and disappointment—with the woman's body always at fault. In a larger sense, it provides a potent masculine weapon. A husband's critique of his wife's body can be a useful and devastating means of venting other hostilities. She is defenseless against it. She has heard repeatedly that she should be physically near-perfect, or at least working on becoming so. The failed body reveals a failed soul.

For all these reasons, the slim ideal has tremendous power over us. Yet it contains not only philosophical, but also physical, contradictions and distortions. We are incessantly told that if we just diet and exercise enough, we can look like the ideal. But for most people, the new standard of slenderness is too extreme for any kind of normal life or impulse. We cannot achieve it unless we fight the natural tendencies of our flesh through ascetic and punishing—and ultimately, impossible and self-defeating—rituals of diet and exercise. We don't see this trap in our new ideology, a trap that makes failure inevitable.

Very few women, unless they're starving or naturally thin, gravitate to the weights now considered "ideal." We often hear that fatness has never been considered beautiful. Hugh Hefner insisted that young, slender maidens have always been the only paragons of erotic beauty. This, of course, is untrue historically, and it is certainly untrue when we look at other cultures. What most people, like Hefner, do not realize, and what I have tried to underline in this book, is that although slenderness has been in vogue since the turn of the century, the definition of "slender" has changed dramatically, as have the definitions of "plump" and "fat." They are relative terms. In our own time, slim has come to border literally on an anorexic body type. When Twiggy burst upon the scene, even fashion pros were shocked by her emaciation. The Twiggy days may be behind us, but the visual standard of normalcy they established is not. Our new ideal is not as achingly skinny as Twiggy, but she is not much bigger, either, and she is virtually devoid of body fat. For this reason, the beauties of the fifties still look voluptuous to us, and someone once called "pleasingly plump" is now deemed fat. We have, in effect, a collective distortion in our image of what the female body should look like. Recent estimates suggest that our models and actresses are all at the slimmest end of the weight-distribution curve for American women: Only 5 percent of the female population falls into this category. These weights are hardly normal, let alone even close to average. The other 95 percent of us must diet and exercise fervently in order to be "thin enough."[3]

A glance at the habits of our beauty professionals is evidence of what extreme measures must be taken to meet these standards. Victoria Principal, Jane Fonda, Donna Dixon, and others proudly report their near-starvation diets and their hours of punishing exercise—and assure us that with the same efforts, we can look as good as they do. Perhaps it is even more significant that Miss America contestants are following the same course, since the Miss America competition represents a symbolic heartland of acknowledged "normality." *People* described the habits of Kylene Barker, the 1978 Miss America. After an exhausting day of public appearances, she sat down for a dinner that consisted of "a pair of appetite suppressing candies with a black coffee chaser" and then "she permitted herself a salad and a Perrier." In 1983 Miss California, Shari Ann Moskau, was having a harder time. She had gained 20 pounds since winning the state title. The local pageant committee was distraught and, in accord with popular orthodoxy, accused her of lacking discipline. Shari had lost 10 of the 20 pounds but was told to diet and exercise more strenuously to lose 8 more pounds in just four days. Shari was a victim of our extreme slenderess standard: Though she stood at 5'7", she was being urged to get down to 115 pounds—a weight that even the very conservative MLIC deemed desirable for a woman four inches shorter than Shari.[4]

These, and others like them, are the physical models most women try to emulate. They are well below the weights established by the MLIC, but even the MLIC "desirable" weights are substantially below the national average. Once again, both popular and official spheres are colluding in the creation of an unrealistic standard. And because acceptable body size has become so rigid and narrow—we don't even have the old choice between being a voluptuous Playmate or a thin *Vogue* type—our only options seem to be "fatness" or neverending rituals of semistarvation and exercise.

Thin can never be thin enough in part because exterior standards keep moving toward an extreme. Our current variation of this ideal—the taut, fat-free, muscled female—is also an impossible extreme. It resembles the body of a sixteen-year-old athletic boy, of a youthful Apollo. It is not the body of a woman. And the effort to get it, to put on muscles—even just enough of them to make every ounce of flesh taut and firm—catches us in a similar vise. We must battle our own biologies, our anthropometric typology. Few can develop this look without strenuous, punishing exercise and diet. And even then, it is hard to shed the telltale traces of softness and curves common to the female form.

Female bodybuilders are acutely aware of this problem. The press is full of tales about the rigorous low-calorie diets they follow to get their fat-to-lean ratios low enough for their muscles to show through. Many also restrict their liquid intake to avoid the fluid retention that puffs out flesh. And still others also use the dangerous and controversial drugs, steroids, to help build muscle mass and shed their female traits. They may have a superhealthy look but they certainly do not use health-promoting techniques to get it. Much as it is promoted as a panacea for physical transformations, exercise—even when pursued as a full-time occupation, as it is by many competitive bodybuilders— cannot easily masculinize the female body, nor can it even significantly alter the bulges, cellulite, flab, and other flaws that inevitably seem to adorn female flesh.

These failures stem from an even deeper trap in our lean ideal, one that has dogged women since boyish slenderness came into vogue. The effort to shed fat stores, whether to achieve a straight and sleek form or a muscled and taut one, sets women on an unrealistic quest. Although some women are born with this body type, physical anthropology suggests it is more typical of males than females. The idea that biology is destiny is not very popular today, but it is a reality that cannot be ignored. Nature seems to demand that the female of our species keep a supply of extra adipose tissue and, in this respect, females are inherently different from males. They simply were not genetically programmed to look like young Apollos or to be as fat-free as males. Our masculinized female ideal forces us into a campaign to reorganize our own biologies. For this reason, women who try to shed fat face insuperable odds: They are squeezed between ever-leaner body standards and a biology that favors fat storage.

From birth, girls generally have a higher fat-to-lean ratio than boys and, by the prepubescent stage, they have 10 to 15 percent more fat than boys, a finding that cuts across geographic and ethnic boundaries. These differences become most dramatic at puberty. Boys' puberty is characterized by gains in lean body mass and decreases in fat to about 10 to 15 percent of their body weight. For girls, just the opposite occurs: Their fat-to-lean ratio increases. In fact, a certain fat-to-lean ratio, estimated at about 22 percent, must be established for menstruation to begin and continue. Although the mechanisms are not clearly understood, it appears that as women proceed with maturation, their metabolic and endocrine systems tend to conserve or add to fat stores. Each pregnancy reinforces this tendency. By the time she is in her forties or fifties the normal woman has about 38 percent body fat and has gained about twenty to thirty pounds. These anthropometric changes are not unique to the industrially advanced Western nations. They are norms characteristic of the female of the species.[5]

These biological facts have very visible effects. The extra padding or fat added at puberty is what keeps women's skin smooth and soft, unlike the skin of adult males. It is also why women's body shapes are so much more variable than men's. "Fat," physical anthropologist Anne Scott Beller explained, "is an almost infinitely expandable and plastic tissue" and causes the greater "plasticity in women's shapes and sizes as opposed to men's" as well as the greater "modulation and relief of the female figure." This fact is reflected in clothing manufacturers' methods for standardizing sizes. In the United States, sixteen different sets of measurement sites are needed for women's garments, while only two to six are needed for men's. Few of us can avoid the fleshiness that comes with puberty and maturity.[6]

Biology confounds women in another way as well. That extra adipose tissue is deposited not only as an extra layer—or as extra bulges—under the skin, but also accumulates in very well-known spots: the breasts, hips, and thighs. For some women, this fat has a particular kind of dimpled connective tissue, known today as that cursed blight, cellulite. It is easy to see why 73 percent of the respondents in *Glamour*'s study of women's body attitudes complained most about their hips and thighs. The whole "weight" of our culture has combined to convince us that what is normal for women is abnormal and excessive. In 1985 fashion writer Eugenia Chandler, in her book *The Venus Syndrome,* went so far as to argue that big hips and thighs were a "medical problem" and even pointed to the Paleolithic statue, the Venus of Willendorf, to prove that "the problem has troubled women ever since." The Willendorf Venus and other female statues from the Paleolithic have troubled many modern observers. They are essentially globular, with fat, pendulous breasts, stomachs, and thighs. They assault our faith that these are unnatural flaws caused only by modern excesses in eating and inactivity. And, like Chandler, many cannot accept the possibility that such statues might have been fertility or erotic symbols. They have so internalized our modern ideal that they forget well-fleshed behinds and thighs adorned with dimples have been considered natural as well as erotic and beautiful until our own century.[7]

There is another way in which biology makes our current standards insidious. If men's weights and appetites can remain stable from month to month, women's are typically unstable. The menstrual cycle causes monthly fluctuations on the scale and can create irregular appetite patterns. Just before menstruation, when progesterone levels are high, many women feel a voracious hunger that does not abate until the cycle passes into its next phase. And many women retain fluids prior to their menses, which produces unnerving upward trends on the scales. Nor do men have to confront the dramatic weight gains and hormonal changes that accompany pregnancy. For many women, these gains can only be lost with great effort, and their effects are often irreversible, no matter how much we diet and exercise. With each pregnancy and lactation, skin and muscles lose a little more of their tone and elasticity, stretch marks deepen and spread, and breasts sag just a little lower. These are not regarded as marks of maturity, trophies of a body that has fulfilled its destiny and been marked with a fascinating map of its odyssey. Instead, they are regarded with shame. Hard as we work on them, our lived-in bodies refuse to be recycled into pristine neophytes—and they defy efforts to make them as predictable and regulable as machines.[8]

Oddly, these facts have led very few to question, let alone denounce, the creed of slenderness. Ever shaped by exterior impulses, few advocate standards of health or beauty that coincide more with women's systems, or condemn our punishing current standard. One of the saddest testaments to this blindness is *The Woman Doctor's Diet for Women* by Barbara Edelstein. After convincingly showing how female biology makes women's weights and appetites inherently unstable and their bodies plumper than our ideal, Dr. Edelstein doesn't conclude that women should learn to accept their extra fat. Instead, she simply presents yet another diet that is different "because it accounts for these changes." Even she doesn't point out that there is nothing natural about a woman who has shed, or tries to shed, every layer of fat from her body. If the women's press headlines, "Those Extra 5 Pounds—Don't Lose Them, Use Them," it has not really freed women from an impossible quest. Most of us have more than 5 pounds to lose to match this ideal, and it is as difficult for us to convert this fat to muscle as it is to lose it. The woman who tries to live up to our standard is likely to meet disappointment.[9]

Perhaps the cruelest trap of all is the notion that women should retain the bodies of youth even as they age. Health authorities insist that we keep the ideal weights of twenty-five-year-olds; fashion does the same. Yet, historically and cross-culturally, weight gain with age has been a normal phenomenon for both sexes. We didn't need the culinary plenty of modern times to make it happen. Health officials were always well aware of this tendency, as we have seen, but rather than allowing us to yield to it, they began to insist we combat it. The mature woman today believes she can and should retain the body of a teenager or a twenty-two-year-old. The same holds true for our effort to maintain low fat-to-lean ratios. Again, both men and women exchange muscle for fat as they age. Even the most avid exercisers cannot reverse this process, though they can slow it down. The average woman doubles her percentage of body fat as she hits forty or fifty. So does the average man—even when both manage to retain their youthful weights. Yet women—and men—are desperately trying to fight this tendency.

Maintaining a youthful form is not just difficult because of fat-to-lean ratios. In addition, the shape of the body changes with age. Physical anthropologist Anne Scott Beller, among others, observed that the silhouettes of young boys and girls are similar. With puberty, their silhouettes deviate radically, with women developing small waists and curving hips, thighs, and breasts, while boys become lean and narrow-hipped with big shoulder mass. But with middle age, they begin to resemble one another again. Waists thicken, male shoulders soften as lean mass diminishes, and women lose the slenderness of waist that characterized their early adult years—Joan Collins notwithstanding. We don't accept these changes. Despite all our reverence for the "natural," we feel compelled to fight passionately all these signs of aging. We see them as evidence of our failure to combat or "negotiate" with them. It takes even more effort for an older woman to meet the fashionable ideal. We are trapped precisely because we feel we can and should control this process. Just as we veered toward a unisex society in the sixties, so we veered toward a uni-age society. No one was supposed to look or act like they were over thirty-five. We welcomed this as liberation, but we have had to pay a price for it. Now all women, no matter what their age or social standing, believe they should resemble the nubile acrobats of the fashion pages. How successful can they be?[10]

Today's unrealistic body ideals came in tandem with, and perpetuated, obsessive regimens that are based on equally unrealistic premises. We traced the emergence of the idea that the amount of food people need can be determined by their weights: If they are overweight, then they are eating too much. And, just as our body standards moved to extremes, so did our notions about human caloric needs: We came to believe that "overweight" people do not need food to function. Americans who want to lose 5, 10, or 100 pounds believe their bodies can run on stored fat and on noncaloric nutrients and supplements like vitamins. This distorted premise leads us to try "undereating"—and to fall into yet another trap in our creed. Undereating does not make us healthier, happier, or thinner. It is physically and psychologically punishing and, as a result, also usually self-defeating.

Food deprivation triggers food obsessions and cravings for both physical and psychological reasons. People get hungry. Historical and current descriptions of dearth and famine, and scientific studies about the biology of human starvation have shown repeatedly that when calorie intake is reduced, even if all essential nutrients are present, several dramatic things occur. The undernourishment produces lassitude, depression, and irritability. Body metabolism slows down in order to conserve energy stores (the "plateau" of stabilized weight dreaded by so many dieters); sensitivity to cold increases; and energy expenditure declines either through reduced activity levels or less efficient movement. And hunger drives the hungry person to obsess about food.

The classic semistarvation study was conducted by physiologist Ancel Keys at the University of Minnesota near the end of World War II. Keys hoped to find what the condition and needs of populations in war-torn Europe would be after liberation. He began an experiment with young, healthy, conscientious objectors who volunteered to live at the University for six months and to eat prescribed rations similar to the meager, monotonous diets forced on the victims of war. These young men, all with strong moral commitments, changed dramatically. From being pleasant, well-adjusted, and active, they became withdrawn, depressed, and lethargic. Their interests narrowed and they were obsessed with food even in their dreams. When the experiment ended, they could not control their ravenous appetites. Not until their prediet fat-to-lean ratios had been restored did they finally return to normal. On 1,700 calories a day—more than many modern diets recommend—and on a diet much like those advocated today—lots of fresh vegetables, complex carbohydrates, and very little meat—these men were slowly starving.[11]

Hilde Bruch was one of the few researchers to see the remarkable parallels between these starvations studies and the vast literature on the overweights' dieting problems. It repeatedly chronicled behavior and reactions like those of Keys's subjects. Researchers found them among dieting obese patients, and Bruch found them especially among what she called "thin fat people"— women who managed to maintain their stylish figures only through compulsive dieting. Dr. Albert Stunkard described "dieter's depression," and some researchers found obese people veering toward psychosis during stringent diets.[12]

After reviewing both sets of literature, Bruch astutely concluded that starvation and semistarvation trigger primitive physical and psychological responses. Morals and taboos are forgotten in the drive for survival. The cannibalism of the Donner Party during their entrapment in a snowbound mountain pass in 1880 is only one extreme example of the powerful compulsions hunger unleashes. Bruch noted that with progressive degrees of semistarvation, there is a coarsening of emotions, sensitivity, and other humane traits. One of her most interesting observations was that anorexic patients exhibited remarkably uniform behavior and emotional patterns until they gained some weight. Only then did their individual problems and personalities emerge. These had been submerged beneath responses typical of the starving human organism, even though their starvation was self-imposed.[13]

Most dieters don't reach these extreme states precisely because food is available to them and they eat it. But they are essentially no different than the victims of externally imposed hunger. They are often trying to subsist on the same number of calories and they, too, are chronically hungry. They are expected to function cheerfully and competently on the starvation or semistarvation rations we now deem appropriate for overweight people. When they complain of lassitude and depression, of obsessions about food, doctors accuse them of lack of motivation and weakness of character. Quite simply, they are hungry. And they usually succumb, voraciously, to their very human need for food. Like Keys's subjects, many are unable to stop their weight gain until they restore their former fat levels—and then some. This pattern of behavior has been described widely as the *yo-yo syndrome,* and it has been blamed for many cases of obesity. Experts call it *diet-induced obesity,* and today many suggest that physiological and psychological mechanisms are responsible for it.

There are other, more exclusively psychological reasons dieting is self-defeating. Bruch suggests there is a primitive psychological terror of hunger which, at least throughout most of human history, has proved to be a fortunate survival instinct. Even after hunger has ended, the nagging terror of it remains. She noted that a disproportionately large number of concentration camp victims became obese once they resumed normal lives. Some orphans adopted from poverty-stricken countries cannot control their compulsion to smuggle and hide food, sometimes even after living for years in secure culinary environments. Researchers have even reported that some people exhibit the emotional traits of semistarved individuals just at the prospect of a diet, before caloric deprivation could have triggered them. The terror of hunger seems to run deep in the human psyche in ways modern researchers do not yet understand.[14]

Recent research has shown another nemesis in dieting, one common among comfortable Americans. The very effort to avoid food triggers cravings for it. Banned foods become the focus of intense inner conflict as would-be reducers struggle between the urge to eat them and the compulsion to avoid them. Keys's volunteers became terrified of going outside the experiment environment where they would be tempted by the foods they had agreed not to eat. When they did succumb, these once normal young men returned to the researchers with hysterical, half-crazed confessions about their lapses, their failure at control. Dieters who yield after a similarly bitter struggle often find themselves plunged into eating binges which they feel they cannot control.

A landmark study conducted in the 1970s at Northwestern University shed new light on the psychological dynamics that cause these patterns. Psychologist Peter Herman did not investigate the behavioral differences between fat and thin people, as his colleagues had been doing, but rather the differences between slender people who dieted to keep their weights low and those who were "naturally" slim. He used as subjects a group ideally suited to mirror the diet compulsions of the era: sorority girls. He found a startling difference between the girls who constantly tried to diet, whom he called *restrained eaters,* and those who didn't, the *unrestrained eaters.* When the former felt they had "blown" their diets by eating the ice cream required in the experiment, they ate far more than hunger would dictate and far more than their unrestrained sisters. They explained that since they had broken their diets anyway, they had decided to splurge and enjoy all they could before resuming them.[15]

It is not surprising that women who binge report binge-eating on high-calorie sweets and snack foods. These are the very foods they struggle to resist in order to "get thin." It is also not surprising that many in the seventies theorized there was something addictive about sugar and other "junk" foods. They are prohibited on most diets. The problem is, they taste good. Many struggling dieters find themselves doing what the restrained eaters in Herman's study did: splurging, even gorging on taboo foods once they have yielded to the temptation to eat them. They attribute the ungovernable voracity they feel to some addictive quality in the foods rather than to the more likely cause: They have violated their self-imposed controls, and in a frenzy of release, tried to satisfy their bottled-up urges before resurrecting those controls. Feminist psychotherapists such as Susie Orbach and Kim Chernin discovered the same phenomenon. Once women felt they were entitled to eat what they wanted, when they wanted, and as much as they wanted, their obsessions about food diminished. With this "permission" to eat, their conflicts about food dwindled, and the crazy careening pattern of alternately binge-eating and starving also subsided.[16]

There is nothing inherently abnormal about people eating in spates of gluttony, but culture imposes limits on behavior, especially on how basic bodily functions are carried out. In earlier times, voracious eating was considered normal, and a gargantuan appetite was often associated with nobility. With the rise of courtly and bourgeois manners, from the Renaissance on, more and more self-control over bodily functions was required for people who had any pretension to good breeding. Each time new constraints were imposed on these once innocent functions, new areas of psychic conflict emerged as individuals battled against their impulses to meet the standards of their class and culture. Gluttonous eating was one practice, among many, that ceased to be acceptable. Today, with our anorexic body ideal, we have set up a standard of eating behavior that compels millions to exert tremendous control over their hunger and their appetites. Just as fat appears to us as a physical symbol of unrestrained, uncivilized behavior, so does the self-indulgent, abandoned eating we believe produces it. We have turned eating into a conflict-ridden issue. Our very system of culinary moralism—with its healthy "good" and unhealthy "bad" foods—invests food and eating with extraordinary symbolic significance.[17]

This powerful conflict explains why so many normal women have turned eating into a pathologic problem and why so many have developed eating disorders. Feminist psychotherapists, among others, have come up with mythopoetic explanations for this modern epidemic. In her most recent book on the subject, *The Hungry Self,* Kim Chernin argued that women's complicated relationships with their mothers are the cause. Women want to be like their unliberated mothers, yet they don't want to be like them at all. They want to devour them, to absorb their identities, but they also want to reject them. Because mothers are our physical and emotional nurturers, these conflicts are expressed around our source of nurture, food. Undoubtedly, feminism has made the mother-daughter relationship more complicated, but such psychoanalytic theories continue to regard food exclusively as a symbol and eating exclusively as a metaphoric act and thereby miss the more likely reason eating disorders have become widespread.[18]

Neither anorexia nervosa nor bulimia are modern inventions, but eating problems have become widespread precisely because our society has set up control of appetite as the new virtue. Authorities tell us how many calories we should eat and how many should make us feel full. They also tell us what our body size should be. Women's food problems seem to stem, not from ambivalence about their mothers, but from their effort to get an ultralean body, one that every cultural authority assures them is normal, accessible, and a badge of good breeding. They have internalized this cultural value in the same way they internalize other values. But the only way women not genetically endowed with this body type—more than 95 percent of them—can hope to meet it is by putting themselves on deprivatory diets. They inevitably are whirled into the mind-set of the restrained eater, and sometimes beyond it. Or, following the pernicious dicta of our era, that we virtually do not need food, they are whirled into the physical and emotional state of people who are semistarved. And their perpetual cycles of defeat—in binging and weight gain—take a terrible toll on their psychological well-being and on their feelings of self-esteem and self-worth.

Psychological problems unrelated to food undoubtedly do contribute to eating disorders. Nonetheless, it seems likely that these problems are manifested through eating because it has become the conflict-ridden instinct of our era, much as Victorian women manifested their problems through sexual dysfunction, the conflict-ridden instinct of that era. Their specific problems with food, like those of their psychologically healthier sisters, derive from the battle they are waging against their appetites and their bodies.

Indeed, some researchers now suggest that stringent dieting may trigger anorexia nervosa in individuals with particular biochemical make-ups, which would explain why only a few women cross the line from dieting to pathology. For them, chronic undernutrition may cause neuroendocrine abnormalities which in turn create involuntary addiction to starving. Such dynamics—a biological predisposition interacting with a certain behavior—now often are also used to explain why only some drinkers become alcoholics. But in both cases, exposure is essential. Alcoholics must have their first taste of liquor; anorexics must go on their first diets. In short, the inordinate value we place on 'undereating' and on skinniness has not solved our weight problems. It has created pathologies with food.[19]

Of course, not all dieters fail. There are probably millions of women—at least 5 percent of us—who manage to diet their weights down permanently but who never appear in the statistics because they do not join official weight-loss programs. But they, too, often careen between binge-eating and dieting. And they have other problems. To maintain a body weight below what was natural for them, such fashionably thin women kept themselves on painfully low-calorie diets. Bruch found them irritable, tense, fatigued, and full of vague emotional complaints, not unlike those of Keys's undernourished subjects. And they were strained by their ritual of self-control, by their fear that one slip-up would make them fat. Like fugitives, they could not shed the feeling they were being shadowed by a sinister force. Doctors prescribed tranquilizers for them; Bruch suggested that three square meals a day would have been a much more effective prescription. By 1980 more and more researchers were acknowledging the considerable emotional and physical consequences of chronic dieting, including "symptoms such as irritability, poor concentration, anxiety, depression, apathy, liability of mood, fatigue and social isolation . . ."[20]

Bruch justly complained that fat people were condemned for their selfishness and thoughtlessness when it was really these dieting women who had sacrificed their calm, their sense of well-being, and their productivity at the altar of Dame Fashion. Yet today, both men and women boast about their self-imposed undernutrition—a value perfectly captured by the new diet product, "Undereat," which is advertised with the venerated resolve: "I will undereat at breakfast; I will undereat at lunch; I will undereat at dinner. I will undereat"—and expect the world to applaud them for it. They certainly look good by our modern standards, and we, looking at them, cannot see the price they pay to get their weight down just a few more pounds. They don't see it, either. They are so blinded by the promise of how good they will feel if they undereat that they don't recognize how badly they really feel—or if they do, they attribute it to other problems. Dieting, even when it is called "a permanent change in eating habits," as it is today, is counterproductive.[21]

Women are sabotaged by their efforts to diet for another reason as well. Despite the changes wrought by feminism, most women are still the nourishers, the preparers and servers of the daily family meal. Mothers cannot ignore food and they cannot minimize its importance. They plan the family meals, stay up on the new nutritional rules, pack the children's lunches, and make sure the kids have nutritious, tasty snacks around. All this puts women dieters in a painfully vulnerable position. It is as hard for them to get the kitchen out of their minds as it is for them to get out of the kitchen.

What has been displaced is not only our sense of what constitutes normal eating but also what constitutes normal bodies. Women strive for a high degree of physical perfection and magnify their flaws into failings that merit self-hate because our whole culture has been seduced by the idea of physical perfectibility.

It is not surprising that we have unrealistic expectations. Today we have come to believe that the ideal body is the norm. In contrast to the past, when disease, disabilities, deformities, and discomforts were an accepted fact of everyday life, modern Americans are indeed privileged, a group of body aristocrats. While science certainly hasn't managed to cure all suffering and disease, it has radically changed our experience of our bodies. We expect to feel healthy and we expect to look good, and we have come to integrate techniques and disciplines that produce them—orthodontia, plastic surgery, and diets—into our idea of normalcy. The belief that we should dominate and even legislate our own biology has become standard.

Americans' egalitarian ideology, particularly in its present variation, contributes to these expectations. We don't just believe that everyone should have the same opportunities. We also believe that everyone can and should have the same achievements, and we try to alter the social conditions we believe prevent this. The same principles apply to body build. We are convinced everyone can meet the new beauty ideal.

Armed with these expectations, we compare ourselves to beauty professionals whose nude or seminude bodies are prominently displayed by our ever more pervasive and influential media. We assume there should be no gulf between them, the celebrities, and us, the average people. The media stars are as familiar to us as our next-door neighbors and, in this therapeutic, confessional age, they confide publicly about their personal and medical problems—though only a few decades ago, such information was shared only among intimate friends. The distance between us and them is constantly denied. They seem to be our peers, to people our immediate world, and we take them as our standard of normalcy.

This breeds grandiose expectations and a curious self-deception. We forget that models are chosen precisely for their unusual beauty, for their approximation of the ideal, their blemishes minimized by cameras, lights, angles, and touch-ups. We certainly know from home photographs and movies how some angles, hair styles, makeup, postures, and settings can make us look more attractive than others do—yet we forget to apply this knowledge to these models. We still expect our mirrors to reflect images that look like theirs.

Such expectations are especially unrealistic because they apply to the naked body. A recent issue of *Glamour* magazine brought home to me how much the near-naked models distort our notions about our own bodies. An article appeared about how to choose a bathing suit that would highlight strong points and camouflage flaws—no easy task for a bathing suit since it hardly covers anything. What was most striking was that the six girls who modeled the "right" and "wrong" suits happened to look like real women, the kind you see at the beach or in a locker room. They were not picture-perfect models. They were not fat, but they had all the ordinary flaws: One was top heavy, one was hippy, one had skinny, shapeless legs, one had a big stomach and no waist to speak of. These women were real. It is not clear whether *Glamour* intends to continue this policy. After all, fashion magazines are supposed to present ideals—albeit ones we can strive to meet—and to create a fantasy world of sorts, and the means for us to enter it. The problem today is that clothes will not bring this fantasy world into our own reality. Only the body underneath those clothes will.[22]

But efforts to achieve this perfect body are doomed because we are trapped in the dilemma of the naked versus the nude. The naked is the human body undressed. The nude is an art form, the naked body idealized, its flaws erased. The art historian, Sir Kenneth Clark, underscored the profound difference between the two. "A mass of bodies does not move us to empathy (i.e., artistic inspiration), but to disillusion and dismay. We do not wish to imitate, we wish to perfect." Art historians might shudder to hear these commercial pictures compared to the nude, but they have become our only stylized images of unclothed females. Modern artists no longer present us with competing, alternative images. Instead, they depict abstract forms or else, like Willem De Kooning and others, they incorporate pinups and modern movie stars into their works. But the distinction between the naked and the nude underscores why so many women have distorted body images and loathe their own shapes. They compare their naked bodies to these modern nudes, the advertisers' and filmmakers' images. When they scrutinize their mirrored reflections, they see only the imperfections and remain oblivious to the fact that in making beauty the body itself, our culture has blurred the distinctions between the naked and the nude, between the natural and art. The naked is not perfect. And our effort to make it so is a virtually Sisyphean task.[23]

This effort has had another disturbing effect. Much as we proclaim a unity of mind and body, much as we believe that how we look is how we feel, we end up disassociating ourselves from our very flesh. Just as we have distanced ourselves from food and hunger, so we have distanced ourselves from our bodies. We do not live harmoniously in them but rather in conflict with them. We don't mildly condemn their flaws, blaming ancestors who bequeathed us unfashionable genes, and then calmly accept this fate as we might accept the freckles or straight hair or height with which we were endowed. Instead, we fight our heredity and treat our bodies as things, raw forms that must be molded. We have developed an almost schizophrenic separation from our bodies, one endorsed by the whole culture. And we have come to regard them, not as the vessels through which we live and try to realize happiness and meaning in life, but as objects whose perfection will give us that happiness and meaning.

Our beauty celebrities may have legitimate reasons for seeking a high degree of physical perfection: Their bodies are the instruments of their trade. But it is puzzling that ordinary women also pursue it intensely—or feel that they should—even though they are not going to be captured on film and viewed and judged by millions, and even though their livelihoods do not depend on it. Certainly, appearance has always been crucial for men and especially for women—indeed, in every society, how an individual looks is a vital aspect of social interaction. There is an equally long history of outward appearance signaling inner worth. In our own era, however, there seems to be an unusually strong emphasis put on appearance and unusually strong pressure to make it perfect. This has occurred not only because we have pared appearance down to skin level and have adopted unrealistic body standards, but also because of the larger cultural and social changes we traced in the preceding chapters.

Strangers cannot help but judge us by our external appearance. But in societies where there is a clear-cut social hierarchy, people are defined as much, if not more, by their backgrounds and inherited status as by their looks. These "dress" them more than their clothing does. In societies where there is geographic and/or social stability, people rarely meet strangers, and those they do meet usually do not have a significant influence on their personal lives. Their social interactions occur primarily among people who are familiar with their personalities, their private histories, their strengths and weaknesses. Their physical appearance is simply one of their accepted traits, as familiar and unremarkable as the looks of family members and old friends. In the industrially advanced Western nations, the dilution of a firm social hierarchy and of geographic stability was part of the modernization process. This dilution was particularly pronounced in America, in part because of its ideology, which denied the legitimacy of social hierarchy and which encouraged geographic and social mobility. Appearance has become more crucial for Americans because they live, more than ever, in a world of strangers.

Americans have always been a peripatetic group, moving without qualm from one neighborhood, city, or state to another. But today such migrations occur more frequently and include more and more people. We keep moving farther away from our home bases, transferred by giant corporations, by new educational opportunities, or by the desire to try new options. Each time we move we have to introduce ourselves anew and impress others anew. Our social lives are also affected. We tend not to live around the people we grew up with, nor do we search for romance and mates among old and familiar groups. Instead, we thrust ourselves into the fiercely competitive environment of strangers and hope we can establish new ties. Women especially have put themselves "out there," leaving the relative intimacy of home and community for the public world of the marketplace. We have been as stripped of a given social identity as of concealing clothing. We are acutely aware that the image we project—our appearance—will be used to define us and will influence our success or failure. Our media-saturated experience reinforces this conviction. We have learned that visual image is vital: Even our presidents must be telegenic. As we live in a world increasingly peopled by strangers, our physical appearance becomes correspondingly more important. It is perhaps not so surprising, then, that ordinary women feel that they, too, will be scrutinized as carefully as the beauty professionals.

Part of our absorption of ideal physical standards is based on other expectations as well. Americans today have extraordinary expectations for themselves in all facets of life. They seem to regard the traditional avenues to happiness—a good job, a nice home, and family—as inadequate. They want to excel, to be stars at whatever they do. Historically, America had a powerful Perfectionist movement, which gradually unmoored itself from its religious roots and became an increasingly secular concept, one that merged with the ideology of the self-made man, the man who seizes social and economic opportunities and makes something of himself. Today we believe the individual can be perfect, not in a moral or spiritual sense, which seems to interest us very little, but in a worldly sense. We all aspire to do our personal best—to win health, wealth, beauty, and fame.

This is particularly true for the generations born after World War II. Their high expectations reflect their privileged childhoods and the promises of capitalist America. Children born in the middle classes and above, blessed with all that modern America has to offer—health, leisure, education, unlimited professional opportunities, and doting parents—see little reason to expect less than the best from themselves. *Vogue* recently captured this mood: "The moment we're born, our parents count us perfect. And perfect we try to continue to be . . . . " We don't accept limitations, partially because we have had so few of them. We don't believe in accepting fate with either graciousness or dignity.[24]

Our advertisement-saturated, consumer-oriented society further encourages us to search for perfection and to feel dissatisfied with what we have achieved. We have been assaulted with messages promising that personal problems—boredom on the job, conflicts at home and at work, ennui, and inner inadequacies—can be solved by ownership of various commodities and, indeed, that ownership of them will give us the "good life." We have come to identify inner feelings with commodities and so can believe that possession of things can magically affect us. As Christopher Lasch astutely pointed out, " . . . mass culture encourages the ordinary man to cultivate extraordinary tastes, to identify himself with the privileged minority against the rest." But it also breeds discontent and self-contempt, precisely because it fosters "grandiose expectations" that cannot possibly be met and that leave the consumer restless, ready to search for another product, another way to satisfy the longings it has created. A perfect female body is one of the central images in this iconography of commodities and the good life—almost as though it indeed were another commodity. Men have been led to believe that having this "thing"—a woman with a perfect body—will make them happy, and women have been led to expect that having it will make them happy, too. But just as the good life is never quite achieved, neither is the perfect body—or the satisfaction it is supposed to bring.[25]

These pressures toward perfectionism seem particularly acute among women, and the women's movement inadvertantly may have contributed to them. We saw how this movement and the rise of eating disorders seemed to follow a parallel course. Hilde Bruch and recent psychotherapists have speculated that as women's social role and very nature were being redefined, new and sometimes confusing expectations emerged. A young girl no longer feels it is enough just to be a pretty, nice, intelligent woman who settles comfortably into marriage and childrearing within her social circle. Instead, she feels she must excel and be something more than just what her mothers or peers are. So do adult women. They expect to be superachievers—professional successes, supermoms, superlovers, superwives, super–wage earners—and superlooking. Even more than men, they cannot settle into the life routines of their parents or accept traditional limitations. They have to improve their lives and their bodies. They can never be thin enough because they can never be perfect enough.

Their passion for physical perfection may also stem from another effect of both feminism and current social conditions. Women, like men, are curiously alone. Feminism's ideology of self-sufficiency—that women should need neither physical nor emotional nurturing, that they should be dependent on no one for their happiness, fulfillment, and financial support—encourages an individualism that borders on isolation. The extent of our prescriptive isolation is perhaps best encapsulated by some feminist justifications for abortion: The fate of the fetus is entirely a woman's choice because it is seen as affecting *only* the woman's body. The woman who carries a child need recognize no larger obligations to the prospective father, grandparents, other relatives, community, or society at large. She refuses to see her reproductive capacity as vitally significant to anyone but herself.

But this ideology also seems almost a legitimate response to new realities. Social and geographic mobility, the adversarial relations that now prevail even within businesses, the heightened competition for limited numbers of jobs, and, above all, the instability of personal relationships leave individuals feeling that they are indeed alone in a hostile world. Women have even been told that childbearing and childrearing alone are not worthy or fulfilling life goals. They are not to live passively through their children's accomplishments, but through their own—a principle that encourages them to leave home for the market-place and that may stand them in good stead if they end up among the growing ranks of single mothers whose living standard plummets while their divorced mates' improves. In any case, they are trying to raise children who will be independent enough to seize the geographic and social opportunities of a mobile society—and so, to leave them. In such insecure, competitive social conditions, a perfected body can be a form of insurance. But more importantly, these conditions have encouraged women to believe that fulfillment must come from what they provide for themselves. And one seemingly reliable avenue for such happiness is self-perfection—including a perfect body.

The saddest trap in our quest is precisely this expectation that physical perfection will make us happy. It is not surprising that 42 percent of the respondents in the *Glamour* survey cited earlier reported they would rather lose 10 or 15 pounds than find success in romance or careers—the very things that weight loss supposedly brings. We seem to believe it can transform our personalities and open possibilities we never imagined, as though extra pounds were barriers to some sense of inner worth and accomplishment—whether they are 100 or merely 5 pounds. We have already seen Hilde Bruch's sobering caution about such expectations. The thin person within is not different than the fatter person without. But as long as women believe the equation thinner/ fitter = happier, thin can never be quite thin enough, for how many of us manage to reach a state in which we can say we are happy and fulfilled? And how many of us can resist the hope that losing just a few more pounds, or firming up a flaccid thigh, will bring us the vague something that is missing in our lives? The myth itself is precious. To relinquish it would be to relinquish the very dream of self-transformation. We would be forced to accept ourselves as we already are.[26]

As long as we regard control of appetite and the battle against fat as morally virtuous, we are doing more than striving for self-transformation when we faithfully follow diet and exercise rituals. We are fulfilling our culture's pre-scriptions about civilized behavior and appearance, thereby earning respect from others and self-respect, for we are being good. We are engaging in a moral effort.

We have developed a mystical numerology in which fewer is always better, whether it be inches, pounds, dress sizes, or calories. This definition of good-ness is powerfully reinforced by the whole culture, particularly the people closest to us. The greeting, "You've lost weight," is always a compliment, especially because it is invariably accompanied by an admiring look. The comment, "You're so thin," is answered with a thank you and usually also with a full rendition of the methods that made it happen. It is these inter-changes that are the most powerful force leading us to try, perpetually, to become ever-thinner. It is through such social interactions that cultures pass on their values and imprint them within our very souls. This is yet another reason thin is never thin enough. How can we ever feel we have been good enough? And so we keep trying for ever-lower weights and ever-tauter bodies, never noticing that our culture has set up a female body standard that is antithetical to female biology.

In essence, we have come to value as "good" efforts to control the natural female form. We have already seen how feminist ideology contributed to a masculinized female ideal. Just as women were to suppress the soft and nurturing traits traditionally associated with them, so they were to suppress their soft and nurturing physical traits. Ironically, "oppressed" women seemed to want to resemble their male "oppressors." But we have also seen deeper impulses at work: The female body seems to remain the terrain on which cultural ambivalences are played out. As though following some primitive law of balance, our society gave women new freedoms and simultaneously, chained them to a neverending ritual of self-control.

In this exchange, there is a cruel historical consistency. More stringent controls are required of the female body than of the male. As we have seen, with the civilizing of manners, the unembarrassed, humorous acceptance of animal functions—belching, nose-wiping, farting, table manners, gluttonous eating, defecating, urinating, sweating, scratching, spitting, sex, masturbation, bawdy jokes—declined. Particularly among the middle classes, these behaviors were relegated to the private sphere or were buried in elaborate refinements. Curiously, however, these demands were much more stringent for women than for men. Today, in the male subculture, there is jocularity about and acceptance of them: Among boys, for example, farting, urinating, belching and masturbation are a common source of humor and even of playful contests. Men are entitled to these behaviors which do not compromise their masculinity, but, rather, often seem to confirm it. The reverse is true for women. When in all-female groups, and even when alone, such physical freedoms remain embarrassing, sources of shame, not playfulness. They compromise femininity, even femaleness. They are not accepted as natural to the female body. Not only does this difference profoundly divide men and women but, more important, it means that women have a very different sense of their bodies and natural functions than men do. Stringent self-control of the physical body lies at the heart of femininity. The diet-exercise imperative is simply another manifestation of this cultural rule.

A paradox seems to lie here, for women traditionally have been identified with nature, men with culture, yet men are afforded these physical liberties. But the paradox is superficial, for our masculinized ideal reflects a deeper impulse as well. Certainly civilization, and especially fashion, has always tried, to varying degrees, to mold the human animal into a human being through suppression or disguise of what are considered animalistic traits. But today the female body must be "dressed" with masculine characteristics precisely because female nakedness and all it symbolizes strikes us as vulgar and conflicts with some of our most cherished ideals about human beings.

The natural female body, with its primordial rhythms, transformations, and odors—evident during menstruation, pregnancy, lactation, and sexual excitation—and with its fleshy plasticity, seems primitive, almost an evolutionary anomaly in our technological and sanitized age. We have managed to so dominate nature that we fear we have irreversibly harmed the planet itself. We have even managed to engineer pregnancy without sexual intercourse. Our current social ideology even makes pregnancy an incidental, not a central, function of the female body. The naturally functioning and natural-looking female body, then, seems to be our last primitive vestige, an insult to our ability to control nature—and especially, to exert conscious, rational control over ourselves. The woman who disciplines this unruly physiology and form until it functions as predictably and smoothly as a machine—or as a male body—is indeed being good. She is civilizing her biology.

The desire to control nature also contributed to the imperative that all adults maintain the bodies of twenty-two-year-olds. We refuse to accept death or its ominous symptoms—aging. Those who "let themselves go" disturb us not so much because they look ugly as because they seem to be surrendering to nature—and so, ultimately, to death and decay. We place as much value on diet and exercise as on a lean body itself because we believe they are rituals for not surrendering, no matter how ineffective they are. Again, the female body holds a special place in this context. The ripe and fecund female is a symbol of fertility and regeneration, but as such, she is also a reminder of our humble animal origins, and of time, of the cycle of decay and death. Our current social ideology encourages us to live primarily for ourselves, which makes us recoil from reminders of new generations who pressage our own aging and death. With our current technocratic mentality, we also recoil from images of nature and death triumphant. Naked, fleshy female bodies then, strike us as vulgar and offensive. And women, absorbing these sensibilities, try to tame them, to "dress" them in masculinized form in order to fulfill modern civilization's deepest commands.

But the imperative to discipline this female body has taken its toll on women, and for good reasons. There are traps hidden in the new dogma which make failure inevitable. Our lean/fit standard has become extreme and overexacting. Few women can meet it. They don't see that it pits them against their own biology. The "healthy" look doesn't bring health. It brings hunger, and a dogged sense of failure. We can't see that the liberated fashion has enslaved us. Ironically, we also can't see that as liberated as we aspire to be, we have come to put our energies into perfecting our bodies, not our souls, minds, or character. We have not been freed from preoccupation with appearance.

Most women would deny they are perfecting their bodies just to be beautiful or good. Invariably, they claim they are doing it—or their disgruntled mates insist they are demanding it—for health. But the penultimate irony in our lust for leanness is that the very premises on which it is based are beginning to crumble. Thinner/fitter is not healthier. And thinner/fitter is not necessarily more beautiful. The very scaffolding of our war on fat has been a myth.

13

The Prejudice Exposed

Our society and our behavior are suspended in a paradox. All about us is a culture that sustains the fundamental belief that thinner and the techniques for thinning are healthier, sexier, happier, and more beautiful. It maintains with equal fervor the inverse: Fatter and the behavior that produces it are unhealthier, unhappier, and uglier. Yet, despite these convictions, high-level medical, sociological, and psychological studies, as well as the evidence we see at the popular level, indicate that these, the very pivots of our new religion, are based on fiction, even myth, not on scientific fact.

As we have seen, the principle source of our belief that thinner is healthier is life insurance studies, particularly as they were interpreted by Louis Dublin and the Metropolitan Life Insurance Company (MLIC). From them we derived six convictions:

1. There is a narrow weight range for each height that correlates with longest life expectancy, called "ideal" or "desirable" weight. Those whose weights are above this standard are overweight.
2. Thinner is always healthier. The graph plotting the relationship between weight and mortality is linear: The more one deviates above "desirable" weight, the higher the chances of premature mortality; the more one deviates below, the lower the chances. We have a sense that nobody can be *too* thin to be healthy.
3. Overweight is a primary cause of shorter life expectancy and of the most prevalent modern killer, cardiovascular disease. Although the original actuarial data did not link obesity and cancer, later studies associated obesity with uterine and breast cancer in women.
4. "Desirable" weights are well below average weights, so being normal is not healthy, and a vast number of adult Americans are unhealthily overweight.

5. It is unhealthy—and there is no reason—for adults to gain weight after the age of twenty-five, though this is the normal pattern. Here, too, normality and health are not equivalent.

6. Finally, and most important, weight loss prevents degenerative diseases and improves life expectancy.

Two presumptions underlie all these convictions: that fat is not a useful or protective tissue, but rather a pathogenic one, and that people can control their body weight. Dublin and the actuarial data provided the evidence and the justification for the national campaign for weight loss.

We have already discussed the flaws in these insurance studies and the experts who questioned or disagreed with their conclusions, but not until 1980 were there enough other, meticulously researched, large-scale, long-term, national and international studies to test the MLIC dicta. They came from Sweden as well as Oakland, California, from Yugoslavia and Macon, Georgia, from autopsy reports as well as from studies of different occupational groups. The results were startling: Whether evaluating scale weight or fat-to-lean ratios—and even when people who were thinner because of smoking, cancer, or some other pre-existing condition were carefully screened—they flatly contradicted all six convictions. None of them showed that thinner was healthier.[1]

One of the most thorough and respected of these investigations was the Framingham Study, begun in 1950. In order to determine the causes of cardiovascular disease, 5,209 men and women between the ages of thirty and fifty-nine were monitored for thirty years. In 1979 three of the Framingham researchers measured their data against the dicta of the MLIC. The result: The thinnest men in Framingham had the *worst* life expectancy and, otherwise, weight seemed irrelevant. The women in Framingham had a slightly higher mortality only if they were very thin or very fat. However, the belief that thinner is healthier was so deeply entrenched that some Framingham researchers, while acknowledging that these results were not unique to their study, could not accept their own findings with equanimity. They concluded that "... despite considerable exploration of the data, we do not have a comprehensive explanation for this finding." This kind of conservatism—and disbelief— continued to mark many weight-mortality studies.[2]

One of the most ambitious studies of the causes of cardiovascular disease was directed by low-cholesterol campaigner and internationally respected researcher, Dr. Ancel Keys. Over a twenty-five-year span, he and his associates evaluated populations in Japan, Greece, Italy, Yugoslavia, the Netherlands, Finland, and the United States. Their results, published in 1980 in *Seven Countries: A Multivariate Analysis of Death and Coronary Heart Disease,* also flatly contradicted the MLIC presumptions. Keys, reviewing his own and other data, observed: "The idea has been greatly oversold that the risk of dying prematurely or of having a heart attack is directly related to relative body weight. For middle-aged men, the best prospect for avoiding death in ten or fifteen years is to be about average, or a bit over, in relative weight. The risk rises somewhat with departure in either direction from the happy middle ground, but risk increases substantially only at the extremes of under- and overweight."[3]

The data contradicted all our convictions. The notion of a narrow range of "ideal" weights appeared to be a statistical fiction. None of the studies showed a direct linear relationship between overweight individuals of 10, 20 and 30 percent and excess mortality. In a series of articles, Dr. Reubin Andres, Clinical Director of the National Institute on Aging, one of the National Institutes of Health, reviewed the accumulating weight and mortality studies, and concluded that weight-mortality graphs should not be linear, but rather, U-shaped curves. Best longevity correlated with the broad range of average weights at the base of the U; worst longevity only with the weight extremes in a population: the thinnest and the very heaviest.[4]

Thinner was not better. Indeed, to the extent that there was a linear relationship between weight and mortality, it went in the *wrong* direction: Life expectancy was worst among the leanest in the populations, and in many instances best among the fattest. The MLIC's desirable weights were too low. In all the studies, weights substantially *above* the MLIC's figure correlated with longer life expectancy. In Framingham, men 25 to 40 percent above "desirable" weight lived longest. A fourteen-year study of 1,233 employees of the Chicago People's Gas Company, published in 1975, concluded that the optimum weight for a 5'9" man in his fifties was 198 pounds—49 pounds *more* than the MLIC deemed desirable.[5]

The evidence also undermined the idea that overweight causes cancer, heart disease, diabetes, and hypertension. Dr. Andres sensibly pointed out that if this were true, then it should show up in the mortality data, with fatter people dying earlier of these mortal illnesses—and clearly, just the reverse tended to occur. Dr. William Bennett and Joel Gurin, reviewing the same evidence in their book, *The Dieter's Dilemma,* pointed out that although American men have continued to get fatter, the disastrous effect predicted for so many years is not occurring: Since mid-century, there has been a consistent decline in the age-adjusted rate of deaths from cardiovascular disease, not an upsurge.[6]

Diabetes and hypertension are associated with overweight, but the debate about whether it is a cause or, particularly in the case of diabetes, either a symptom or a complicating factor, is tending toward the latter explanation. Certainly weight loss does not cure them, but rather helps control them. As Bennett and Gurin concluded, except, possibly, for morbid obesity—when over half of body weight is composed of fat, a condition that affects only 600,000 Americans and is probably caused by metabolic abnormalities—and for people with diabetes and hypertension, "fat is not hazardous to your health." This may explain why researchers have had such difficulty discovering the actual physiological processes by which overweight causes pathology.[7]

The data also explode our deeply held convictions that the typical American is overweight. Like Keys, Andres concluded that to the extent that weight plays any role in longevity, it is best to be at the national average or 20 to 30 percent above the MLIC's "desirable weight." He even reminded us of a fact that had not been widely appreciated: The MLIC mortality statistics themselves had been based on how much individuals were above *average*, not *desirable*, weight. Yet, in all the publicity and even in many medical articles and pronouncements, this distinction had rarely been made. Normal weights may indeed be the healthy weights.[8]

The data also revealed that it is not best to maintain the weight of a twenty-five-year old throughout one's mature years. When Andres used data from these emerging studies—including the hallowed MLIC data—and correlated weight, mortality, and age, he found that optimal life spans for people without diabetes or hypertension occurred when they gained about 10 pounds with every decade. It appeared that even in the MLIC sample, middle-aged spread did not augur shorter life spans, and adults who maintained the "desirable" weight of twenty-five-year olds were certainly not winning better life expectancy for themselves. Andres even cautioned physicians to beware of urging healthy middle-aged patients to drop 10 or 15 pounds. They might be doing them a disservice.[9]

Not one of these highly respected studies, which evaluated different groups from all over the world and in the United States, could duplicate Dublin's finding that weight loss improved life expectancy. Indeed, to date, his study is the only one that supports such a hypothesis.

Andres courageously went on to propose the formerly unthinkable. He recommended that research begin to focus on how and why some fat and mature weight gain were beneficial, on how and why they offset the harmful effects generally associated with them. In short, he was suggesting that fat might not be a pathogenic tissue at all, but, rather, a useful one. Nature may not have been playing a dirty trick on us by making weight gain a common feature of middle age or by making some people plumper than others.

These investigators were not the only ones finding flaws in the overweight-mortality link. In 1979 the Society of Actuaries published their most recent actuarial data in an update of the 1959 *BBPS*, the *Build Study 1979*, and in 1983 the MLIC issued new height and weight tables based on this data. Both events shocked the American public, albeit briefly. The weights that correlated with best mortality now were as much as 10 to 15 pounds *heavier* than they had been in the 1959 tables. More than 16 million Americans—whose weights had not budged an ounce—suddenly discovered that they were no longer unhealthily fat.[10]

The new tables were radical: They suggested that fat was not so dangerous after all and that thinnest was not best for the low end of the recommended weights had also been raised. Other radical implications were evident in the MLIC article explaining the tables. The MLIC tried to disassociate itself from all the myths that had accumulated around the notion of "desirable weight."

It stressed that its new recommended weights did not "optimize job performance nor [were they] the weights for best appearance" or "the weights that minimize illness or the incidence of disease." It literally tried to deny any responsibility for—or perpetuation of—the thinner-is-better myth. All the ideas put together so carefully by Dublin were being dismantled.[11]

What, then, were the new tables all about? According to the MLIC, they indicated the "weights at which people should have the greatest longevity," but they did not insure that longevity. They were simply a "guideline." The company no longer called its tables either "ideal" or "desirable" because, it explained, these terms had "caused all the misinterpretation of meaning and purpose" of the earlier tables. Now, it called them simply the Metropolitan Height and Weight Tables. In a very real sense, the MLIC had abdicated from the weight-loss campaign.[12]

Considering the wealth of evidence that contradicts the thinner-is-healthier idea, we may well ask why the general public and so many professionals seem oblivious to it. One obvious reason is that no one has launched a public information campaign about it like that launched by the MLIC and the Public Health Service in 1950. In addition, much of this evidence accumulated only in the seventies and eighties, and some time must elapse before it can be absorbed and accepted, particularly by scientists bred and trained with the implacable rule that fat is pathogenic. And the scientific community, particularly the medical profession, tends toward a praiseworthy conservatism, accepting new theories only when ample evidence justifies them. In addition, the MLIC minimized the radicalism of its findings by insisting it was still "wiser to weigh less than the average rather than more" and by reconfirming the bleak news that Americans were still getting heavier—though, oddly, as in 1959, this fact applied to men, not women. The century-long trend for insured women was toward weight loss, not gain. This, too, the MLIC glossed over in its by now ritualistic warning about the national epidemic of obesity.[13]

Furthermore, many authorities simply rejected the new evidence and the new tables. Ironically, authorities who had embraced the MLIC "desirable weight" standards wouldn't accept the new ones even though they had been derived by identical methods. The American Heart Association objected, insisting that fatness still correlated with higher incidences of chronic diseases. The American Cancer Society also objected and charged that smokers, who tend to be leaner and to die younger, had not been properly screened in the studies. Weight Watchers and Diet Workshops also refused to accept the idea that thinner was not better.[14]

This resistance probably stemmed not just from a praiseworthy conservatism but also from the fact that the conclusions threatened an enormous network of beliefs, morals, and rituals. Had the MLIC revised its recommended weights downward instead of upward, they no doubt would have been accepted without demur: It would not be surprising to learn that fat was even more pathogenic than we had thought. But by revising them upward, the

MLIC undermined the very idea that fat was pathogenic. In addition, there seemed to be a lurking fear that with relaxation in the rule to watch their weights, Americans might fulfill the nightmarish vision haunting health reformers and gorge until they really did become obese. The new evidence also undermined the whole moral system of the health ethic: It suggested that rigid control—even suppression—of appetite were not virtues after all. It even demanded a revision of our national self-image: The nation might not be guilty of the sin of avaricious appetite. Even more disturbing was the void it created: If weight and eating habits were not very important, how could Americans control their health? What rituals would they use instead to make them feel they were combating death, disease, and old age? Resistance to the new evidence was inevitable.

The evidence that thinner is not healthier seemed to confirm other new research indicating that for most overweight people, fat is not an "unnatural" growth caused by overeating and inactivity. It is becoming clearer that nature genetically programmed people to have different weights and fat-to-lean ratios, just as they have different heights and other varying characteristics. Certainly, experts have long known the vital role of heredity in body weight, but from the fifties on, they stressed that environmental factors—nurture, not nature— determined whether people would fulfill an unfortunate genetic tendency to overweight, and they warned that those so inclined simply had to diet and exercise harder.

However, in the seventies and eighties evidence accumulated about the tenacity with which the human body clings to a "preferred weight" regardless of diet and exercise habits, and researchers began to lean toward nature, and to revive and recast outdated theories about *luxuskonsumption* and metabolism. Whether called *setpoint, homeostasis,* or *thermogenesis,* they described the same phenomenon. The body seems to defend, vehemently, a preferred weight and fat-to-lean ratio. When caloric intake is reduced, many mechanisms—most notably, lowered metabolic rates and other subtler changes now being analyzed—mobilize to conserve fat stores. The reverse happens when caloric intake increases.[15]

This was most persuasively demonstrated in the seventies by researcher Allen Sims when he tried to get his subjects to *gain* weight, not lose it. Startlingly, his subjects had considerable trouble adding even 20 to 25 percent to their starting weights. One man did go fairly easily from 110 to 138 pounds, but he had to force himself to eat 7,000 calories a day to maintain it. All of the subjects became increasingly lethargic and apathetic as they hit their peak poundage, and many began to dread meals. When the experiment ended, all but one of them returned rather rapidly and spontaneously to their pre-experiment weights. Reviewing this and similar studies which demonstrated that it is as difficult to raise the body's "preferred weight" as to lower it, Bennett and Gurin justifiably observed that if fashion now favored fatness, the thin would have as hard a time getting their weight up as the fat have reducing theirs—and they, too, might be accused of lacking self-discipline.[16]

Such findings undermine the linchpin of our war on fat: the idea that people have absolute control of their body weight. It appears that our mechanical model—that intake of 3,500 calories over energy expenditure always equals a pound of fat—cannot explain a complex biological organism like the human body. Indeed, other studies are also revealing that eating and exercise habits are not the primary determinants of body size. While starving people, of course, do get emaciated and well-fed ones do not, in a secure culinary environment, personal habits may cause only narrow weight fluctuations, not the difference between obesity and slenderness. Body size may not be an index of self-control and character.[17]

The fat do not have a unique relationship to food. If fatter people eat when they are depressed, nervous, or happy, or if they binge, they are not doing anything normal-weight people don't do. Nor do infant feeding and weight patterns determine adult body size: A fifteen-year study at U.C. Berkeley revealed that obese six- to twelve-month-olds were most likely to be normal or lean by age nine, and some lean infants become chubby. More shockingly, despite the confessions of ex-obese authors of diet books which suggest the fat eat alarming quantities, most of them do not, a fact Jean Mayer discovered in the early sixties. Recently, two leading obesity experts acknowledged the growing consensus that "obese persons do not, in the long run, eat much more per unit of lean body mass than nonobese persons." They hastened to add that these people are not defying the laws of thermodynamics. Their bodies do maintain a stable balance between energy intake and expenditure—but at levels we call "obese."[18]

Indeed, other evidence suggests that even how much we eat and exercise is not determined solely by external cues, cultural conditioning, and conscious choice. Experimenters are finding that some still undetermined biological mechanisms influence our caloric intake. One study found that both humans and rats, when kept on liquid diets, spontaneously altered—within a matter of days—the amount they drank when the caloric density of the liquid was changed, so that their average intake remained constant. Bottle-fed infants were found to do the same. Intriguing new evidence even suggests that tendencies toward activity or lassitude may also be inborn. And most normal people maintain remarkably stable average weights for years without any conscious effort. The human body seems to balance energy intake and expenditure with superhuman, exquisite precision, which suggests that, even without the pressure to diet, most Americans probably would *not* end up eating themselves into gross obesity.[19]

Many experts are beginning to agree that "preferred" or physiological weight is, as J. Lercy defined it, an "individual's average weight which remains constant," at which he feels well and healthy, and which is maintained without undue attention to diet and exercise. And they argue that people whose preferred weight is high are not necessarily unhealthy. Indeed, critics of the MLIC dicta have argued that to define "unhealthy" overweight simply as deviation above a norm is both intellectually sloppy and misleading. Like slim people, some obese people are in excellent health while others are not. Already in 1963 an international conference on overnutrition had concurred that there were different types of overweight and that "obesity" as a clinical condition represented not just an extreme on the normal distribution curve for weight, but was a true disorder with metabolic and anatomic features of its own." For these people especially, diet and exercise tend to have little effect. But other people who maintain a stable physiological weight—even at levels we might call obese—are neither unhealthy nor abnormal.[20]

However, it does appear that there *is* something abnormal and potentially unhealthy in people who struggle to maintain weight below what is natural or comfortable for them. As early as 1886 a leading obesity authority had observed that "there are some people to whom it is essential to be fat; they become weak and sick the moment one reduces their fat . . . . Not every person can be lean." Modern scientists are beginning to agree. Researchers at the prestigious Rockefeller Institute examined some formerly obese women from Overeaters' Anonymous who had reduced to "normal" weights. They looked healthy but had symptoms usually seen only in women with anorexia nervosa: Their fat cells were shrunken, they were amenorrheic, their pulses were 50–60 beats per minute instead of the normal 70–80, their blood pressures were abnormally low, and they were always cold. In addition, cruelly enough, they burned 25 percent fewer calories than their heights and weights indicated they should. They literally were semistarved and had to stay that way to maintain their "normal" weights.[21]

The OA women are not unique. Many successful dieters also reduce their body metabolisms so that they need almost 25 percent fewer calories to maintain the same weight as a naturally lean person. Researcher Dr. Robert Eckel recently warned that "the only way to maintain their lower weight is to bite the bullet and realize they cannot allow themselves to return to normal food-intake patterns." Indeed, behavior modification programs may have their weight-loss successes not because they re-educate the body, but because, as Albert Stunkard postulated, they train "someone who biologically should be obese to live in a semistarved condition." In short, successful reducers must be like the "thin fat people" so vividly described by Hilde Bruch.[22]

Efforts to get overweight people below their "preferred" weights create not only abnormalities and emotional and physical distress but other problems as well: The wide weight swings characteristic of the chronic dieter *are* unhealthy and, ironically, they also often exacerbate what they are supposed to cure. The syndrome of diet-induced obesity, which we discussed earlier, has physiological as well as psychological causes. Experts now concur that the body becomes geared to the fluctuations of feast and famine and, with each diet, defends itself by becoming ever more efficient at storing calories. The overweight might indeed find that though they eat like birds, they look as if they were eating like stevedores.[23]

Certainly the concept of "preferred" weight explains many of the puzzles that have dogged obesity research, such as why so many weight loss efforts fail (especially considering that many dieters are trying to reduce to what the leanest 5 percent of the population weighs) and why so many sincere dieters end up fatter than when they started dieting. Millions of research dollars were spent to find out why Americans could not reach and maintain "desirable" weight—but it appears something was wrong with the concept, not with all those who couldn't succeed. The millions of Americans who faced defeat after defeat in the weight-loss game simply were fighting a losing—and emotionally and physically costly—battle with their own quite benign biological tendencies.

These facts underscore how distorted our current food ideology is. We believe that if someone is "overweight," he or she is "overeating." Food has become a total abstraction, disconnected from how we feel. But if bodies respond differently to the same number of calories, and if people were meant to come in different weights, then the number of calories people need cannot be determined solely by their body size. It certainly seems much more likely that, as Hilde Bruch pointed out, some people may need more calories than others to keep them functioning at a happy, productive level. Appetite may be as individual a matter as weight, and both most likely will vary from one person to the next.

Even more pernicious is our underlying assumption that food is not really a necessity. The number of calories deemed necessary for human health kept getting lower over the decades, and some scientists, like Roy Walford at UCLA, argue that the healthiest and longest-lived people are those who fast regularly and keep their caloric intake to the barest minimum. The facts, of course, are quite different. People do need the energy supplied by food, and food deprivation, as we have seen, causes severe emotional as well as physical distress and can create neurotic obsessions like those typical of eating disorders. Bruch observed that in her thirty years of practice, patients with weight-gain disorders did not die prematurely, but those with anorexia and bulimia did. Recent estimates suggest that between 5 and 19 percent of diagnosed anorexics die from the disorder, one of the highest fatality rates for any psychiatric diagnosis. Starvation and weight-loss disorders, not overeating, cause death.[24]

There is also the often-concealed issue of food as a physiological and psychological pleasure. Over the decades we have denied that it is acceptable to regard food in this way. Yet, when researchers actually documented scientifically people's emotional reactions before, during, and after a meal, they found that common wisdom had been right: People of all weights become somewhat irritable before meals, eagerly anticipate them, reach a peak of happiness when they sit down to eat them, and subsequently experience a soothing sense of relaxation. Americans have become so confused about their relationship to food, so preoccupied with trying to control or find symbolic reasons for the pleasures associated with it, and so distrustful of that pleasure that they persist in referring to food disparagingly as an "escape," a "cheap drug," or a "sedative." Food may indeed serve this function, but given the new evidence, this hardly seems reason for concern, let alone repressive measures.

Recent studies also suggest that the negative characteristics we associate with fat people are based more on prejudice than on any objective, scientific facts. The biological differences that dispose some to be plump and some thin may indeed cause differences in temperament and behavior, but to date we have little evidence to this effect.

As we saw, when weight preferences changed at the turn of the century, there was an about-face in the traits associated with the amply fleshed. From being regarded as cheerful, well-adjusted, productive types, they came to be seen as depressed, emotionally disturbed, and nonproductive. Psychoanalytic explanations for obesity, which began to prevail in the forties and fifties, validated these estimates and reinforced them. It was postulated that overeating was caused by neurotic neediness and unresolved infantile conflicts. Oddly enough, when researchers shifted their attention from psychiatric patients to the general population, they almost consistently found that the overweight were as—or less—neurotic, anxious, and impulsive as normal-weight individuals. More surprisingly, they were also found to be less depressed than people of normal weight, which might explain a well-known mortality statistic: Overweight people rarely commit suicide. Such data led the American Psychiatric Association to define obesity in its 1980 *Diagnostic and Statistical Manual of Mental Disorders* as a "physical disorder . . . not generally associated with any distinct psychological or behavioral syndrome."[25]

These negative associations persist nonetheless, in part because of inconsistencies in the data itself. There are a variety of psychological disturbances that cause appetite derangements and obesity, but Hilde Bruch underlined that such clinical abnormalities could not be applied to average, overweight Americans. Nevertheless, both popular and professional psychologists continued to extrapolate from these clinical cases, often using a form of reasoning—unfortunately common to the psychotherapeutic mentality—that makes disproving a phenomenon almost impossible. When Dr. Robert Simon found in 1963 that overweight airmen were rarely depressed, he concluded that this proved overeating was a successful defense mechanism against depression. It was inconceivable to him that his findings might need no such explanation, that the overweight airmen in fact were *not* depressed either consciously or subconsciously. Such thinking, so powerfully shaped by prevailing theories and prejudices, has continued to dog research about the overweight and perceptions of them.[26]

The final reason for the persistence of these associations is the data we saw in earlier chapters: the despair many overweight Americans described. However, it appears that in most cases, their depression or emotional problems did not cause their overweight but rather were caused by the agony of having a body society deemed grotesque, and by their very efforts to shed their "excess" weight. Bennett and Gurin justifiably argued that all studies of the overweight must be refracted, not through their fatness, but through their probable experience as chronic dieters. "If dieting is the crucial variable," they write, "then the fat do not eat because they hurt inside; rather, they hurt because they are trying not to eat, to make their bodies conform to social norms," and their psychological and personality profiles must be interpreted in light of the constant struggle in which they are engaged.[27]

Our belief that the fatter are mentally and physically slow also merits re-examination. When a series of IQ tests were administered in the forties obese youngsters, almost consistently, had higher IQs than thinner youngsters. Other tests indicated that the overweight were better at memorizing lists. When Mayer and his coinvestigators evaluated the college board scores of overweight girls in the sixties, they found that body size did not interfere with intellectual achievement. In other words, the presumption that the plumper are mentally lethargic is based on prejudice, not fact.[28]

The same holds true for our belief that the overweight must be unathletic and unfit. Certainly in the nineteenth and early twentieth centuries, a large, robust body was deemed a stronger, more energetic body, one well-suited for difficult physical labor. Around the turn of the century, the idea began to develop that the bigger body was clumsy, awkward and weak, and as standards of normal body size became slimmer, this judgment was brought upon ever-slimmer bodies. These are prejudices that developed in tandem with the thinner-is-healthier idea. Hilde Bruch observed that obese youngsters generally have larger muscles and bones than slender ones, which hardly suggests weakness, and she cited studies that indicated there was little noticeable difference in activity between overweight and lean youngsters in school playgrounds.[29]

And, as with depression and overweight, what lethargy is found is often a result, not a cause, of overweight. As we saw, Bruch drew a different conclusion than Mayer about why some obese youngsters often were sedentary. Aware of the shame, depression, and self-consciousness that they feel, she suggested they avoided athletic activities, or participated only half-heartedly, because their bodies were an acute source of shame and embarrassment. With every move, they could feel the hated fat moving with them. They were, in a sense, crippled by the awareness—not the fact—of their fatness.

Today, magazines devoted to big women are pushing hard to overturn this prejudice. *Big Beautiful Woman* regularly features very big women, many well over 200 pounds, water skiing and snow skiing with grace and skill; *Radiance* magazine is filled with ads for gyms run by and for big women. They are shown in their leotards and headbands leaping with as much energy as any slim exerciser. The pages of these magazines are filled with stories of how these women learned their former inactivity was caused by shame, not incapacity. "Fat can be fit" became one of their slogans.

One of the most potent and persistent myths about fat people, particularly fat women, is that they are less sexual than the slender. We believe thinner-is-sexier with the same vehemence that we believe its converse that fatter-is-unsexier. This belief also developed with the growing preference for slenderness; as the plump came to be seen as sexually unappealing, they also came to be perceived as having diminished or disturbed sexual appetites. Psychoanalytic theories also reinforced this perception. It was presumed the fat overate because they were stunted in the infantile stage of sexuality in which gratification came from sucking and swallowing and that they were unable to cope with mature, genital sexuality. A related psychoanalytic theory, nicely summed up by Stanley Conrad in 1954, argued that obesity was an unconsciously motivated choice, designed to make the overeater sexually unattractive so she could avoid sex.[30]

Although official psychoanalytic theory has dismissed such explanations, the idea that oral fixation or fear of sex cause obesity has proved remarkably durable. Just recently, feminist psychotherapists have presented them in updated guises. As discussed above, Kim Chernin argues that the conflict-ridden mother-daughter relationship spawned by feminism has caused oral fixations and eating disorders, and Susie Orbach argues that fat women often unconsciously opt for obesity because through the "protective aspects of fat," they can appear as people, not sex objects. Such ideas persist, too, because of our food ideology. We believe people virtually do not need food; therefore, hunger and appetite have ceased to be regarded as independent and powerful urges that can shape behavior. With the pervasiveness of popularized psychoanalytic thinking, we have come to see erotic drives as primary. All others, including food and eating, are symbolic erotic substitutes.[31]

As we have seen, history defies the equation that fatter is less sexy. To eroticize a female form that is "close to the bone" is a peculiarly modern phenomenon. And evidence does not confirm that the overweight are sexually abnormal. Studies in 1977, 1978, and 1979, some of which evaluated morbidly obese patients and some of which reviewed the profiles of obese psychiatric patients, all arrived at similar conclusions, nicely summarized by psychologist Colleen Rand: "There are no data which indicate that the obese individual has significantly greater or fewer sexual problems than [the] nonobese individual." To the extent that sexual problems did exist among the overweight, a 1979 study concluded, it appeared that "their fear of rejection because of their body size may be the inhibiting factor."[32]

Indeed, the persistence of the stereotype can be attributed to the same bending of facts to fit theory that we encountered with neurosis. Two researchers at Michael Reese Hospital in Chicago attempted to demonstrate that thinner women are more sexually appetitive. They found just the opposite.

They matched and compared pairs of fat and thin married women and found that all had sexual relations about nine times a month, but that the fatter women wanted to have sex more often than the thin, and that on scales of erotic readiness and general sexual excitability, fat women outscored thin ones by a factor of almost two to one. The researchers did not conclude that their hypothesis had been wrong. Instead, they theorized that "an underlying psychic hunger must be what lies behind the otherwise merely symbolically related appetites for (sexual) love and food." They did not seem to realize, or were not able to accept, the fact that their findings undermined the theory that food was used to avoid sex. Instead, they attached unpleasant, neurotic qualities to fat women's sexual desires—something they certainly would not have done had their slender subjects shown these responses. The fat simply could not win.[33]

The Michael Reese study, however, may have uncovered a startling truth. Certainly thin people who get that way through stringent dieting are unlikely to be more sexually appetitive than the plump. Studies consistently show that with dietary deprivation, sexual interests dissipate. Keys's subjects, on 1,700 calories a day, ceased having sexual fantasies and ceased masturbating. The amenorrhea of many dieters and exercisers also points to an intimate link between fat stores and hormone levels. And Dr. Domeena Renshaw, director of Loyola University's Sexual Dysfunction Clinic, recently reported that weight-loss disorders have a more severe effect on sexual function than weight-gaining disorders. "The obese women were more eager to date, more eager to mate . . . . ," while those with weight-loss disorders "were so concerned with their bodies that they had fewer sexual fantasies, fewer dates and less desire for sex."[34]

Some experts have even postulated that fatter women are physiologically sexier than thin ones. Beller speculated that because bigger women have bigger fat cells, and since fat cells produce some estrogen, the bigger woman may actually be more "feminine" than the thin. She further hypothesized that since sex is a need state like hunger, people are likely to respond to these needs in similar ways. A hearty eater might indeed also be a more hearty lover. Once again, much of this speculation may be more accurate when we distinguish, not between the fat and the thin, but between those who maintain a "natural" weight and those who have shrunk themselves down to stylish standards. The evidence suggests, and common sense would confirm, that a hungry, undernourished animal is less, not more, interested in the pleasures of the flesh.[35]

As this evidence should indicate, the idea that thinner is happier is also fictive. Certainly people who maintain low weights only by stringent diet and exercise cannot be said to feel better, as Hilde Bruch so trenchantly pointed out in her discussion of thin fat people. Even experts most intimately involved in obesity research confirm that the pathway to permanent slenderness does not produce a sense of well-being. Dr. Jules Hirsch told *Time* in January, 1986, that for the formerly overweight, keeping at a normal weight "requires not only constant vigilance . . . but often the acknowledgment of persistent discomfort."[36]

It is not only that dieting and trying to maintain weights below what is normal for us often produces distress but that weight loss rarely brings the longed-for happiness to the vigilant. Despite all their expectations, reducers rarely find there was another self submerged beneath the "excess" weight. Nothing is quite as compelling as the romance of personal transformation, and, like control, it is at the heart of the religion of slenderness. As we saw, Bruch cautioned against these unrealistic expectations. Weight loss is not quite a metamorphosis: All that changes is the body, not the personality, the mind, or the soul. These unrealistic expectations also prompted the MLIC to warn in 1983 that its charts did not correlate with greater productivity, better appearance, or a more successful life.[37]

How then can we explain why so many people say their are happier, more energetic, and sexier when they lose weight? There are good reasons. They are proud of themselves. They feel they have mastered *the* American problem: control of appetite. Through will power, they have come closer to being one of the body aristocrats. This sense of accomplishment easily extends into other areas of their lives—while it lasts. If our culture placed little value on the feat of weight loss, the act of controlling calories would seem banal and would not have this halo effect.

Successful dieters feel good also because they are no longer at war with society, a struggle that can be very wearing. Fat people get little praise. They are accorded even less dignity, and they can rarely escape the uttered or unuttered question: When are you going to do something about your weight? They face, daily, the excruciating pain of living in a body that their society regards as grotesque and believes they have created through overeating and underexercising. Those who reduce end this war, and they also begin to earn rapt praise and admiration from acquaintances, friends, and family.

Palpably absurd as it is, there is evidence to suggest that even extremes of thinness, like anorexia, can be viewed as admirable by our society. Psychologists have found that some families of anorexic patients actually admire their offsprings' ability to get so thin. A commercial greeting card pictures a 300-some-odd pound woman. Inside the card are the words: "Anorexia. Where can I get it?" A woman writes to Ann Landers distraught about her close friend who once weighed 180 pounds but who is steadily losing weight because she has terminal cancer. Uninformed acquaintances and friends run up to her and gush, "You look wonderful. How did you lose all that weight?" In this environment, slenderized people cannot help but feel good—no matter how they really feel.[38]

A similar dynamic explains why a woman believes she has more libido when she's dieted down to the bone. In our culture, all but the leanest are considered—and consider themselves—sexually unattractive. People who lose weight know they look sexier, so they often feel sexier. A svelte woman doesn't have to fear rejection because of her body size, and she can be proud of her body and proudly show it to her lover. No more sex under the covers for her. She indeed feels sexually energized—not because fat submerged her sexuality but because it made her feel sexually undesirable.

If the myths about thinness can be exploded, what of fitness? Advocates vaunt exercise for its fat-burning powers and argue that fitter is healthier and happier. But here, too, we have been seduced by unrealistic expectations. Now that the fitness craze has been with us for several years, more evidence has accumulated about its actual effects, and some of the disenchanted are beginning to expose its underside.

Like all the weight-loss panaceas that have come and gone over the years, exercise has proved to be less effective as a weight-reducing technique than everyone had hoped. It can help people reduce—but only within the limits of their "preferred weight." Jean Mayer had argued that moderate exercise would help the formerly sedentary lose weight but that vigorous exercise is balanced by increased appetite. Even fitness guru Covert Bailey had not promised that exercise would bring down scale readings. Rather, he claimed that fat would be exchanged for muscle, so novice exercisers would *look* slimmer. The theory that exercise will increase metabolic rates enough to reduce "preferred weight" is still controversial. Certainly, it has not worked effectively in diet-exercise programs. Reviewing the results of such programs, psychologist M.R.C. Greenwood warned prospective dieter-exercisers not to expect too much. "It is feasible," she told a journalist in 1986, "to think of losing 5 to 10 pounds and keeping it off." But the prospects for those who want to lose 20 pounds or more are "dismal—less than 5 percent."[39]

Exercise can also help us resculpt our bodies only up to a point. As early as 1971 researchers dismissed the cherished maxim that "fat doesn't form over a working muscle." Even Covert Bailey reported that when he noticed a roll developing around his midsection, he started doing 300 sit-ups a day. His stomach did become as strong as "cast iron"—but there were still "three inches of marshmallow on top of the muscles." He, like many other exercise advocates, insisted that only with intense aerobic exercise could fat stores really be depleted and that this, with spot exercising, would produce physical transformations. But, as we have already seen, such transformations are not easily achieved. Biology is, to a large extent, destiny, and flaws have a stubborn way of resisting change. Few of us have the time and money necessary to resculpt ourselves, and few have the already near-perfect forms that make such resculpting gratifying.[40]

If exercise cannot make us beautiful, can it at least make us healthier by protecting us from heart disease? Just as evidence does not support the notion that thinner is healthier, so both research studies and the cases of well-known individuals indicate fitter is not necessarily healthier. Winston Churchill was a rotund, ruddy, cigar-smoking man who enjoyed the affluent diet of an advanced Western nation and who had one of the most anxiety-ridden jobs known in the modern world. Productive to the end of his life, he died at the age of ninety-two. Running guru, James Fixx, who eschewed fatty meats, alcohol, and cigarettes, was lean and ran marathons for several years, but he dropped dead of a heart attack at the age of fifty-four. Survival does not always go to the fittest.

Two examples, of course, are not scientific proof, but our surprise over them underscores how much we have come to believe we can control our physical fates. They also reflect the controversy on exercise in the medical literature. Reviewing this vast literature, cardiologist Henry Solomon remarked how odd it was that studies supporting exercise were not subject to more critical peer review. Their flaws were evident, and they reflected a problem common in the epidemiological method: When is the variable studied a cause, not just an associated characteristic? Solomon also observed that the evidence linking better health to more strenuous occupations, to vigorous exercise, and to exercise programs for cardiovascular patients is matched by an equal volume of evidence that shows either the reverse—more strenuous activity linked to *higher* incidences of cardiovascular and other deaths—or shows no relationship at all. He argued that this was probably because no absolute relationship exists. Even Bennett and Gurin, who wanted to find a positive correlation between exercisers and lower rates of heart disease, admitted the evidence was inconclusive.[41]

Fitness developed its positive reputation because it came to be regarded as synonymous with health, even though many scientists explained they are quite different. Fitness refers to the body's ability to do work: A fit body is one with muscle strength and with muscles that are more efficient at getting oxygen out of the blood stream. But muscles are simply an outer layer and have little to do with health, that is, with whether or not the body is diseased. The fittest body remains vulnerable to a cold or the flu, and it can have cancer or cardiovascular disease, even while it continues to act with endurance and strength. And fitness is not likely to protect one from heart disease by strengthening the heart muscle: Most cardiac disease involves the coronary arteries, not the heart itself, and exercise tends to strengthen the voluntary muscles, not the involuntary ones.[42]

As the fitness craze continued, researchers also began to examine whether exercise was beneficial, not because of its effect on the heart itself but because of its effect on risk factors for heart disease. Many argued that exercise could reduce high blood pressure and either raise HDL—the "good" cholesterol (though how good it is remains controversial)—and thus lower the ratio of LDL—the "bad" cholesterol. The accumulating evidence is disappointing. The Chairman of the Joint National Committee on Detection, Evaluation and Treatment of High Blood Pressure concluded in 1980 that "there are no convincing data that systematic exercise, even if performed vigorously three to four times a week, resulted in significant continuous lowering of blood pressure." A series of studies published between 1980 and 1982 all indicated that exercise did not significantly alter HDL levels; in some cases it actually lowered them; and one researcher was surprised to find high total cholesterol levels and low HDL levels among competitive long-distance runners. He concluded that vigorous physical activity "does not . . . guarantee low total cholesterol or high HDL-cholesterol values."[43]

Indeed, we have little evidence to suggest that strenuous exercise is beneficial or that competitive athletes have better life expectancies than the rest of us, though we presume this to be true. And one can't help but wonder whether the enormous stresses put on the superathlete's body, and the injuries sustained, might not be more harmful than beneficial. Dr. Solomon observed that the characteristics of what physicians call the "athlete's heart" are unnervingly similar to those of people with cardiovascular disease. The heart of the superfit may not be the healthiest. Similar cautions must apply to patients with a history of cardiac disease who are encouraged to exercise: Dr. Solomon warned his colleagues that for many cardiac patients, exercise *strains,* not strengthens, the damaged organ.

Even more surprising, perhaps, strenuous exercise can *cause* deaths that might otherwise have been avoidable. Solomon commented, "Observations that incriminate exercise as a precipitating factor in cardiac event are old and established." A 1973 study, in which more than half of twenty-eight deaths occurred during or immediately after severe or moderate physical activity, caused Dr. Meyer Friedman (formulator of the Type-A personality theory) to conclude that "the close temporal relationship observed between severe or moderate physical activity and more than one-half of the instantaneous coronary death cases makes us question whether it is worth risking an instantaneous coronary death by indulging in an activity the possible benefit of which to the human coronary vasculature has yet to be proved." Our belief that superexercise protects from cardiovascular diseases is based more on hope than fact. We seem to be grasping at straws in the hope that we indeed do have some control over this surreptitious killer.[44]

But we do not exercise strenuously just to be healthier. We are lured by the promise that fitter is happier, by the romance not just of physical transformation but of spiritual regeneration. Here, especially, we are being seduced by unrealistic expectations. Some fitness fanatics are beginning to report the disappointing results of their pilgrimages for physical excellence, such as Blair Sobol in her 1985 book, *The Body of America.* After beginning a rigorous fitness regimen, Sobol had repeated aches and pains from muscles that too often had been pushed to the burn and beyond. Her love life and her social life were not better: They had all but evaporated. She had no time for friends and lovers. She collapsed into bed by 8:00 P.M. so she could be up early the next morning for her prework workout. Her sex drive hadn't increased. It, too, had evaporated somewhere between her morning workout and her evening run. Her interests had indeed changed—they had narrowed to her nutrition, vitamins, workouts, pulse rate, fat-to-lean ratio, and methods for treating sundry injuries. She *was* more in control of her life—now that it consisted primarily of tending to her body. And she was disenchanted. Somehow, her life, as life is usually understood, had disappeared.[45]

Sobol's experiences are not unique. Sports physicians increasingly are alarmed about the number of injuries sustained by avid and not-so-avid exercisers. They are particularly alarmed by those who, spurred by the spiritual promises of exercise, strive to get beyond the "wall" of their endurance limits by ignoring pain and resolutely carrying on. They tend to sustain the most serious and irreversible injuries precisely because they ignore warning symptoms.[46]

And Sobol is not alone in finding her life vitiated, not enhanced, by her devotion. Both the lay and professional press are beginning to talk about a strange new addiction—to exercise—and about fitness fanatics who are obsessed with their exercise routines. Like all addictions, these hardly improve personal lives. A 1984 *New England Journal of Medicine* (NEJM) article on compulsive male runners revealed that they resembled Sobol. Their lives and thoughts, too, were structured around their exercise routines which led to neglect, not enrichment, of their personal lives. And the new superwomen who follow Jane Fonda's advice and let nothing interfere with their workout schedules often find themselves in frazzling, helter-skelter routines that produce not energy, calm, and happiness, but, rather, exhaustion. The Holy Grail they seek has produced a strange generation of fitness ascetics, of whom Blair Sobol is only one vocal example.[47]

And, like slenderness, fitness does not enhance libido. Far from becoming eager, supple, sexual athletes, exercisers seem to lose interest in sex. Considerable evidence is accumulating about the altered menstrual and hormonal patterns of even noncompetitive athletic women. The *NEJM* article indicated that one symptom of the compulsive runner was a dwindling interest in sex, and it reported there were suggestive hormonal changes among the men. But even if such changes prove to have no effect on libidinal impulses, it takes little more than common sense to recognize that a fatigued, overexercised body is not likely to be a more sexually energized body. Certainly, for almost a century, strenuous exercise had been advocated not to fire sexual energies but to defuse them, particularly among adolescents. Sadly, common sense rarely has been used to evaluate the complex of beliefs that today make up our health ethic.[48]

I am not trying to suggest that exercise cannot be invigorating, or make us feel good, or be fun. I am objecting to the extremes encouraged and to the exaggerated and unrealistic expectations we have set up about what strenuous exercise can do. It is not the panacea we so desperately want it to be, and very often, like all extremes, it delivers the opposite of what we seek from it.

Just as our ideas about body weight and exercise are flawed, so are the new nutritional guidelines we follow religiously and the expectations we attach to them. As we saw, they evolved from the thinner-is-better conviction, and like the fitness craze to which they are linked, they now are advocated and sustained for benefits independent of their weight-reducing properties. We are convinced that the standard American diet is not only too caloric but also unnutritious and even pathogenic: We get too much cholesterol, saturated fat, sugar, salt, and additives and too little calcium, fiber, vitamins, and trace nutrients. We have also attributed remarkable powers to a proper diet. We believe that somehow the "right" foods are the secret to a longer, healthier life. We have set up the same unrealistic expectations about nutrition that we have about thinness and fitness.

In our eyes, average Americans are overfed but undernourished because they eat the "wrong" foods. This is a prejudice, not a fact. Government nutrition studies conducted in the seventies and eighties revealed that Americans are not suffering from nutritional deficiencies. The only groups who have some nutritional inadequacies are premenopausal and pregnant women, whose stores of iron may be low. Nor, surprisingly, despite our image of Americans as a people who are gluttonously consuming ever-greater numbers of calories, over the century there has been a decline in the average number of calories consumed. Between just 1965 and 1977 the FDA reported a 10 percent reduction in per-capita intake of calories. Nor do health statistics support the contention that the standard modern diet has caused a deterioration in Americans' health: Life expectancy has continued to improve as the standard diet has modernized.[49]

We saw in chapter 9 the distortions and misconceptions that inform our indictment of the standard American diet, and today more and more experts are trying, as the Food and Nutrition Board has, to provide the public with accurate nutritional information and to dispel the shibboleths that have developed about sugar, salt (a recent study suggests that only 10 percent of the American population is sensitive to this substance), "junk food," additives and preservatives, natural or organic foods, and vitamin needs. Diet reforms have been based on considerable historical and nutritional misinformation.[50]

Again, I am not suggesting that we should forego monitoring the new techniques used to produce and process our food, nor that further nutrition research cannot yield critically important results. I am arguing that we have gone to irrational extremes. We have constructed a system of beliefs about food that resembles the dietary laws of a religion more than the sensible conclusions reached by scientists after long and painstaking study. We have invested food with supernatural powers and, in this respect, despite our highly rational scientific age, we have returned to a form of magical thinking. This tendency most alarms experts. They try to point out that no diet, food, or vitamin is magical or the secret to a longer life.[51]

The warning against diets high in cholesterol and saturated fats is one of the new food rules that seems to be waxing, not waning, in popularity. Yet, the campaign launched in October, 1987, by the National Heart, Lung, and Blood

Institute along with the federal government and twenty other health organizations urging Americans to lower their serum cholesterol levels to 200 or less has an unsettling similarity to the campaign against overweight launched thirty-seven years ago—and seems to have similar flaws. Once again, conflicting evidence was cast aside, what was average was deemed unhealthy—average cholesterol levels were deemed too high, just as average weights had been—and Americans were exhorted to make rather drastic changes in their personal habits.

Reviewing the ongoing cholesterol saga in the *Annals of Internal Medicine,* Public Health professor Marshall Becker cautioned against what seemed to be another unjustified—or certainly premature—public-health effort. He outlined the multiple studies that undermined the new guidelines and their presumptions. The diet-heart disease link was weak. Seven important epidemiological investigations about the relationship between health and high consumption of cholesterol, fat, and calories went in the "wrong" direction. The high-cholesterol-heart disease link was equally tenuous. Numerous major studies continued to report no relationship between serum cholesterol levels and mortality from heart disease, and the benefits of lowering cholesterol promised to be minimal: A team of researchers reported that if Americans between the ages of twenty and sixty who were at low risk for heart disease met the guidelines, they could expect to live three days to three months longer; those at high risk might gain eighteen days to twelve months. In short, serum cholesterol levels were a weak risk factor, far less important than smoking or high blood pressure. And, just one month after the announcement of the new campaign, Soviet researchers reported that among 8,000 Soviet men, those "with extremely low total cholesterol levels had higher death rates from heart disease than those with average cholesterol levels" and that high HDL (the "good" cholesterol) was associated with "an increase in the overall death rate." Dr. Becker, too, noted that in each of the five studies linking dietary change to reduced mortality from heart disease, the reductions were "balanced by *increases* in death from other causes: life expectancy therefore remained unchanged." He wryly commented that "this observation suggests that the effects of our intervention are analogous to stewards rearranging the deckchairs of the Titanic."[52]

Becker went on to quote multiple studies that disputed the crucial link: that diet determined serum cholesterol levels. Researchers at Texas A & M University argued that for as much as 80 percent of the population, serum cholesterol levels are unrelated to dietary cholesterol. Cholesterol is produced endogenously, and the body maintains a stable level, increasing or decreasing production in response to dietary intake. Genetic or constitutional makeup factors seem to account for most of the variance in cholesterol—just as they do for body weight.[53]

The low-cholesterol campaign seems to be just a new manifestation of our thirty-seven-year war on heart disease. Like its predecessors, it has been launched by eager health reformers and embraced by a frightened and trusting public. Becker rightfully urged his colleagues to be more moderate and judicious: "We have advocated too many important alterations in lifestyles in the absence of sound medical and epidemiological groundwork . . . . Some advice is subsequently considered to have actually been harmful." And he voiced an opinion rarely heard today: Health officials should not interfere with private habits and pleasures unless clear evidence confirms that they are dangerous. He implicitly condemned the puritanism that seems to dog our current health campaigns.

The continuing mystery about what causes cardiovascular diseases and cancer is probably responsible for the overeager health campaigns of recent decades. Researchers have tried to identify personal habits that might be "risk factors," but, except for cigarette smoking, they have not had great success. In 1978 the results of six major investigations of the causes of heart disease were discouraging. Only about 10 percent of the men who had two or more risk factors developed heart disease, while 60 percent of those who had either one or no risk factors did. In 1980 the FNB reported that only 50 percent of cardiovascular diseases could be attributed to currently recognized risk factors.[54]

Clearly, our knowledge about the causes of heart disease remains rudimentary at best. Yet we have developed the notion that personal habits are of primary importance, and so we believe we can control our health. In this respect, we have been misled. Becker trenchantly observed that "personal control over health is often substantially limited by heredity, social class, environment, culture, and chance." Fate and chance are not aspects of life that we, in our secular, technocratic age, are willing to accept. And so we continue to promote and embrace health precepts that, in the last analysis, are ascetic, magical rituals for earthly salvation. One can only wonder if the enormous time, energy, and resources focused so exclusively on these risk factors have diverted efforts to uncover other, more crucial but still unknown causes of cardiovascular diseases and cancer. And one can only regret the fear, asceticism, and unfounded hopes being foisted on the American public. And, at the root of all these campaigns lies our venerable war against animal fat. Yet, it may be that, beyond certain limits, we can no more control our physical fate than we can control our weight.[55]

We can expose many of the current "truths" that underlie our weight obsession for the myths that they are, but a more potent one remains, and it lies at the core of our war on fat: our belief that a lean, taut, muscled body is beautiful. Though a complex structure of beliefs motivates them, women do not follow the new dietary rules religiously to fend off death, they do not exercise every obscure muscle group to live a year or two longer, they do not hate themselves when they gain 5 or 15 pounds because they fear they have shortened their lives. They do it because they want beauty.

If thinner-is-healthier is a prejudice, can the same be said for thinner-is-more-beautiful? Beauty, of course, is an aesthetic value, and scientific proof and common sense are unlikely to alter it. Yet fashions and tastes do change—sometimes rather rapidly. In the space of five years, female muscles became desirable, though women had never before worn them with pride. This development did not significantly change the ideal we sought—fat-freeness and exposed musculature were just another form of skinniness—but it does indicate that our tastes are not immutable. We must re-evaluate whether looking like Giacometti sculptures, like anorexics with barbells, or like the metamorphosed Jane Fonda herself really constitutes beauty.

If we step back a moment and look at our ideal of beauty from a more distant perspective—perhaps that of a future historian or an anthropologist—we might at least consider revising our judgments. The look we admire is not just close to the bone; it is the bone. The media are full of models who look like skeletons with thin parchment stretched over them as skin. Seen in a half-light with their gloss and color dimmed, *Vogue*'s bathing-suited models resemble photos of starving Biafran women and children, or even those of concentration camp victims only their postures are better. But they are every bit as scrawny as these unfortunate victims and look as undernourished. Their leaping stances and colorful garments do not make them seem embodiments of youthful energy: They seem rather more like parodies of life, sticklike figures bouncing about in a grotesque dance of death.

Future historians might conjecture that Americans had fallen in love with death, or at least with mortification of the flesh. They might speculate that terror of nuclear destruction had made fashion play with cadavers and turn them into images of beauty. Or they might argue that we had been so influenced by modern art, Bauhaus aesthetics, and contemporary steel architecture that our ideal human body also had come to consist only of the scaffolding that holds it up and of the machinery that makes it move. Or they might suggest that we had come to see technology, not human beings, as the prime force in history and so had chosen to resemble our conquerors. Alternatively, they might argue that our fascination with the unconscious, and our new awareness that scientific reality is concealed from us—that the universe is made of particles we cannot see and governed by laws that defy the logic of our senses—led us to strip the outer body of any meaning or significance and of any possible beauty. Or, more simply, they might conjecture that in an era of population density, it was more practical and economical to have skinny people: They would need less room, so more of them could be squeezed into the spaces on mass transit and in workplaces, and they could live in smaller houses. It certainly also might be interpreted as democratic: No one had the right to take up more space than another or to command respect through the imposing grandeur of body size.

They might also conjecture that late-twentieth-century America had so confused its image of women that what looked female could no longer be considered beautiful. Even more, they might contend that we had dehumanized, not just masculinized, the human form. We had reduced it to its smallest, least imposing form. They might argue that we had come not only to idealize technology but also, in our secular age, to distinguish humans from other animals and the civilized from the uncivilized, not by the presence of consciousness, a soul and conscience, but by suppressing animal fat. They might even suggest that we had become so terrified of what makes us human—especially our passions and our vulnerability—that we didn't want our bodies to betray any softness, curves, or idiosyncracies. Or they might think we had suppressed tender flesh because we no longer saw human beings as sources of comfort and nurture. Certainly they would sense a remarkable terror of abundance.

From a purely aesthetic perspective, our fat-free beauties might come out no better. Their faces are gaunt and angular, their necks steeples of bones. Their unfleshed arms and legs, full of sharp angles, look gangly and disproportionately long for their shrunken heads and torsos. Their clothes hang shapelessly from their shapeless forms. At the April, 1988, Academy Awards, actresses in décolletage proudly showed off protruding clavicles and ribs, knobby shoulders, and scrawny necks. Even tiny Nancy Reagan and the lovely Princess Diana, when dressed in their finery, cannot dispel this pinched, skeletal aura. Indeed, dieted women look as though all the life and color have been sucked out of them. Nor, for all the paeans to strength, do these scrawny, narrow women look strong, stable, or as if they have a stature to be reckoned with.

In striving to be fat-free, women also lose more subtle and animated forms of beauty. They sacrifice their faces and skin tone for their slender bodies, especially as they enter middle age. The late-nineteenth-century fashion of calling fat a "silken layer" was justified. It is subcutaneous fat that fills out the skin and gives it a silky, smooth texture and that gives babies' and children's skin its wonderful softness. Boys lose this layer when they hit puberty; mature women used to have skin that was different from men's precisely because they didn't lose it. Yet, this is the adipose tissue women now try so desperately to shed. With this divestiture, the neck, arms, and especially the face tend to become dried-out, gaunt, and peaked with loose skin, unsupported by adipose tissue, hanging somewhat forlornly. Facial features become exaggerated and lose all softness—noses stand out with alarming sharpness, chins look angular and harsh, eyes protrude, cheeks become sunken. When slenderness came into fashion in the early 1900s, beauty manuals consistently warned about being too thin because of these attendant flaws. Today, diet advisers often warn dieters not to be deflected by criticism about how peaked they have become. They promise that once the redistribution of weight is completed, faces fill out again. Judging from the looks of many dieting women, one can only take this reassurance with a grain of salt.

The lean body looks as repressed and controlled as the spirit that must have gotten it that way. In the movie *Desperately Seeking Susan,* Madonna was a voluptuous contrast to her costar, Rosanna Arquette. Her carefree indulgence in junk food, her exuberance for life, and her fuller body formed a cheerful contrast to Arquette whose appetite for food was as depressed as her appetite for life. When her character finally did rebel, her puritanically disciplined body didn't fit the transformation. She simply could not convey the joie-de-vivre, expansiveness, and humor of Madonna.

If eroticism is a component of beauty, and sex is a pleasure of the flesh, it is odd that we have an erotic ideal that suppresses flesh and minimizes sexual characteristics. There is little to linger over, to explore, to discover. When the body has been efficiently reduced to a flat surface, it offers no softness, no warmth, no tenderness, no mysteries—qualities once integral to images of sexuality. Our erotic ideal has become as hard and unyielding, perhaps, as the love relationships that dominate our social life. Certainly, it does not convey the wonderfully rich and multifaceted sensuality of a Sophia Loren, a Bette Midler, or a pre-diet Dolly Parton or Madonna.

Although maternal fulfillment and maturity were once an important aspect of more varied notions of beauty, our ideal leaves no room for the full-fleshed body of a mature woman who has borne children. Nothing is inherently ugly about the mature body, unless one values only youth. It can be an object of desire and even transformed into the beauty of the nude, depending on who is looking at it. There is no reason an older woman cannot have a place in the hierarchy of erotic beauty, as she did at the turn of the century. While slenderness can be charming on an adolescent boy or girl, or on someone who is naturally slim, it looks silly on the average full-grown woman: She appears incomplete and unfulfilled, ensconced in a body that has artificially preserved immaturity or that, spinsterlike, has never earned the fullness and the scars, the dignity and mystery of a body that has matured and lived.

Ironically, contrary to current beliefs, many men do not find leaner and thinner more attractive. In a recent study of 500 college-age men and women, women indicated their ideal body weight was even thinner than they thought men liked most, and men reported preferring female bodies that were even heavier than women thought they would like most. I have known several educated, single men who insisted they wouldn't even go out with a plumpish woman—only to find them marrying women who, according to current standards, would have to be deemed plumpish. The men didn't seem to notice. Male definitions of "lean" may be as different from ours as those of the MLIC are.[56]

And men rarely seem to notice the flaws that women find disfiguring. In general, they are much less critical than women of women's appearances. They seem to form an overall impression about whether a woman is attractive and leave it at that, while women set much higher standards and scrutinize every detail, carefully appraising strengths and weaknesses. It is not surprising that this is so: For the past 150 years, fashion has been primarily women's game, and they are experts on female beauty. A person who rarely looks at paintings would not notice subtleties that an artist or art historian would pick up at a glance. Someone only slightly familiar with a sport would be unable to appreciate the finer points of the game that give fans their pleasure. The same holds true for women and female bodies. They are the experts at the art or game of female physical perfection. They notice every weak point or flaw in others and in themselves. And when they strive for physical perfection, they are not just trying to please men. Indeed, women have pursued fashion's whims regardless of what men say—which is why they so often have dismissed men's ridicule of new styles. They have more serious purposes than pleasing the uninitiated of the species: They are trying to meet their culture's ideal of female beauty.

Our rigid and distorted beliefs about health and beauty have led us to see only polarities. We believe our choices are thinness or fatness, gluttony or starvation, vigorous exercise or lethargy, ascetic rituals or self-indulgence, youthfulness or old age, beauty or ugliness. We seem to have forgotten that there is a middle ground, one much more likely to promote happy, healthy, and productive lives and one that allows us to make peace with our human flesh and its frailties. We need to restore moderation, to restore the golden mean.

14

A Look to the Future: The Golden Mean Restored?

In criticizing our new religion, I am not suggesting that we gorge until we are buried beneath layers of fat, that we stop exercising, neglect our bodies and our health, or ignore our physical appearance. This would merely be a surrender to the polarities that dominate our thinking. What I am arguing is that we have gone to the opposite extreme. Thinness and leanness are neither inherently healthy nor inherently beautiful. Nor are they usually natural—except for people who are starving. I am suggesting that we revise our standards and recultivate our tastes, that we find a happier middle ground where our bodies can round out with more life and flesh, where we can relish the fruits of our prosperity without self-punishment, and where we understand that the nourishment that is one of life's greatest pleasures is also one of its most basic necessities. There is a golden mean. We need to find it again.

We need to find it again because our new religion, evolving as it has from obsession and myth, is sadly wanting. It does not produce physical or emotional well-being nor reasonable guidelines by which to live. Our bodies, our fitness, and our food should not be our paramount concerns. They have nothing to do with ethics, or relationships, or community involvements, or with the human soul or spirit. They have nothing to say about the meaning or purpose of life except that we should survive as well and as long as we can. They leave us with no wisdom to pass on to our children—save the injunction to take care of their bodies. They give us no purpose beyond ourselves. It is a religion appropriate only for a people whose ideals do not extend beyond their own physical well-being and whose vision of the future—and of the past—is strangely empty. Surely Americans can produce a worthier creed.

Already, there are indications that we are edging away from our new religion. Recent medical and actuarial evidence demonstrates that thinner is not healthier. There is more general acceptance of the theory that nature programmed varying weights and fat-to-lean ratios for people of the same heights and that trying to alter "preferred weight" can be both insuperably difficult and emotionally and physically damaging. The epidemic of eating disorders is making the women's press more cautious about exhorting people to reduce, and it is making the public reconsider its standards of slenderness. It has even provided us, finally, with a pejorative adjective for excessive thinness: If women always assumed the comment, "You're so thin," was a compliment, they do not do so with the much more barbed comment, "You look anorexic." Nutritionists are trying to check the extremes of our food faddism, and the popular press recently ran a spate of articles letting us know that sugar is not a poison and "junk food" is a misnomer. Even fitness fanatics are beginning to confess that vigorous daily exercise does not invigorate, but vitiates.

More significantly, perhaps, resistance against the lean ideal is mounting. Carol Shaw's *Big Beautiful Woman* magazine paved the way for change by letting dress manufacturers and advertisers know there was a vast clothing market that had not been tapped. By 1980 department stores had opened sections for the bigger woman, *Stores* magazine reported on "Sportswear Gains in Large Sizes," and agencies for big models had opened in New York City. By 1984 some southern California stores had big manikins in their display windows, and lingerie and other specialty shops for the bigger woman were opening. Large women were being enfranchised into the fashion game. For the first time in decades, they were told fatness did not make them ugly and dowdy, but their self-loathing and consequent neglect of their appearance did. With the growth of this fashion subculture, advertisers found positive adjectives about bigness with which to woo customers and so forced the first wedge in our implacable belief that only slim could be beautiful. Big women were being given a chance not only to dress well but also to look at their bodies in a new, positive way.

In 1983 a group of California feminists staged an anti-Miss America pageant. They exposed the grotesquerie hidden behind the radiant smiles of our beauty celebrities by making their theme "gorge and purge" on junk food, thereby underlining the connection between our current ideal—thinness at any cost—and bulimia. In March of the same year, the big, or at least, bigger, can be beautiful idea pervaded even the sacrosanct pages of *Playboy*. Several pages were devoted to a display of naked, well-fleshed women, artistically posed like nudes in Impressionist paintings, with their measurements and weights boldly detailed. The following year *Glamour* made an editorial decision to start including fashion and beauty strategies for women who didn't "fall into that 'model perfect' category." In February, 1987, the CBS "Morning Show" included an interview with a New York modeling agent who reported women could now gain some weight because a fuller body was in style. She even brought models along to demonstrate. The same month *Cosmopolitan* announced on its cover, "The Voluptuous Girl. She's Bouncing Back"—even though Helen Gurley Brown, the magazine's editor, had often been heard to declare fat was abhorrent. Inside were the remarkable words, "Do you have swelling hips, a lush bosom, Rubenesque thighs? If the answer is yes, you may have been feeling a trifle out of favor lately." After this masterpiece of understatement, *Cosmo* continued, " . . . those long, lean, not-an-ounce-of-fat figures are terrific of course . . . but not to mope if you don't have one! Keep in mind that the voluptuous body is the quintessentially female ideal of many, many men—and learn to make the most of yours . . . . " Accompanying this revolutionary judgment were photos of a fuller-bodied beauty in underwear and reminders of other well-endowed beauties such as Ann-Margret, Sophia Loren, Mae West, Ursula Andress, and Jayne Mansfield. Tastes seemed to be changing, slowly, tentatively opening up to include the fuller female body.[1]

It would, however, be foolish to conclude from these examples that we are about to accept a bigger body ideal. Even in these instances, there were strong qualifications: Seeing the "bigger" models, the CBS interviewer couldn't help blurting out, "Bigger? You call that bigger?" and *Cosmopolitan* warned that "lush ladies . . . must hold the line with light, constant-dieter fare . . . or run the risk of turning a voluptuous figure into a (gasp!) frankly fat one . . . . " By and large, society and its most visible role models are still dedicated to slimness.

The fitness crusade is still going full-steam ahead—more a part of the daily routine than eating for many people. Younger physicians often have been front-runners in this fitness fair and, like their cohorts, they cannot hear above its din the possibility that thinner/fitter is not healthier. And even as nutritionists are trying to correct our demonology of food, the public and some overeager reformers are taking it to further extremes. Mothers and teachers conscientiously tell their children that candy, fast foods, and snack foods are dangerously unhealthy. More and more of the rich are hiring their own private nutritionists, many of whom have dubious qualifications. They have come to believe that there is a secret alchemy in food, and nutritionists are emerging as their alchemists. They are being asked to produce the magic elixir that will give permanent youth, health, and beauty. It might be easier to make gold. Bona fide nutritionists have an uphill battle ahead of them. Americans are becoming more, not less, phobic about food.[2]

But we also cannot dismiss totally these hints at a relaxation of our rigid body standard, hints that we may be in the process of recultivating our tastes. In part, this relaxation may be a reaction to how extreme our body standard has become. It may also be the slow stirring of reaction against the frightening epidemic of eating disorders. It may also be due to the fact that the very circumstances that helped create our lean standard are changing.

Demographics are different. The generation that brought in the radicalism of the sixties and Twiggy is hitting middle age: Many are inching past fifty. They can't continue to identify with or idealize the slim, youthful look of the

"Pepsi generation." And advertisers who intend to tap this market, which still constitutes the largest and richest consumer block in the nation, will have to find ways to appeal to and flatter the now older, somewhat plumper, middle-aged consumer. In the process, they will help reshape our images of beauty.

There is also a trend toward reintegrating traditional roles into women's richer and more complex lives, and with these changes could come changes in beauty aesthetics. The liberated women who opted for careers instead of children have begun having second thoughts as their biological clocks tick away. They, and younger women as well, are beginning to have children again and are as enthusiastic about it as if they themselves had discovered the process. The baby boomlet is restoring maternity to a position of respect and even of envy. A more maternal, fecund female ideal could certainly emerge in this environment. The successes of feminism may also help erode our masculinized ideal. Women are more confident about being accepted than they were not very long ago, when they were the token females in male territory. To be accepted as professional equals, they had to downplay whatever made them seem traditionally female. Today, particularly among the younger generation of women, these problems are much less formidable. Just as women came to take their right to vote for granted, forgetting the dedicated battle their forebears fought to win it, so this younger generation can take their places in male occupations without having to fight the battles their mothers or older sisters fought. Women may now feel they can be treated as equals even if they obviously have the bodies of females. They may no longer feel so compelled to prove themselves by suppressing their curves.

The sexual promiscuity of the sixties and seventies has also taken a different turn with the epidemics of herpes and AIDS and with the new trend toward social traditionalism: Weddings are back in style and divorce rates are edging down from their all-time highs. Even the Playboy empire is beginning to flounder. In the eighties Playboy Clubs were closing in several major cities. Perhaps Americans have become too sophisticated for the sophmoric titillation provided by the Playboy gestalt. Even *Cosmopolitan,* which for so long glamorized recreational sex and pre- or extramarital affairs, is beginning to change its tune. A recent article was entitled, "Love Him, Don't Leave Him." Its argument: Sex is better with a well-established lover than with someone new. This indeed was a new position for the Cosmo woman. Intimacy may once again mean more than a promiscuous sexual encounter. With the return to more traditional behavior and with the waning emphasis on the mechanics (as opposed to the emotions) of sex, the pressures that made women focus so intensely on their bodies may also begin to wane.

And the fashion industry, while it continues to promote slenderness and body-hugging styles, has been unable to impose overall body-baring styles like the miniskirt. In a show of independence, women—particularly professional women, the "most powerful new force in the marketplace" as *Time* recently dubbed them—rejected the mini, much as they had rejected the midi twenty years before. As one professional woman explained to *Time:* "I have worked very hard to reach a point where I am taken seriously in the business community . . . . A short, short skirt is not going to help that." Conservatism may continue to mark future styles. Variety may as well for, in deference to women's refusal to bow to their dictates, designers are providing a wider array of styles and skirt lengths. This trend may allow women to seek clothing that suits their bodies and relieve them from feeling they must make their bodies suit prevailing styles.[3]

And finally, fashionable beauty, even when it's called health, cannot stay long at one extreme. Fashions change in response to large historical developments, but they also evolve in accord with their own internal dynamics, like any plastic art. Historically, styles have tended to move toward one extreme and then rather quickly rebound away from it, leaving only a vestige that eventually disappears. No stylistic fad can last forever, simply because it becomes boring and loses its novelty. Fashions in body shape and size, of course, change much more slowly and are more deeply rooted in a complex of cultural values and beliefs. But, to the extent that they are subject to fashion's dynamics, we can hope that the fashion for the slender body, which began at the turn of this century, and the trend toward ever leaner female forms, will have spent itself by the century's end.

I certainly am not suggesting, as many current feminists have, that we do away with beauty and fashion standards. It would be a bleak world if we did not celebrate beauty and if we did not allow ourselves the pleasure and play involved in bedecking ourselves and molding our own images. The impulse toward adornment and self-beautification runs deep in human culture and is connected to humanity's most profound and finest aspirations. Nor am I trying to suggest that the fashion standards of past eras were always benign. Each era exacts its own price for beauty—though it appears that only our era has produced a beauty standard based exclusively on the bare bones of being with such disastrous effects. Rather, I suggest that we cultivate more catholic tastes so a slender woman can be appreciated for her assets, and a Rubenesque woman for hers, so we can see the beauty of youth as well as the beauty of maturity.

Our current religion has distorted our perception about health and our health goals. We have developed a remarkably elastic—and sloppy—definition of obesity, one that has obscured the fact that clinically abnormal and dangerous obesity is not merely a matter of being at the heavy end of the normal weight-distribution curve but a condition with particular metabolic and anatomic features. The conviction that body weight is largely a mechanical matter of diet and exercise has led many researchers to subject the obese to painful, and, upon occasion, life-threatening, regimens and operative procedures. A more disturbing effect has been that what is normal is no longer perceived as healthy. Our presumptions have obscured the fact that for the large numbers of people who do not fall into the slenderest end of the weight-distribution curve, "overweight" is healthy for their body makeup and not in the least abnormal.

In some sense, the campaign against overweight has been an ambitious national experiment to get everybody down to a standard size, to get them to look the same, a goal perhaps fitting for a society that reveres equality. But it appears that in our zealotry, we have been guilty of confusing medical and political goals and of confusing equality and uniformity. People, proscriptively at least, are equal in social and political life, but they cannot be made physically uniform, without suffering.

Indeed, our new religion has generated a myth about health and beauty that functions much like nineteenth- and early twentieth-century ideas about poverty, which was presumed to be the result of individual flaws. Today, we believe that fatness and even ill health are also the result of individual flaws, of failure to discipline personal habits. We have so minimized the importance of heredity, body constitution, disease, and sheer luck—of the unpredictable vagaries of nature itself—that we believe people are responsible for their physical status. Sadly, the overweight and to a somewhat lesser extent, the sick, now must feel the double insult not only of their body condition but also of insinuations that it is their fault.

Our new religion has also distorted our attitudes and our behavior. Its underlying presumption is that what is normal in America is unhealthy, whether it be body weights, cholesterol levels, dietary patterns, or exercise habits. This view, pushed by eager health reformers and disseminated by our news-hungry media, powerfully affects us. It has spawned a negative national self-image: We do not see Americans as robust and resourceful but rather as self-indulgent, lethargic, weak, and diseased. It has also spawned a pervasive sense of dread and hypochondria: We believe that to live a typically American life-style is to court premature death, and we attribute serious illnesses as well as minor malaises to this life-style and to our inability to reform the personal habits it encourages. We have lost, unnecessarily, faith in our culture—and in the resilience and capacities of the human body.[4]

These views have led millions of us to behave as though we are invalids for whom one slip-up in our controlled regimen can mean disaster. Like frail little old people, we fret about every twinge in our bodies, every minor malaise, and every morsel we put in our mouths. Like T. S. Eliot's timid and repressed J. Alfred Prufrock, we ask, "Do I dare to eat a peach? Do I dare and do I dare?" and we measure out our lives, not in coffeespoons, but in doses of calories, vitamins, and exercise units. We have swung to such extremes in these preoccupations that instead of adopting habits that are natural extensions of the body's own inclinations, we have dominated the body with unpleasant and often debilitating regimens. In our lust for health, we have fallen into the trap described by François de La Rochefoucauld in the seventeenth century: "To preserve one's health by too strict a regimen is itself a tedious malady." We are encouraging a dour and ascetic way of life.

Perhaps the most deleterious effect of our new religion and of the fat-phobia that underlies it is how it has contorted our relationship to food and appetite. We have come to believe that people need only minimal amounts of food, that eating is a self-indulgence, and that eating abundantly does not nourish—it kills. Here, too, we have gone to unrealistic extremes. Human beings, like all living things, need nourishment to live. It is as essential as air and water. Better nourishment, both in quality and quantity, produces better health. At what point better becomes excess and causes debility or death is not clear: We do know that formerly starving or semistarved people—whether yo-yo dieters, anorexics, or famine victims—who suddenly begin to stuff themselves and gain weight rapidly often die. Apparently the body cannot tolerate such radical extremes. But as we have seen, our presumption that Americans are "overnourished" is not borne out by the evidence—yet we continue to insist that they should "undereat" and that they need very little food.

We have turned control of appetite, denial of hunger, abstemious eating, and their physical manifestation, thinness, into our primary virtue. In this respect, our "religion" is unique among the major religions of the world, if not of certain sects. While there is a long history in religion of fasting for spiritual purity or cleansing, no religion has set it up as a virtue, and most have frowned upon it. Buddha tried fasting but rejected it because he did not find it was the way to Enlightenment. Judaism prescribes a few fast days a year, from sundown to sunset. Otherwise, it proscribes such deprivation because, the Talmud explains, people must be well-nourished so they can do what is most important in life—follow God's commandments and perform *mitzvot,* that is, good deeds. The early Church fathers, too, condemned fasting, and the Church exacted higher penances for the sin of not eating than it did for the sin of gluttony. The fast days of Catholicism did not require abstinence from all food but rather from meat or from rich and delicious foods. Even the Muslims, during their great fast of Ramadan, do not abstain from food. They are merely proscribed from eating during certain hours in this period, and the nonfast hours are given to feasting, especially on delicacies associated only with the holiday. For these religions, food has not been seen as a temptation put in humanity's path but rather as a vital necessity for people to carry out their larger spiritual tasks.

Indeed, our distrust of food and appetite has led to a curious perversion of common sense. We seem to ignore the rather striking fact that the pleasures of the palate are nature's way of ensuring that we will eat. It seems more than fortuitous that things have been arranged so that humans find great pleasure in sex and in eating. They are the two voluntary functions that ensure survival, the former of our species, the latter of the individual. Hearty appetite is not a symptom of derangement but rather a sign of health and life. Indeed, loss of appetite characterizes people who are ill—which is why so many women today are half-grateful for bouts of illness: They make dieting effortless. Loss of appetite, not excessive appetite, characterizes old age: The most commonly undernourished group in this country is the widowed elderly who have lost their interest in life and in food. Loss of appetite, not excessive appetite, characterizes those who have lost their urge to live. Hilde Bruch observed that one type of psychologically induced obesity, reactive obesity, occurs among people who have suffered severe emotional loss—the death of loved ones, the end of a love affair—and who respond to these events not with suicidal despair but with overeating. She suggested that food was a comfort for them and a reminder that life still held pleasure and meaning.

The well-nourished person, not the undernourished one, grows strong and healthy. Today, experts warn that youngsters on "healthy" low-fat, low-cholesterol, nonsugar diets may suffer from failure to thrive and, possibly, irreversibly stunted growth. The well-nourished person, not the undernourished one, is more productive and better able to function, and more free, possibly, to be creative. One of the developments that preceded the eighteenth- and nineteenth-century industrial advances in the Western nations was improved nutrition. Several historians have suggested that this was a prerequisite for those advances.[5]

Yet our new religion distorts these rather obvious facts. The diets many of us try, or are exhorted to follow, are as low in calories as those in impoverished countries. And while we deplore their tragic effects on such populations, we regard our own adherence to them as virtuous and energizing. We subscribe to dietary rules that resemble older prescriptions that we have sex only at certain times and then only in the missionary position. But perhaps our sensual life has designed us to burst such constraints. Certainly it would seem that those of us who eagerly anticipate meals and who relish them exhibit not a lack of self-control but, rather, a passion for life.

Women are especially susceptible to the contorted beliefs about food and appetite because they try so hard to meet our emaciated female ideal. Men are less so because their body standards are not as thin as women's and because bigness and hearty appetite never became totally separated from masculinity. These contorted ideas have been largely responsible for the spread of eating disorders.[6]

I am not trying to suggest that every case of eating disorder—whether obesity or anorexia or bulimia—is culturally induced, but certainly cultural attitudes are critical. When the eighteenth-century philosopher, David Hume, suddenly went from very lean to quite heavy, he wrote to his physician that "in six weeks time I passed from the one extreme to the other, and being before tall, lean and rawboned, became a sudden the most sturdy, robust, healthful-like fellow you have seen with a ruddy complexion and a cheerful countenance." Notice how happy he was about his transformation and contrast it to how we today would regard such a change. We would be distraught, and for each of his positive adjectives, we would plug in its opposite. We would think we had some very serious psychological or physical problem and would hastily begin efforts to exorcise this deadly new fat. It is in this way that cultural standards shape our mental life.[7]

The primary reason one can only hope that our current religion will wane is because of its inadequacies as a religion. It provokes us to place extraordinary importance on physical appearance despite all our lip service to health. Ironically, the generation that spurned fashion for being frivolous and superficial now sacrifices sleep, time, money, and even physical well-being to get the body proportions idealized today. The moralism we attach to body size has even encouraged the belief that the shape of the body reveals a person's character, his or her capacity for self-discipline, and moral strength.

Our new religion does not produce better people. We might be able to run farther, do a few more jumping jacks, and lift some heavier weights. We might even have learned to say no to succulent meats and rich desserts. But whether we are worrying about how good we look or whether we are avoiding disease, the emphasis is always and exclusively on us and, more precisely, on our bodies. We are so self-absorbed, and so preoccupied about the possibility of dying, that we cannot lift our heads away from our body chemistries, pulse rates, muscle tone, or fat-to-lean ratios to ask what the purpose of these rituals—and of longer life—is.

It is one thing to follow a rigid dietary code and rituals of behavior in accordance with the laws of a God we worship. In such instances, the faithful are trying to fulfill God's commandments, not only for their own salvation, not only to help sustain His system of morals and laws, but also to hasten the arrival of a more perfect world. It is quite another thing to follow rigid dietary and behavior codes only to improve our physical selves. Such actions are not part of a larger system of morals. They don't place value on giving to others. They have no vision of a higher good or of a better future that their rituals might help create. This is a solipsistic religion in the narrowest and strictest sense in that it is not about meaning or wisdom or harmony, or kindess or human ethics, but only about the literal bare bones of being. If avoiding death and disease are our primary concerns, the main preoccupations of our lives, then what are we living for?

The religion has so trivialized our sense of morality that we have come to believe personal purity is connected only to the food we put in our bodies, to bare physical realities. Recently, a homosexual published his "diary" in which he described the sexual encounters he had on an average weekend. They consisted of an unending series of orgies with strangers in parks and in gay bars, sometimes with four or five men at a time performing oral, anal, or masturbatory sex on one another. The diarist happened to mention that he took time off to grab something to eat. He would not eat "junk food," he explained, because he did not want to sully his body. This is the kind of morality our new religion condones.[8]

Our new religion has also distorted our sense of what we should appreciate.

Women are particularly swept up in this distortion. Historically unprecedented numbers of us are healthy, able to enjoy sex without fear of unwanted pregnancy, to go through childbirth without the once-omnipresent threat of death, to treat easily once-mortal infectious diseases, and to alleviate the minor aches and pains that caused discomfort to our forebears—from toothaches to earaches to headaches to skin eruptions to upset stomachs. Advances in technology, medicine, and food production, wrought by painstaking human efforts have given us a well-being rare in previous centuries. We should be grateful for the condition of our bodies, but we hate them because they bulge here or are flabby there or because they are too fat. Surely this is the worst form of hubris—overweening pride and arrogance—to despise our bodies because they are not quite beautiful enough. And indeed, our new religion neither puts checks on this kind of vanity nor underscores how very trivial is the accomplishment of weight loss and of physical perfection. Instead, it leads us to believe that the quest for such perfection is the worthiest of human goals.

At the heart of our religion and of women's quests for lean bodies is a terrible fear of abundance. We have become so frightened of our plentiful food supplies that we have forgotten food once was tied to humanity's most sacred rituals and beliefs, that food and drink were the first offerings put on the altars of the gods. It has also been the traditional focus of festive life and of social relationships: how much so can be seen from the very roots of the word *companion.* It derives from the Latin *com,* which means together and *panis,* which means bread—a companion and an intimate are those with whom we break bread. And, indeed, from the Biblical days of Abraham until quite recently, offering food to those who enter one's home has been an indispensable gesture of hospitality.

Today, many authorities argue that such attitudes are historical vestiges, inappropriate for industrially advanced nations with secure and cheap food supplies. Modernization has ended the ancient rhythm of alternating periods of feast and famine, and fear has mounted that without natural or economic restraints on appetite, feasting could become permanent. And with the modern pestilences—cardiovascular disease and cancer—experts have fastened on this overabundance as a pathogenic agent. We have come to seek nutrients without calories; to fear food, and to regard it as a luxury, not a necessity. And oddly, we seem to believe that because we live in an environment of plenty, we as individuals do not need to eat much. But the fact that food is plenteous does not make it any less essential for individual human survival and should not make us value it less. Indeed, as with women and their bodies, hubris lurks here. We have been so befuddled by how much we have that we spurn it instead of being grateful for it.

Our new religion also reflects a terror of abundant flesh. Those who argue that our food attitudes are an evolutionary anomaly argue the same about bodies prone to fatness. Presumably, such a body was well adapted to survive the dearth or famine that often followed periods of plenty (though one cannot help but wonder if this is an anthropological fiction: The fat do not seem to tolerate dietary deprivation better than the thin). Since we no longer have natural periods of dearth, the argument goes, the tendency to add fat stores has become maladaptive. Fatness therefore strikes us not only as ugly and unhealthy but also as primitive and uncivilized. Of course, this argument holds true only for the small portion of humanity that lives in industrially advanced nations. The rest of the world still faces an unremitting cycle of feast—or at least of adequate food supplies—and famine.

The idea that people should go hungry and reduce their body size to its minimal elements is peculiarly modern. Only in the late nineteenth century do we begin to find total fasting elevated to a virtue. Perhaps in an age when religion began to lose its hold and God, as Nietzsche proclaimed, was dead, people had to find virtues to replace those that flowed from His presumed existence or from a divine reason in man. They had to find other ways to demonstrate that they were above the uncivilized. What could be more dramatic than total abstinence from food—proof that they could defy the most elemental animal need of all, the need for nourishment and proof that they did not even need to rely on animal matter to live? Such an act could indeed seem superhuman, could indeed attract and satisfy the religious impulses of people who live in a secular age.[9]

Perhaps our secular worldview also spawned our fervence for prolonging life. Certainly, humanity has always feared death and adopted rituals to avoid it, but religions provided the comforts of an afterlife and helped make some sense of the apparent senselessness of human mortality. All religions have denied the finality of death, whether through concepts of reincarnation, of a lifelike heaven, or of an awaited Messiah who would raise the dead from their graves. We, with our philosophical materialism, do not permit the luxury of such beliefs. We generally assume that when our bodies die, so does whatever comprises our souls. All we have is what we have here on earth. If we cannot prolong our lives, we do have nothing.

Our values about human appetite and flesh also reflect changes in our attitudes toward nature. The rise of modern technology and the kind of thinking that came with it implied not human harmony with nature, but human control of it. We applied to the body the principles we used, to tame the wilderness and to reach outer space. Nature seemed subject to our intellectual and physical control. It could be brought to submission. Perhaps we turned the skinny body, the repressed appetite, and the refusal to yield to aging into virtues precisely because they symbolize penultimate control of the human machine itself.

Our conviction that we can determine our fates personal habits may also stem from this new view of nature. Human beings have always lived with dread of both death and of the world coming to an end. But today, we believe that the source of such cataclysms will not be natural disasters and pestilences nor divine wrath, but, rather, people. We believe human beings and their technology alone threaten our survival: They can destroy the natural environment and they can unleash nuclear war. As a result, we are persuaded that longer life can be achieved simply by resisting the hazards that modernization has strewn before us: processed food, culinary abundance, and inactivity.

We focus on our daily habits also because this view has led us to minimize nature's power. Indeed, we now believe it is our responsibility to save the natural environment. We no longer think that nature victimizes us, but rather that we victimize it. With this emasculation, nature has come to seem beneficient and kindly, and we ignore its brutality and capriciousness. Consequently, we refuse to accept the power biology and chance wield over our fates and instead put all our faith in reforming our behavior.

The awesome power we now perceive human beings to have may also have led us to favor an unfleshed body. Symbolically, our urgent demand for control of appetite and body size may reflect our fear that if human impulses are not restrained, catastrophe could result. We may idealize the scrawny form precisely because it signifies a human being who is in total control.

Perhaps our new religion derives not so much from our fear of uncontrolled human impulses as from a loss of faith in humanity itself, in its capacity for goodness and reason. This loss may stem not only from disillusionments with politics and with modernization, but, on a more personal level, from the instability of even our most intimate relationships. A social ideology that advocates commitment to the self and to self-realization over commitments to others, including spouses and children, is an ideology that carries individualism to the extreme. We may desperately seek health and strength and feel compelled to "take care of ourselves" because we are afraid that if we don't, no one will be there to take care of us. And indeed, we may have stripped our human ideal down to bare bones because we believe we should not regard others—especially women—as sources of emotional and physical security, comfort, and nurture.[10]

Certainly, our current body standards are based on a peculiarly hostile view of humans and of the flesh that gives them life. We have all gone to our local malls and have seen those dumpy, lumpy "fat" Americans who have caused us such distress. But they are less abnormal than our standard of what they should look like and what clothing styles they should wear. Indeed, if we look at images of human beings from earlier periods, such as Breugel's painting, *The Wedding Dance,* the men and women have the same kinds of bodies we see in the mall, yet their amplitude bespoke their fertility and vitality—as the men's erections (camouflaged in many later reproductions) demonstrate. Ample flesh signified humanity's indomitable will and ability to survive in an often hostile world.

To suggest that we allow more latitude in our standards of body size and that we return to a philosophy that celebrates food and flesh instead of dreading it may seem at best utopian. But I am not suggesting that we ignore our health or that we overthrow all food rules: Cultures must provide coherent and meaningful patterns for us to satisfy our needs. I am not suggesting that we become militantly inactive. Exercise can be fun and make us feel good, and feminism's accomplishment in encouraging women to be athletic must be applauded: It's wonderful for those inclined to athleticism. But we have gone to extremes, and it has taken its toll—particularly in the distorted values it has spawned. We need to return to a golden mean and to more worthy values.

We need to end the rigidity of our skeletal body-size standards both in medicine and in fashion. We should replace them with body types more suitable to our life-style, more in keeping with the normal variety of body sizes, and more congenial to life itself. And we need to distinguish more carefully between moral and health issues. Certainly, in the case of our health ethic, we have fallen into the confusion described so well by Susan Sontag: We have used illness as a metaphor for larger cultural concerns and prejudices.[11]

Even more, we need to correct the distorted values of our new religion. To elevate physical perfection into our primary goal is to trivialize human life itself. We need to restore a more humanistic vision in which self-improvement means cultivating the mind as well as enlarging the soul, developing generosity and humor as well as dignity and humility, living more respectfully and graciously with our own biologies and with aging and death—and even with our own limitations. We need to restore a more meaningful concept of self-improvement, one in which we remember that we have the obligation and the opportunity to learn from the past, to build on it, and to bequeath this knowledge and, especially, wisdom to future generations. Instead, we stand poised between a past for which have lost respect and a future we do not even try to envision. We place all our energies and thoughts into trying to prolong our own lives and perfect our bodies. Is this a philosophy to bequeath to the future?

Recently, a journalist for the *New York Times Magazine* described some of the dangers of liposuction, one of which is death from surgical complications. She remarked that she had toyed with the idea of having the procedure done but was repelled by the thought that if she were one of those who died, her young daughters would have to be told that she had risked death to make her thighs a little more becoming. Perhaps only with the awareness that the young depend on us for sustenance and moral guidance can we really begin to see the folly of our new religion.[12]

We have been victims, not of a conspiracy, but of a confluence of developments that created a taste for shrunken, fat-free bodies, and that unleashed a war on one of humanity's most basic needs and delights: food. It is time we worked our way out of this web of cultural myths and prejudices. We must make peace with our abundance. Without the feast and without human flesh, there is no celebration, no reconfirmation of life.

Notes

CHAPTER 1

1 "Dieting: The Losing Game," *Time,* Jan. 20, 1986, 54; *Tufts University Diet and Nutrition Letter,* Aug. 1985, 1; "Fat Chance in a Thin World," PBS Nova program, broadcast March 22, 1983, WGBH transcript; Gallup Survey reported in "Working Out in America," *American Health,* March 1985, 42–47.

2 On studies of San Francisco children done by nutritionist Laurel Mellin and on other studies, see Jeannine Stein, "Why Girls as Young as 9 Fear Fat and Go on Diets to Lose Weight," *Los Angeles Times,* Oct. 29, 1986, V:1; also see "Fear of Obesity Hits Youngsters," *Los Angeles Times,* June 29, 1986, IX:10.

3 Theodore Berland and the Editors of Consumer Guide *Rating the Diets,* Consumer Guide (New York: Beckman House), 1983.

4 "Dieting: The Losing Game," loc. cit., 54; *Tufts University Diet and Nutrition Letter,* May 1986, 3.

5 Berland, op. cit., 148.

6 *Tufts University Diet and Nutrition Letter,* Aug. 1985, 3.

7 *Tufts University Diet and Nutrition Letter,* Jan. 1985, 1.

8 The numbers of people exercising regularly vary considerably from source to source. The 60 percent figure is from Hillel Schwartz, *Never Satisfied: A Cultural History of Diets, Fantasies and Fat* (New York: The Free Press, 1986), 255; the number of joggers, from *Stores,* Feb. 1984, 8; also see figures of National Sporting Goods Assn. and National Running Data Center of Tucson, Ariz., reported in Joe Domanick, "Sport of Running Is Taking a Different Direction in LA," *Los Angeles Times,* Feb. 24, 1987, V:1.

9 Jim Seale, "Exercisewear," *Stores,* June 1984, 13–16.

10 David P. Schultz, "Selling the Newest Trendy Pastime: Exercise," *Stores,*

Feb. 1983, 10; Julia Vitullo-Martin, "The Business Education of Jane Fonda," *Fortune,* Feb. 20, 1984, 130.

11 Harvey Green, *Fit for America: Health-Fitness-Sport and American Society* (New York: Pantheon Books, 1986); Number of marathon runners cited in William Bennett M.D. and Joel Gurin, *The Dieter's Dilemma: Eating Less and Weighing More* (New York: Basic Books, 1982), 244 and in Joe Domanick, loc. cit., 1; On numbers of joggers and triathalon, see Janet Wallach, "Triathalon," *Stores,* Feb. 1984, 5–9.

12 *People,* Jan. 6, 1986, 37.

13 Jim Seale, loc. cit., 13.

14 NIH position and the fact that Americans are the fattest population in "Dieting: The Losing Game," loc. cit., 55.

15 Ibid.

16 Mayer cited in *Time,* Sept. 10, 1973, 75; White cited in ibid., 80.

17 Hirsch cited in "Dieting: The Losing Game," loc. cit., 55.

18 McGovern committee report comment cited in Patricia Hausman, *Jack Sprat's Legacy: The Science and Politics of Fat and Cholesterol* (New York: Richard Marek Publications, 1981), 191.

19 Jane Fonda, *Jane Fonda's Workout Book* (New York: Simon and Schuster, 1981), 49.

20 Robert M. Cunningham, Jr., *Wellness at Work: A Report on Health and Fitness Programs for Employees of Business and Industry* (Chicago: Blue Cross/Blue Shield Association, 1982); *Healthy People: The Surgeon General's Report on Health Promotion and Disease Prevention,* U.S. Dept. of Health Education and Welfare (Washington, D.C.: USGPO, 1979), vii; Secretary of Agriculture's statement and other departmental reorganizations cited in Jurgen Schmandt, Rose Ann Shorey, and Lilas Kinch, *Nutrition Policy in Transition* (Lexington: Lexington Books, 1980), 17–19.

21 Robert Half, "Fatter Execs Get Slimmer Paychecks," *Industry Week,* Jan. 14, 1974, 21, 24; Sylvia Auerbach, "Obesity: An Obstacle to Managerial Success," *Computer Decisions,* 14, 1982, 166–68.

22 Information on comparative weights of models was cited by Dr. C. Wayne Callaway, director of the Center for Clinical Nutrition at George Washington University at the 17th annual California Council Nutrition Conference at Newport Beach, California, in May, 1987 and was reported in Verne Palmer, "Where's the Fat?" *The Outlook,* May 13, 1987, C-1.

23 Mrs. Richards Hughes quote in *Ladies' Home Journal,* Oct. 1968, 147.

24 Benton quoted in *People,* Jan. 6, 1986, 34.

25 Cover, *Ms.,* May 1986.

CHAPTER 2

1 Kim Chernin coined the term the tyranny of slenderness in Kim Chernin, *The Obsession: Reflections on the Tyranny of Slenderness* (New York:

Harper & Row, 1981). Statistics on the number of women suffering from eating disorders vary considerably: See Paul E. Garfinkel and David M. Garner, *Anorexia Nervosa: A Multidimensional Perspective* (New York: Brunner/Mazel, 1982); Marlene Boskind-White and William C. White, Jr., *Bulimarexia: The Binge/Purge Cycle* (W. W. Norton & Co., 1983); Jane Brody recently suggested bulimia affects 25 percent of college women, in "Personal Health," *New York Times,* March 18, 1987, C-4; Joan Jacobs Brumberg, who cautions about using the term "epidemic" to describe the incidence of eating disorders, nonetheless confirms that they have increased dramatically in recent years and argues that it was "the disease" of the seventies, to be eclipsed only by AIDS in the mid eighties. She presents what seem to be the most reasoned estimates of their incidence in Joan Jacobs Brumberg, *Fasting Girls: The Emergence of Anorexia Nervosa as a Modern Disease* (Cambridge: Harvard University Press, 1988), 12. See also Hilde Bruch on the increasing prevalence of anorexia nervosa in Bruch, *The Golden Cage* (New York: Basic Books, 1978), Introduction.

2 The mortality rate from anorexia nervosa is cited in Jacobs, op. cit., 13.

3 *Newsweek,* Dec. 13, 1982, 84.

4 Erving Goffman cited in B. J. Kalisch, "The Stigma of Obesity," *American Journal of Nursing,* 72 (1972), 1124–1127.

5 McDermott case cited in "Dieting: The Losing Game," *Time,* Jan. 20, 1986, 54.

6 NAAFA example cited in Marcia Millman, *Such a Pretty Face: Being Fat in America* (New York: Berkeley Books, 1982), 17. There is an enormous amount of literature on the suffering of fat people in both the popular and professional press. See also, A. Harmetz, "Oh How We're Punished for the Crime of Being Fat," *Today's Health,* January, 1974, 21–24; Lisa Schoenfielder and Barb Wieser (eds), *Shadow on a Tightrope: Writings by Women on Fat Oppression* (Iowa City: Aunt Lute Book Company, 1983); Hillel Schwartz, *Never Satisfied: A Cultural History of Diets, Fantasies and Fat* (New York: The Free Press, 1986); Anne Scott Beller, *Fat and Thin* (New York: Farrar Straus & Giroux, 1977); William Bennett, M.D. and Joel Gurin, *The Dieter's Dilemma: Eating Less and Weighing More* (New York: Basic Books, 1982); J. Mayer, J. Dwyer, and J. J. Feldman, "The Social Psychology of Dieting," *Journal of Health and Social Behavior,* 11, (1970), 269–287; Kalisch, op. cit. The best examples of our culture's contempt for fat people can be found in the language of diet books themselves which, in exhorting readers, describes the repulsiveness of fatness and of the personal weaknesses that allowed it to grow.

7 Examples cited in Schoenfielder and Wieser, op. cit. and Millman, op. cit.

8 On children's reactions, see sources cited in note 6 above, particularly J. Mayer, J. Dwyer, and J. J. Feldman, op. cit. and Kalisch, op. cit.

9 Millman, op. cit., 216.

10 Mayer, Dwyer, and Feldman, loc. cit.; Bennett and Gurin, op. cit., espe-

cially chapter 2; Hilde Bruch, *Eating Disorders* (New York: Basic Books, 1973).

11 Bruch, *Eating Disorders,* op. cit., 142.

12 Robert M. Cunningham, Jr., *Wellness at Work: A Report on Health and Fitness Programs for Employees of Business and Industry* (Chicago: Blue Cross/Blue Shield Association, 1982), 76.

13 Monaghan story in *People,* Jan. 6, 1986, 37; Goldberg cited in Chris Chase, *The Great American Waistline* (New York: Coward, McCann & Geoghegan, 1981), 231; Hirsch cited in "Dieting: The Losing Game," loc. cit., 60.

14 See, for example, Michael Pugliese, Fima Lifshitz, Gary Grad, Pavel Fort, and Marjorie Marks-Katz, "Fear of Obesity: A Cause of Short Stature and Delayed Puberty," *New England Journal of Medicine,* Sept. 1, 1983, 513–18; and Rose Dosti, "Nutritionists Express Worries About Children Following Adult Diets," *Los Angeles Times,* June 29, 1986, 6.

15 Bruch, *The Golden Cage,* op. cit.; Garfinkel and Garner, op. cit., 100–112; On the remarkably female character of group dieting programs, see Hillel Schwartz, op. cit., 202–213; and Brumberg, op. cit.

16 Rubin cited in Chernin, op. cit., 35; "Feeling Fat in a Thin Society," *Glamour,* Feb. 1984, 198–201, 251–53; Geoffrey Haynes (AP), "Study Shows Men Unhappy as Women About Weight Gain," *Lansing State Journal,* Jan. 18, 1988, 4B.

17 Robin Lakoff and Raquel Scherr, *Face Value: The Politics of Beauty* (Boston: Routledge, & Kegan Paul, 1984), 141–42, 168–69.

18 "Letters," *Ms.,* Jan. 1984, 10.

19 Dalma Heyn, "Why We're Never Satisfied with Our Bodies," *McCall's,* May 1982, 80, 114–16; "How to Make Peace with the Body You've Got," *Glamour,* Oct. 1984, 276–81.

20 For a good, brief discussion of this with the major references cited, see William Bennett M.D., and Joel Gurin, op. cit., 139–41; see also Hillel Schwartz, op. cit., 279–80.

21 "When Heavy Exercise Halts Menstruation," *Tufts University Diet and Nutrition Letter,* Vol. 4, No. 7, Sept. 1986, 2; On amenorrhea in dieting overweight women, see Gina Kolata, "Overweight and Where It Begins," *Smithsonian,* Jan. 1986, 94; Iris F. Litt, "Amenorrhea in the Adolescent Athlete: Exploration of a Growing Phenomenon," *Postgraduate Medicine,* Vol. 80, No. 5, 1986, 245–53.

22 "When Heavy Exercise Halts Menstruation," loc. cit., 2.

23 Ibid.

24 Chernin, op. cit., 34; Bruch, op. cit., 13; C. Branch and L. Eurman, "Social Attitudes Toward Patients with Anorexia Nervosa," *American Journal of Psychiatry,* 137 (1980), 631–32.

25 "Breslow Prescription" cited in Robert Cunningham, Jr., op. cit.; for the original description, see Nedra B. Belloc and Lester Breslow, "Relation-

ship of Physical Health Status and Health Practices," *Preventive Medicine,* Aug. 1972, 409–20.

26 Bruch, op. cit., 194–211; Albert Stunkard, "The 'Dieting Depression'," *American Journal of Medicine* 23 (1957), 77–86; idem., *The Pain of Obesity* (Palo Alto: Bull Publishing Co., 1976); Bruch, op. cit. 9–23; David W. Swanson and Frank A. Dinello, "Severe Obesity as a Habituation Syndrome," *Archives of General Psychiatry* 22 (1970), 127.

27 J. A. Nichols, "Sports Medicine—Past, Present and Future," *American Journal of Sports Medicine* 8 (1980), 389–94; and a series of articles in the medical press, e.g., W. L. Lehman, "Overuse Syndrome in Runners," *American Family Physician,* Jan. 1984, 157–61. In the early 1980s, considerable debate was carried on in the medical literature about the advantages and disadvantages of exercise and about these less-than-desirable aspects of what some called "obligatory runners," which could also be applied to obligatory exercisers; see, e.g., Alayne Yates, Kevin Leehey, and Catherine Shisslak, "Running—An Analogue of Anorexia?" *New England Journal of Medicine,* Vol. 38, No. 5, Feb. 3, 1983, 251–55 and their citations of other articles describing a similar phenomenon. See also the less convincing rebuttal to their argument in J. Blumenthal, L. O'Toole, and J. Chang, "Is Running an Analogue of Anorexia Nervosa?" *Journal of the American Medical Association,* Vol. 252, No. 4, July 27, 1984, 520–23. While obligatory exercisers may indeed not have the pathology of hospitalized anorexic patients, Yates, et al.'s more general observation remains valid: Obligatory exercisers seem to vitiate, not enrich, their personal lives; see, for example, descriptions of "exercise junkies" in Blair Sabol, *The Body of America* (New York: Arbor House, 1986).

28 For a fuller discussion of these studies and for references cited, see chapter 13 and footnote 1 to chapter 13.

CHAPTER 3

1 "Interview with Hugh Hefner," *Playboy,* Jan. 1974, 68; Frank Harris, *My Secret Life* (New York: Grove Press, 1966).

2 Anne Hollander, *Seeing Through Clothes* (New York: Viking Press, 1978), 106; Kenneth Clark, *The Nude: A Study in Ideal Form* (Princeton: Princeton University Press, 1956), 140.

3 Clark, op. cit., 83.

4 Ibid., 5, 9–10.

5 Shogun comment cited in Fernand Braudel, tr. Miriam Kochman, *Capitalism and Material Life* (New York: Harper & Row, 1973), 235. There are many histories of fashion and of these developments. The best standard work in English is Francois Boucher, *20,000 Years of Fashion: The History of Costume and Personal Adornment,* tr. Harry N. Abrams, Inc., and Thames and Hudson Ltd., (New York: Harry N. Abrams, 1987). A pro-

vocative and informative discussion of many issues considered here, particularly the relationship between the nude and fashion, is in Hollander, op. cit.

6 Quotations and a good description of early Church attitudes are in Valerie Steele, *Fashion and Eroticism: Ideals of Feminine Beauty from the Victorian Era to the Jazz Age* (New York: Oxford University Press, 1985), 13–15, 17.

7 On the development of these theories, see Dr. J. C. Flugel, *The Psychology of Clothes* (London: The Hogarth Press and The Institute for Psychoanalysis, 1930); Thorstein Veblen, *The Theory of the Leisure Class* 1899 (New York: Random House, 1934); Louis Octave Uzanne, *Fashion in Paris in the Nineteenth Century: The Various Phases of Feminine Tastes and Aesthetics from the Revolution to the End of the XIXth Century,* tr. Lady Mary Lloyd (London: William Heinemann, 1901); Max von Boehn, *Modes and Manners of the Nineteenth Century,* 4 vols., tr. M. Edwardes (London: Dent, 1927); Steele, op. cit., Chapter 1; Roland Barthes, *Systéme de la mode* (Paris: Editions du Seuil, 1967); Hollander, op. cit.

8 Lois Banner, *American Beauty: A Social History through Two Centuries of the American Idea, Ideal, and Image of the Beautiful Woman* (New York: Knopf, 1983); Susan Brownmiller, *Femininity* (New York: Simon and Schuster, 1984); Robin Lakoff and Raquel Scherr, *Face Value: The Politics of Beauty* (Boston: Routledge and Kegan Paul, 1984).

9 For a fuller discussion and bibliography of these and the following issues, see Roberta P. Seid, *The Dissolution of Traditional Rural Culture in Nineteenth Century France: A Study of the Bethmale Costume* (New York: Garland Publishing, Inc., 1987), 1–45; also see Yvonne Deslandres, *Le Costume: image de l'homme* (Paris: Albin Michel, 1976); Bernard Rudofsky, *The Unfashionable Human Body* (New York: Doubleday, 1971); Alison Lurie, *The Language of Clothes* (New York: Vintage Books, 1983); Mary Ellen Roach and Joanne Eicher, *Dress, Adornment and the Social Order* (New York: John Wiley and Sons, 1965).

10 Quentin Bell, *On Human Finery* (New York: Schocken Books, 1976), 19.

11 Erving Goffman, "Identity Kits," in Roach and Eicher, op. cit., 46.

12 On profound play, John Huizinga, *Homo-Ludens: A Study of the Play Element in Culture* (London: Routledge and Kegan Paul, 1949); Nietzsche quote in Steele, op. cit., 245.

13 Seminodes cited in Sarah B. Pomeroy, *Goddesses, Whores, Wives, and Slaves: Women in Classical Antiquity* (New York: Schocken Books, 1975), 49–52; Clark cites the young men in the gymnasium, op. cit., 23.

14 On the changing attitudes of the Church, see Clark, op. cit., 313–14; Boucher, op. cit., 191.

15 Emmanuel Le Roy Ladurie, *Montaillou: The Promised Land of Error,* tr. Barbara Bray (New York: Vintage Books, 1979), 141; John McManners, *Death and the Enlightenment: Changing Attitudes to Death Among Chris-*

tians and Unbelievers in Eighteenth-Century France (Oxford: Oxford University Press, 1981), 9–10.

16 On depilation and bleaching hair, see Michael and Ariane Batterby, *Mirror, Mirror: A Social History of Fashion* (New York: Holt, Rinehart and Winston, 1977), 102.

17 Rudolph M. Bell, *Holy Anorexia* (Chicago: University of Chicago Press, 1985); Margaret of Corona quote in ibid., 99; Joan Jacobs Brumberg, *Fasting Girls: The Emergence of Anorexia Nervosa as a Modern Disease* (Cambridge: Harvard University Press, 1988), 41–101.

18 Durability of the phrase, "belle comme une Madone de Raphael," in Kenneth Clark, *Feminine Beauty* (London: Weidenfeld and Nicholson, 1980), 17; The caricature is in Boucher, op. cit., plate 437.

19 Marguerite de Valois story in Batterby, op. cit., 138.

20 Norbert Elias, *The Civilizing Process,* tr. Edmund Jephcott, 2 vols; vol. I (Boston: Urizen Books, 1978); vol. II (New York: Pantheon Books, 1982). Erasmus cited in vol. I, 82–3.

21 Stephen Mennell, *All Manners of Food: Eating and Taste in England and France from the Middle Ages to the Present* (Oxford: Basil Blackwell, 1985), 20–39; Montaigne cited in ibid., 31.

22 For a discussion of Cornaro and his book, see Hillel Schwartz, *Never Satisfied: A Cultural History of Diets, Fantasies and Fat* (New York: The Free Press, 1986), 9–19.

23 Elias, op. cit.; Natalie Zemon Davis, *Society and Culture in Early Modern France* (Palo Alto: Stanford University Press, 1975), 124; Nancy F. Cott, "Passionlessness: An Interpretation of Victorian Sexual Ideology, 1795–1850," in Nancy F. Cott and Elizabeth H. Pleck, *A Heritage of Her Own: Toward a New Social History of American Women* (New York: Simon and Schuster, 1979), 162–82; Gerda Lerner, "The Lady and the Mill Girl: Changes in the Status of Women in the Age of Jackson: 1800–1840," in ibid., 182–93; Thomas Laqueur, "Orgasm, Generation and the Politics of Reproductive Biology," in Catherine Gallagher and Thomas Laqueur (eds.), *The Making of the Modern Body: Sexuality and Society in the Nineteenth Century* (Berkeley: University of California Press, 1987), 1–42; Stephen Nissenbaum, *Sex, Diet and Debility in Jacksonian America: Sylvester Graham and Health Reform* (Westport, Conn.: Greenwood Press, 1980).

24 The Madame de Pompadour example is cited in Barbara Ueland, "Fat or Thin Women," *Saturday Evening Post,* May 10, 1930, 46.

25 David Kunzle, "The Corset as Erotic Alchemy: From Rococo Galanterie to Montaut's Physiologies," in Thomas Hess and Linda Nochlin (eds.), *Woman as Sex Object: Erotic Art, 1730–1970* (New York: Art News Annual, 1972), 93; Lawrence Stone, *The Family, Sex and Marriage in England, 1500–1800* (abr. edition) (New York: Harper and Row, 1979), 283–84.

26 Boucher, op. cit., 335–50; S. Lossignol, "Jacques Grasset de St. Sauveur: Sa vie, son oeuvre iconographique sur le costume regional francais," Master's Thesis, 1976, in Archives, Musée des arts et traditions populaires, Paris.

27 Stone, op. cit., 284.

28 Steele, op. cit., 245; Banner, op. cit., 57–63.

29 Mennell, op. cit.; Gottshalk on Louis XVI cited in ibid., 31.

30 Jean Anthelme Brillat-Savarin, *The Physiology of Taste or Meditations on Transcendental Gastronomy* (New York: Doubleday, 1926 [orig. 1826]), 237.

31 Ibid., 173.

CHAPTER 4

1 Roberta Seid, *The Dissolution of Traditional Rural Culture in Nineteenth-Century France: A Study of the Bethmale Costume* (New York: Garland Press, 1987), 190–91; Francois Boucher, *20,000 Years of Fashion: The History of Costume and Personal Adornment,* (expanded edition), tr. Harry N. Abrams, Inc., and Thames and Hudson Ltd., (New York: Harry N. Abrams, Inc., 1987), 333–64; S. Lossignol, "Jacques Grasset de St. Sauveur: Sa vie, son oeuvre iconographique sur le costume regional francais," Master's Thesis, 1976, in Archives, Musée des arts et traditions populaires, Paris.

2 Frederica of Prussia quoted in Boucher, op. cit., 342.

3 Steel Engraving Lady term used by Lois Banner, *American Beauty: A Social History Through Two Centuries of the American Idea, Ideal, and Image of the Beautiful Woman* (New York: Knopf, 1983); Crowfield (pseudonym for Stowe), cited in Banner, op. cit., 47.

4 Jean Anthelme Brillat-Savarin, *The Physiology of Taste or Meditations on Transcendental Gastronomy* (New York: Doubleday, 1926 [orig. 1826]), 172, 187; Other citations from Banner, op. cit., 45.

5 Gautier cited in Susan Sontag, *Illness as Metaphor* (New York: Farrar, Straus & Giroux, 1978), 29; *Advertiser* quote cited in Hillel Schwartz, *Never Satisfied: A Cultural History of Diets, Fantasies and Fat* (New York: Free Press, 1986), 39.

6 Banner, op. cit., 63–65.

7 Nancy Cott, "Passionlessness: An Interpretation of Victorian Sexual Ideology 1795–1850," in Nancy Cott and Elizabeth H. Pleck (eds), *A Heritage of Her Own: Toward a New Social History of American Women* (New York: Simon and Schuster, 1979), 162–82.

8 Ten percent figure on New York financial leaders in Banner, op. cit., 70; Gerda Lerner, "The Lady and the Mill Girl: Changes in the Status of Women in the Age of Jackson: 1800–1840," in Cott and Pleck, op. cit., 182–97; Carol Smith-Rosenberg, "Beauty, The Beast, and the Militant

Woman: A Case Study in Sex Roles and Social Stress in Jacksonian America," in ibid., 197–240.

9 Stowe quote in Banner, op. cit., 47; On Banting and his diets and their fate, Schwartz, op. cit., 100–101.

10 See note 8, above.

11 Balzac quote cited in Valerie Steele, *Fashion and Eroticism: Ideals of Feminine Beauty from the Victorian Era to the Jazz Age* (New York: Oxford University Press, 1985), 109; Brillat-Savarin, op. cit., 186; Byron quote cited in William Bennett, M.D. and Joel Gurin, *The Dieter's Dilemma: Eating Less and Weighing More* (New York: Basic Books, 1982), 167; L. M. Vincent, *Competing with the Sylph: Dancers and the Pursuit of the Ideal Body Form* (New York: Andrews and McMeel, 1979); See examples in Schwartz, op. cit., e.g., Illustration 5, (1857 cartoon from *Harper's Weekly*).

12 For an excellent discussion of corsets and tight-lacing, see Valerie Steele, op. cit., chapter 9, "The Corset Controversy," 161–92; On tailoring and dressmaking, see Claudia B. Kidwell and Margaret C. Christman, *Suiting Everyone: The Democratization of Clothing in America* (Washington, D.C.: Smithsonian Institution Press, 1974), 25.

13 "Fashions for Old Ladies," *Harper's Bazaar,* March 1902, 249–50; On waist sizes, Helen Woodward, *The Lady Persuaders: Over 100 Years of Women's Magazines—Their Influence on Everything from Fashion to Freud* (New York: I. Obolensky, 1960), 53; Also on age, see Banner, op. cit., 219–20.

14 On physicians' attitudes about what women should eat, see Banner, op. cit., 50; on Sylvester Graham, see Stephen Nissenbaum, *Sex, Diet and Debility in Jacksonian America,* (Westport, Conn.: Greenwood Press, 1980); Harvey Green, *Fit for America: Health-Fitness-Sport and American Society* (New York: Pantheon Books, 1986), 45–53; Schwartz, op. cit., 23–33.

15 On competing images, see Banner, op. cit., 57–63, 91–93; Beecher cited in Green, op. cit., 95.

16 Schwartz, op. cit., 37–43.

17 Quote from 1829 cited in Green, op. cit., 30; on Beecher and Graham, see ibid., 30–53; on meat consumption and French visitor's comment, see Schwartz, op. cit., 41–42; on "thin gluttons," see ibid., 40–43; Dr. Trall cited in Green, op. cit., 31.

18 Graham defense in Schwartz, op. cit., 27; "To feel . . . " quote originally made by Santorio Santorio (Sixteenth century) and used to express Beecher's description of health by Schwartz, op. cit., 64.

19 For this description of nineteenth century fashion, see especially Geoffrey Squire, *Dress, Art and Society, 1560–1970* (New York: Viking Press, 1974).

20 Beauty authority cited by Steele, op. cit., 62.

21 George Ellington on the Greek slave, cited in Banner, op. cit., 60. On the spread of the voluptuous ideal, see ibid., chapter 6.

22 Schwartz, op. cit., 59–60.

23 Harland and Ayer cited in Banner, op. cit., 106; *Pictorial Review,* Oct. 1905, 49; Annie Wolf cited in Banner, op. cit., 114.

24 Steele, op. cit., 218; ad in *Pictorial Review,* Oct. 1905, 49.

25 Cartoon in Schwartz, op. cit., illus. 5.

26 On the three types of beauties, see Steele, op. cit., 220–21; Banner, op. cit., chapters 6 and 7.

27 On Stanton, see Banner, op. cit., 129, in which the physician also indicated that her plumpness was a sign of good digestion: "It would be difficult to find a more perfect sign of digestion than is shown in the fullness of her cheeks"; see also 222–23; Also see Brandeth Symonds, M.D., "The Mortality of Overweights and Underweights," *McClure's,* Jan. 1909, 327 in which he writes, " . . . we must take into account the fact that until recent times overweights were accepted more freely by insurance companies than underweights."

28 On neurasthenia, Beard and Mitchell, see Barbara Sicherman, "The Uses of Diagnosis: Doctors, Patients and Neurasthenia," in Judith Walzer Leavitt and Ronald L. Numbers, (eds.) *Sickness and Health in America: Readings in the History of Medicine and Public Health* (Second edition, revised) (Madison: University of Wisconsin Press, 1985), 22–35; Green, op. cit., 137–67; Schwartz, op. cit., 69–74.

29 Darwin and Walker quotes cited in Green, op. cit., 222–23.

30 *Ladies Home Calisthenics,* 1890, cited in Green, op. cit., 225.

31 For an excellent discussion of this development, see Banner, op. cit., especially chapters 6, 7, and 10.

32 Suffragette cited in Sheila M. Rothman, *Woman's Proper Place: A History of Changing Ideals and Practices: 1870 to the Present* (New York: Basic Books, 1978), 128, as well as her excellent discussion of how this image changed.

33 Woods Hutchinson, "Fat and Fashion," *Saturday Evening Post,* Aug. 21, 1926, 60; Dr. Symonds's refutation of this claim, "Overweight a Burden, Not a Reserve Fund," in op. cit., 327; "How to Get Plump," *Harper's Bazaar,* Aug. 1908, 787; "The Cult of Slimness," *Living Age,* Feb. 28, 1914, 573.

34 "How to Get Plump," loc. cit., 787; On the femme fatale and the vamp, see Patrick Bade, *Femme Fatale* (New York: Mayflower Books, 1979), 6–39; and see discussion and references in Bennett and Gurin, op. cit., 168–209; Banner, op. cit., 194–207; Paula Fass, *The Damned and the Beautiful: American Youth in the 1920's* (Oxford: Oxford University Press, 1977), 291–326.

35 Stephen Mennell, *All Manners of Food: Eating and Taste in England and*

France from the Middle Ages to the Present (Oxford: Basil Blackwell, 1985); Green, op. cit., Schwartz, op cit., 81–88.

36 Schwartz, op. cit., 115–24.

37 Ibid., 115–24; Hilde Bruch, *Eating Disorders* (New York: Basic Books, 1973); for an excellent and precise discussion of these developments, see Joan Jacobs Brumberg, *Fasting Girls: The Emergence of Anorexia Nervosa as a Modern Disease* (Cambridge: Harvard University Press, 1988), 61–100.

38 Norbert Elias, *The Civilizing Process*, tr. Edmund Jephcott, 2 vols; vol I (Boston: Urizen Books, 1978); vol. II (New York: Pantheon Books, 1982), esp. vol. II, 229–319; see also Mennell's use of Elias, op. cit., 20–39.

39 Brumberg, op. cit., 140.

40 On Floradora girls and other earlier ideals, see Ralph Stein *The Pin-Up* (New York: Crescent Books, 1974), 84; see Banner on other show-girl weights in the period, op. cit., 182.

CHAPTER 5

1 Elizabeth Ewing, *Dress and Undress: A History of Women's Underwear* (New York: Drama Book Specialists, 1978), 13; Madame Poiret quote cited in Valerie Steele, *Fashion and Eroticism: Ideals of Feminine Beauty from the Victorian Era to the Jazz Age* (New York: Oxford University Press, 1984), 227; *Vogue,* May 1908, quoted in Steele, op. cit., 227.

2 Steele, op. cit., 227.

3 Ibid., 213–43.

4 "Century of Svelte," term coined by William Bennett, M.D. and Joel Gurin, *The Dieter's Dilemma* (New York: Basic Books, 1982), chapter 7.

5 For a perceptive discussion of some of these trends, see Hillel Schwartz, *Never Satisfied: A Cultural History of Diets, Fantasies and Fat* (New York: Free Press, 1986), 77–81.

6 "The Kinetic Silhouette," *Art-Gout-Beaute,* April 1926 and September 1926, cited in Steele, op. cit., 241; Celia Caroline Cole, "Streamline," *Delineator,* March 1934, 16 cited in Schwartz, op. cit., 231.

7 See Schwartz, op. cit., 80–82; Emma E. Walker, "Pretty Girl Papers," *Ladies' Home Journal,* Jan. 1905, 33; Cocroft ad, 1916, cited in Schwartz, op. cit., 144.

8 Gertrude Battles Lane, *Woman's Home Companion,* 1911, cited in Helen Woodward, *The Lady Persuaders: Over 100 Years of Women's Magazines—Their Influence on Everything from Fashion to Freud* (New York: I. Obolensky, 1960), 6.

9 Ella Fletcher, *The Woman Beautiful,* New York, 1900, cited in Steele, op. cit., 224; quote from *Journal des Dames et Des Modes,* Aug. 10, 1912, 57, cited in Steele, op. cit., 230.

10 Dr. Charles Purdy, "Popular Errors in Living and Their Influence Over

the Public Health," *North American Review,* June 1897, 670 and 664–77; "On Growing Fat," *Atlantic Monthly,* March 1907, 430–31.

11 For a good, brief discussion of the history of insurance companies and their use of weight as a statistical measure, see Bennett and Gurin, op. cit., 123–31; Brandeth Symonds, A.M., M.D., "The Mortality of Overweights and Underweights," *McClure's Magazine,* Jan. 1909, 319.

12 Symonds, loc. cit., 319–27; Actuarial Society of America and the Association of Life Insurance Medical Directors, *Medico-actuarial Mortality Investigations* (New York, 1912–14), cited in Schwartz, op. cit., 156.

13 Critiques of insurance methods in Bennett and Gurin, op. cit., 125–27; Schwartz, op. cit., 156; See also later criticisms leveled against them in following chapters.

14 "The Cult of Slimness," *Living Age,* Feb. 28, 1914, 572–74; Schwartz, op. cit., 88–90.

15 On Atwater, see Schwartz, op. cit., 86–88, 101–102, 131–35.

16 On Chittenden, see ibid., 131–34, 141, 176.

17 Anne Rittenhouse, "Reductio ad Absurdum," *Vogue,* Nov. 15, 1912, 17; ad in *Vogue,* Nov. 1, 1912, 94.

18 On William James and Henry James's interest in Fletcher, see Harvey Green, *Fit for America: Health-Fitness-Sport and American Society* (New York: Pantheon Books, 1986), 297–98; Fletcher quote in ibid., 295.

19 Schwartz, op. cit., 136–39.

20 Dr. Alonzo Taylor, "The National Overweight," *Scientific Monthly,* May 1931, 393.

21 Barbara Gutmann Rosenkrantz, "The Search for Professional Order in 19th-Century American Medicine," in Judith Walzer Leavitt and Ronald L. Numbers (eds.), *Sickness and Health in America: Readings in the History of Medicine and Public Health* (Madison: University of Wisconsin Press, 1985), 219–33; Ronald L. Numbers, "The Fall and Rise of the American Medical Profession," in Leavitt and Numbers, op. cit., 185–97; John C. Burnham, "American Medicine's Golden Age: What Happened to It?" in Leavitt and Numbers, op. cit., 248–59; see also Schwartz, op. cit., 154–55.

22 Figures cited in Schwartz, op. cit., 167; for a more general discussion of scales, see ibid., 164–73.

23 Elizabeth Hurlock, "Youth," *The Psychology of Dress* (New York: Ronald Press, 1929), 165; see also Paula Fass, *The Damned and the Beautiful: American Youth in the 1920's* (Oxford: Oxford University Press, 1979 ed.), 260–326, and Steele, op. cit., 213–42.

24 Florence Courtenay, *Physical Beauty: How to Develop and Preserve It* (1922), cited in Steele, op. cit., 238.

25 Rittenhouse, loc. cit., 17.

26 Norbert Elias, *The Civilizing Process,* tr. Edmund Jephcott, 2 vols; vol I (Boston: Urizen Books, 1978); vol. II (New York: Pantheon Books, 1982);

On early attitudes toward Miss America, see Lois Banner, *American Beauty: A Social History Through Two Centuries of the American Idea, Ideal, and Image of the Beautiful Woman* (New York: Knopf, 1983), 249–70.

27 For example, "On the one hand, it is 'mind the paint,' but on the other, the face that has helped nature holds allure," *Vogue,* Jan. 15, 1920, 27.

28 Christine Herrick, *Lose Weight and Be Well* (New York: 1917) cited in Schwartz, op. cit., 175; see also ads in *Vogue,* eg., "The truth will keep you slim," Health-o-Meter ad, Jan. 15, 1930, 106; for a good general discussion of scales and the advent of private scales, see Schwartz, op. cit., 164–71; Lulu Hunt Peters, *Diet and Health, with Key to Calories* (Chicago: 1917) cited in Schwartz, op. cit., 175; C. C. Cole, "Fat on Thy Bones," *Delineator,* March 1923, 48.

29 Dr. Morris Fishbein, "Pounding Away," *Saturday Evening Post,* Sept. 22, 1934, 18.

30 Ueland, loc. cit., 46; "Wonders of Diet: Systems of Eating, Health Fads, Why You Might As Well Eat What You Please," *Fortune,* May 1936, 91; "Get Thin in Summer," *Literary Digest,* Aug. 16, 1924, 22; On rumored Hollywood deaths, see Schwartz, op. cit., 182–83; J. A. Ryle, "Discussion on Anorexia Nervosa," *Proceedings of the Royal Society of Medicine* 32 (1939), 735.

31 Taylor, loc. cit., 395; Symonds, loc. cit., 319; Bennett and Gurin, op. cit., chapter 5.

32 Florence Courtenay cited in Steele, op. cit., 238.

33 On measurements of early Miss Americas, see Frank Deford, *There She Is: The Life and Times of Miss America* (New York: Viking Press, 1971), 313–15; on Campbell, 116–24; on Ziegfeld, see Ralph Stein, *The Pin-Up From 1852 to Today* (New York: Crescent Press, 1974), 84 and other pages for pictures of reigning beauties; see also Mark Gabor, *The Pin-Up: A Modest History* (New York: Universe Books, 1972); and see Banner, op. cit., for references to measurements of reigning actresses.

34 Lady Troubridge quote in Steele, op. cit., 241.

35 Poiret quote in ibid., 238; Fishbein, loc. cit., 18; Ueland, loc. cit., 46; for a discussion about general resistance to the new styles, see Fass, op. cit., 291–326.

36 Cocroft ad, *Good Housekeeping,* Feb. 1915, 61; Anna Hazelton Delavan, "Exercises to Normalize Your Weight," *Good Housekeeping,* Sept. 1924, 101; Kellogg's ad, *Vogue,* Jan. 18, 1930, 101.

37 Frederick Stare, "Ideal Nutrition," *American Journal of Public Health* 37 (May 1947), 519; Dr. Woods Hutchinson, "Fat and Fashion," *Saturday Evening Post,* Aug. 21, 1926, 58; Ueland, loc. cit., 46.

38 Hutchinson, op. cit., 62, 64; Symonds, op. cit., 327; Taylor, op. cit., 393.

39 Hutchinson, op. cit., 64; Barker quote in Schwartz, op. cit., 158–59; Barker quote and other warnings cited in Hutchinson, op. cit., 64.

40 Davenport idea (1923) cited in Schwartz, op. cit., 226; Ueland, loc. cit., 46; On *luxuskonsumption* theory and its fate, see Bennett and Gurin, op. cit., 80–84.

41 On glandular theories, see Schwartz, op. cit., 135–40; see also chapter 5, where glandular theories are dismissed.

42 Hilde Bruch, "Thin Fat People," *Eating Disorders* (New York: Basic Books, 1973), 194–211.

43 Richard Osborn Cummings, *The American and His Food* (Chicago: Arno Press, 1970 [orig. publication, 1940]), 151.

44 Ryle, loc. cit. 735; "How Not to Be So Thin," *Vogue,* Jan. 1, 1939, 64, 81.

45 Gallup Poll cited in Schwartz, op. cit., 229.

CHAPTER 6

1 Gerald Walker, "The Great American Dieting Neurosis," *New York Times Magazine,* Aug. 23, 1959, 12.

2 "Crazy About Reducing," *Time,* Aug. 6, 1956, 32; Dextrose saga described in Peter Wyden, *The Overweight Society* (New York: William Morrow & Company, 1965), 181–83.

3 Elizabeth Pope, "Why Fad Diets Fail," *McCall's,* Nov. 1956, 187; Ernest Havemann, "The Wasteful, Phony Crash Dieting Craze," *Life,* Jan. 19, 1959, 187; Herman Taller, *Calories Don't Count* (New York: Simon and Schuster, 1961).

4 Alice Payne Hackett, *70 Years of Best Sellers: 1895–1965* (New York, London: R. R. Bowker Co. 1967); "Insurance Ads Pave the Way for . . . Dietary and 'Health' Foods," *Business Week,* Dec. 6, 1952, 48; Walker, loc. cit., 12.

5 "Insurance Ads Pave . . . ", loc. cit., 46–50.

6 "The Big Bulge in Profits," *Newsweek,* July 23, 1956, 61–63.

7 Wyden, op. cit., 41–62.

8 "The Big Bulge in Profits," loc. cit., 61–62; on American Sugar Refining Co. plans, see Wyden, op. cit.

9 "The Big Bulge in Profits," loc. cit., 62; On amphetamines, see Hillel Schwartz, *Never Satisfied: A Cultural History of Diets, Fantasies and Fat* (New York: The Free Press, 1986), 197.

10 "The Big Bulge in Profits," loc. cit., 61; Wyden, op. cit., 215–44; Schwartz, op. cit., 7; Wyden, op. cit., 65–67, 100–19; LaLanne quote in Schwartz, op. cit., 233; Wyden, op. cit., 81.

11 Gerald Weales, "A Family That Prays Together Weighs Together," *New Republic,* March 25, 1957, 19–20.

12 Dior quote in Polly Devlin, *Vogue: Book of Fashion Photography* (New York: Simon and Schuster, 1979), 134; "Fashion Turmoil: Drastic New Styles Will Make Most Existing Clothes Obsolete," *Life,* June 16, 1947, 125–26; "Revolution," *Time,* Aug. 18, 1947, 22.

13 *Mademoiselle,* Nov. 1947, 22; *Vogue,* Jan. 1, 1950, 93.

14 "Newest Styles Give Every Woman's Figure a Chance," *Life,* Sept. 22, 1947, 115–25; *Vogue,* May 1, 1947, 131, 176.

15 *Mademoiselle,* April 1948, 162; *Vogue,* Jan. 1, 1950, 93; Maxwell quote in Walker, loc. cit., 100; Suzy Parker quote in Devlin, op. cit., 138.

16 *Vogue,* May 1, 1947, 138, 150; *Mademoiselle,* April 1948, 14; "Do Husbands Like Plump Wives?" *McCall's,* March 1951, 6, 8; On Gould policy, see Chris Chase, *The Great American Waistline: Putting It On and Taking It Off* (New York: Coward, McCann & Geoghegan, 1980), 199–200; George H. Gallup, *The Gallup Poll: Public Opinion 1935–1971* (Wilmington: *Scholary Research Inc.* 1978), 1126, 1255.

17 "Spring Suited Slenderness," *Vogue,* Jan. 1, 1955, (cover); "Eating Your Way into Fashion," *Vogue,* Feb. 15, 1956, 63.

18 "Big Bulge in Profits," loc. cit., 61.

19 *Vogue,* Feb. 1, 1958, 107; *Vogue,* Feb. 15, 1958, 86.

20 "Making the Bathing Suit Figure," *Vogue,* Jan. 15, 1958, 64.

21 Kennedy Fraser, *The Fashionable Mind: Reflections on Fashion 1970–1982* (Boston: David Godine, 1985), 82–83.

22 On the commercial beauty industry, see Lois Banner, *American Beauty: A Social History Through Two Centuries of the American Idea, Ideal, and Image of the Beautiful Woman* (New York: Knopf, 1983), 208–20; "The Pink Jungle," *Time,* June 16, 1958, 86–90; Elizabeth Ewing, *Dress and Undress: A History of Women's Underwear* (New York: Drama Book Specialists, 1978), 160.

23 Richard A. Kallan and Robert D. Brooks, "The Playmate of the Month: Naked but Nice," *Journal of Popular Culture,* Fall 1974, 328–36; "The Whore vs. the Girl Next Door," *Journal of Popular Culture,* Summer 1975.

24 For information on American attitudes toward beauty queens, see Banner, op. cit.; Devlin, op. cit., 116.

25 Betty Friedan, *The Feminine Mystique* (New York: W. W. Norton and Co., 1963).

26 U.S. Bureau of the Census, *The Statistical History of the U.S. from Colonial Times to the Present* (Stamford: Fairfield Publishers, Inc., 1965), Tables A210–27.

27 For an excellent discussion of the development in the fifties, see Friedan, op. cit., 95–117, 247–70; "Looks That are Better Than Beauty," *Vogue,* Sept. 15, 1960, 225.

28 Albert Ellis, *The Folklore of Sex* (New York: Grove Press, 1961); historian Max Lerner observed that "America has come to stress sex as much as any civilization since the Roman, and David Riesman called sex "the Last Frontier," quoted in Friedan, op. cit., 393, footnote 1, 247–70.

29 See motivational researcher, Dr. Ernest Dichter's, comments in Wyden, op. cit., 32, and discussion on boys' attitudes toward body size in chapter 7.

30 For a good summary of Dublin and other references, see William Bennett, M.D. and Joel Gurin, *The Dieter's Dilemma* (New York: Basic Books, 1982), 131–38; quote on 132.

31 Louis I. Dublin and Herbert H. Marks, "Overweight Shortens Life," paper presented at 60th annual meeting of the Association of Life Insurance Medical Directors of America, New York City, Oct. 12, 1951, printed in *MLIC Statistical Bulletin,* Oct. 1951, vol. 32, no. 10, 1; idem., *Postgraduate Medicine,* Nov. 1951, vol. 10, no. 5.

32 See graphs in Dublin and Marks, "Overweight Shortens Life," loc. cit., 2, and Dublin's more explicit comment about it: "Even among young people, the advantage of a slight degree of overweight is less pronounced than in earlier studies, and at best can now be considered only a temporary advantage," in "New Weight Standards for Men and Women," *Statistical Bulletin,* Nov.–Dec. 1959, 2.

33 Explained in "1983 Metropolitan Height and Weight Tables," *Statistical Bulletin,* Jan.–June 1983, vol. 64, no. 1, 3.

34 Frederick J. Stare, "Ideal Intake of Calories and Specific Nutrients," *American Journal of Public Health,* May 1947, 518; Dublin and Marks, "Overweight Shortens Life," loc. cit., 3.

35 A. L. Stewart, R. H. Brook, and R. L. Kane, *Conceptualization and Measurement of Health Habits for Adults in the Health Insurance Study: Vol. II: Overweight* (Santa Monica: The Rand Corporation, July 1980), 14; see also criticisms of Mayer, op. cit., 28; Ancel Keys and Hilde Bruch expressed the same reservations; see Hilde Bruch, *Eating Disorders* (New York: Basic Books, 1973), 110.

36 Society of Actuaries, Committee on Mortality, *Build and Blood Pressure Study* (Chicago: Society of Actuaries, 1959), vol. I, 24.

37 Mayer, op. cit., 28–29; Bennett and Gurin, op. cit., 133–34.

38 "Big Bulge in Profits," loc. cit., 48; Louis Dublin, "Stop Killing Your Husband," *Reader's Digest,* July 1952, 47–49.

39 John C. Burnham, "American Medicine's Golden Age: What Happened to It?" in Judith Walzer Leavitt and Ronald L. Numbers (eds), *Sickness and Health in America* (Madison: University of Wisconsin Press, 1985), 248–59; Interview with Paul D. White, "Heart Disease: 27 Questions Answered," *Vogue,* May 1, 1947, 182; Louis Dublin, "Foreword" in *Postgraduate Medicine,* Nov. 1951, vo. 10, no. 5.

40 Hundley quoted in "Obesity Called Waste of Manpower and Food," *Science News Letter,* June 16, 1951, 377; Hundley interview in "Danger of Being Too Fat," *U.S. News and World Report,* Nov. 2, 1951, 19; Dr. Sebrell quoted in "Obesity Is Now No. 1 U.S. Nutritional Problem," *Science News Letter,* Dec. 27, 1952, 408; Lester Breslow, "Public Health Aspects of Weight Control," *American Journal of Public Health,* Sept. 1952, 1,117; Louis Dublin, "Overweight: America's #1 Health Problem," *Reader's Digest,* July 1952, 107–09.

41 "Obesity Called Waste of . . . " loc. cit., 19–20; Breslow, loc. cit., 1,119; Jean Mayer, "Overweight and Obesity," *Atlantic Monthly,* Aug. 1955, 69.

42 Breslow results reported in "Study Challenges Obesity-Mortality Link," *Science Digest,* Nov. 1957, 16.

43 "Mortality Among Our Elders Too High," *MLIC Statistical Bulletin,* Oct. 1951, 6–8.

44 Dr. Woods Hutchinson, "Fat and Fashion," *Saturday Evening Post,* August 21, 1926, p. 58; Schwartz, op. cit., 217–21.

45 Dr. Charles Freed quoted in "Food and Fat," *Newsweek,* Feb. 17, 1947, 58; Bruch quoted in "Fat and Unhappy," *Time,* Oct. 20, 1947, 61.

46 Gerald Walker, loc. cit., 100; Lawrence Galton, "Why We Are Overly Larded," *New York Times Magazine,* Jan. 15, 1961, 31.

47 Jean Mayer, "Overweight and Obesity," loc. cit., 71.

48 Bennett and Gurin, op. cit., 139–40; Schwartz, op. cit., 279–280.

49 Schwartz, op. cit., 293–94; "Why We Fatten Up," *Newsweek,* June 8, 1959, 66.

50 Benjamin Spock, *Common Sense Book of Baby and Child Care* (New York: Meredith Press, 1957), 433–34; "Teen-age Gluttons," *Newsweek,* March 14, 1960, 88; Schwartz, op. cit., 271–302; see also "From Fatso to Cool Cat: Story of an 11-Year-Old Boy," *Parent's Magazine,* April 1958; or "Don't Let Your Child Be A Fatty!" *Ladies' Home Journal,* Sept. 1953.

51 Sheldon quoted in Schwartz, op. cit., 223; "Fat and Unhappy," *Time,* Oct. 29, 1947, 61; "Food and Fat," *Newsweek,* Feb. 17, 1947, 58; see also 1950s' psychoanalytic explanations for obesity/overweight summarized in Bennett and Gurin, op. cit., 25–32; "Dear Abby" quote cited in Schwartz, op. cit., 323.

52 See footnote 48; and Bennett and Gurin, op. cit.; Schwartz, op. cit., 194–95, 202–04.

53 "American Food—For Better or for Worse," *Vogue,* Feb. 1, 1950, 169; see also "Good Eater Can Be Too Good," *New York Times Magazine,* Oct. 28, 1956, 48.

54 Mayer, "Obesity and Overweight," loc. cit., 71; "Announcing Vogue's Diet Authority: Edited Here, the Transcript of the First of a Series of Meetings with Nutrition Authorities on the Subject of Overweight," *Vogue,* Feb. 15, 1956, 64, quote on p. 128.

55 George H. Gallup, *The Gallup Poll: Public Opinion 1935–1971* (New York: Random House, 1972), 1255; Later polls cited in Wyden, op. cit., 9–10; Gerald Walker, loc. cit., 12.

56 See examples cited in Mayer, "Overweight and Obesity," loc. cit. 84–89.

57 Dr. Kalb quoted in Lawrence Galton, loc. cit., 44.

58 "Why We Fatten Up," *Newsweek,* June 8, 1959, 66.

59 "Obesity Called Waste of Manpower and Food," *Science News Letter,* June 16, 1951, 377; "The Plague of Overweight," *Life,* March 8, 1954, 120; "Obesity Blamed on Overbuying of Food," *Science Digest,* Jan. 1956, 52;

"Overweight? Blame Our Soft, Lazy Way of Life," *Science Digest,* Oct. 1958, 49–50.

60 George H. Gallup, op. cit., 985.

61 Louis Dublin, "Handicaps of Overweight," *MLIC Statistical Bulletin,* Aug. 1952, 3–5. The litany was frequently repeated; e.g., in *Science Digest* article, cited in note 58: "Finally, the population should be educated with regard to the many advantages that lie in maintaining a desirable weight— agility, beauty, comfort and social acceptability." (p. 6.)

62 Susan Sontag, *Illness as Metaphor* (New York: Farrar, Straus & Giroux, 1978).

63 J. H. Plumb, "The Commercialization of Leisure in Eighteenth-Century England," in Neil McKendrick, John Brewer, and J. H. Plumb, *The Birth of a Consumer Society: The Commercialization of Eighteenth-Century England* (Bloomington: Indiana University Press, 1982).

64 Albert J. Stunkard and Mavis McClaren-Hume, "The Results of Treatment for Obesity," *Archives of Internal Medicine* 102, Jan. 1959, 79–85; White quote in Wyden, op. cit., 18.

65 "Teen-age Dieting Has the Experts Worried," *Woman's Home Companion,* July 1955, 52; Hilde Bruch quoted from *The Importance of Being Overweight* (1957), in "Why Are They Running, Stretching, Starving," *Fortune,* Aug. 1970, 135; Gerald Walker, loc. cit., 12.

66 David Cort, op. cit., 511; Hilde Bruch, "When Not to Diet," *Collier's,* Feb. 5, 1954, 82–83.

67 Hundley quoted in "Danger of Being Too Fat," *U. S. News & World Report,* Nov. 2, 1951, 20–21; Mayer quoted in "Announcing Vogue's Diet . . . " loc. cit., 65; "Why We Fatten Up," loc. cit., 66.

68 *Mademoiselle,* April 1948, 153.

69 Paul F. Secord and Sidney M. Jourard, "Body Cathexis and the Ideal Female Figure," *Journal of Abnormal and Social Psychology* 50 (1955), 243–46.

70 Gallup, op. cit., 1939 poll, 1950, 1965 poll, 1975; Quotes in Wyden, op. cit., 15.

71 Dichter quoted in Wyder, op. cit., 29–32.

72 Miss America statistics in Frank Deford, *There She Is: The Life and Times of Miss America* (New York: Viking Press, 1971), 313–16, 325.

CHAPTER 7

1 "Dietmania," *Newsweek,* Sept. 10, 1973, 74; on the history of high-fat diets, see especially Hillel Schwartz, *Never Satisfied: A Cultural History of Diets, Fantasies and Fat* (New York: The Free Press, 1986), 8, 173; and Theodore Berland and Consumer Guide, *Rating the Diets* (New York: Beekman House, 1983), 113–24; on high-protein diets, ibid., 95–113.

2 Sego story in Peter Wyden, *The Overweight Society* (New York: William Morrow & Company, 1965), 51–52; Schwartz, op. cit., 253; George H.

Gallup, *The Gallup Poll: Public Opinion 1935–1971* (New York: Random House, 1972), 34–36; H. Gallup, *The Gallup Poll 1972–1977* (New York: Random House, 1978), 1200–01.

3 Robert Sherrill, "Before You Believe Those Exercise and Diet Ads Read the Following Report," *Today's Health,* Nov. 1972, 34–36, 68–70; Schwartz, op. cit., 242–43.

4 S. McBee, "Diet Pills: Doctors Who Treat Weight Problems," *Life,* Jan. 26, 1968, 22–28; Chris Chase, *The Great American Waistline: Putting It On and Taking It Off* (New York: Coward, McCann & Geoghegan, 1981), 239–54; Charles O. Jackson, "Before the Drug Culture: Barbituate/Amphetamine Abuse in American Society," *Clio Medica* 11 (1976), 47–58; and a good discussion in Schwartz, op. cit., 196–98.

5 Wyden, op. cit., 79–100; Schwartz, op. cit., 202–13; Berland, op. cit., 143–71.

6 Wyden, op. cit., 100–120.

7 Society of Actuaries, Committee on Mortality, *Build and Blood Pressure Study,* 2 vols (Chicago: Society of Actuaries, 1979); "New Weight Standards for Men and Women," *Statistical Bulletin of the Metropolitan Life Insurance Company,* Nov.–Dec. 1959, 1–4; See also a good discussion of this data in William Bennett, M.D. and Joel Gurin, *The Dieter's Dilemma* (New York: Basic Books, 1982), chapter 5.

8 C. S. Chlouverakis, "Nature and Nurture in Human Obesity," *Journal of Obesity and Bariatric Medicine* 1974 (3), 28–31.

9 "New Weight Standards . . . ," loc. cit., 1–4.

10 See "New Weight Standards . . . ," loc. cit., 1–4; for some of the controversies, see Section 1, "Understanding Obesity and Overweight" in *Overweight and Obesity: Causes, Fallacies, Treatment,* Brent Q. Hafen (ed), (Provo: 1975); and Jean Mayer, *Overweight: Causes, Cost, and Control* (Englewood Cliffs: Prentice-Hall, 1968), 26–44.

11 Reuben Andres, "Effect of Obesity on Total Mortality," *International Journal of Obesity,* 1980, 4:32, clarifies the distinction that is not even clear in the BBPS; Dr. Philip White quoted in "The Crash Diet Craze," *Medical World News,* April 1973, 36; C. C. Seltzer, "Some Re-evaluations of the Build and Blood Pressure Study, 1959, as Related to Ponderal Index, Somatotype, and Mortality," *New England Journal of Medicine,* Feb 3, 1966, 254–59; *BBPS,* vol. 1, Introduction, and Bennett and Gurin, op. cit., chapter 5.

12 Peter Wyden, op. cit.; Peter and Barbara Wyden, "The Doctors' Own Diet—87 Experts Tell the Journal What They Eat to Lose Weight, Live Longer," *Ladies' Home Journal,* Feb. 1967, 61, 127–33.

13 United States Public Health Service, Division of Chronic Diseases, *Obesity and Health,* Publication No. 1485, (Washington, D.C., 1966), 25–26; ibid., iv; U. S. Congress Senate Select Committee on Nutrition and Human Needs, Hearings, 90th Congress, 2nd Session and 91st Congress, 1st Ses-

sion; Parts 3–7, National Nutrition Survey, (Washington, D.C.: U.S. Government Printing Office, 1969).

14 U. S. Public Health Service, National Center for Health Statistics, *Weight, Height and Selected Body Dimensions of Adults, 1960–61,* Series 11 #8, June 1965; Schwartz, op. cit., 246; Kline quoted in Wyden, op. cit., 300.

15 "Why Are They Running, Stretching, Starving?" *Fortune* Aug. 1970, 134.

16 Sidney Abraham and Marie Nordsieck, "Relationship of Excess Weight in Children and Adults," *Public Health Reports* 75 (1960), 263–73; see especially Schwartz's discussion, op. cit., 293–96.

17 Harold Kaplan and Helen Singer Kaplan, "The Psychosomatic Concept of Obesity," *Journal of Nervous and Mental Disease* 125 (1957), 181–201; see also excellent discussion and review of other literature by Bennett and Gurin, op. cit., chapter 2.

18 Mary Moore, Albert Stunkard, and Leo Srole, "Obesity, Social Class and Mental Illness," *Journal of the American Medical Association* 181 (1962), 962–66; see also Stunkard, *The Pain of Obesity* (Palo Alto: Bull Publishing Co., 1976) and the presentation of this material in USPH, *Obesity and Health,* op. cit., 42.

19 On caloric recommendations, see Schwartz, op. cit., 254; on changing standards for elderly people's caloric consumption see Mayer, op. cit., 132–33; on BMR change with age, see Ralph A. Nelson, L. Anderson, C. Gastineau, A. Hayles, and C. Stamnes, "Physiology and Natural History of Obesity," paper delivered in 1972, reprints available through Mayo Clinic; on varying caloric recommendations for normal weights and dieters, see Theodore B. Van Itallie and Sami Hashim, "Obesity in an Age of Caloric Anxiety," *Modern Medicine* 38 (1970), 89–96.

20 See, for example, a popular version of this concern in Bergen Evans's article in *Vogue,* May 1, 1947, 151, where he remarked on the ill-effects on the young of the "growing reluctance of their elders to curl up and die. Dying before 50 has been for millenia one of the most salutary and established human customs," and his quote from Gunnar Myrdal in which he worried that society itself would "take on an administrative, bureaucratic character."

21 See especially *Mademoiselle*'s late fifties' and early sixties' issues, where articles detailed the radical changes in campus culture.

22 See especially "Fashion: Up, Up & Away," *Time,* December 1, 1967, 70–80, which described vividly the changing structure of fashion and the fashion arbiters' response to this change; see also Kennedy Fraser, *The Fashionable Mind: Reflections on Fashion 1970–1982* (Boston: David Godine, 1981), especially 81–91.

23 Marya Mannes, "The New Upper Class—The Kids," *Vogue,* July 1963, 46; photo in *Time,* December 1, 1967, 72.

24 *Vogue,* September 1, 1963, 57; see also "Youth Is Not an Age," *Vogue,* March 1, 1965, 84.

25 On the bikini, see *Vogue,* May 1, 1959, 101; on shorter hemlines, see "Paris Yes and Nos," *Vogue,* March 15, 1961, 62; "Fashion: Up, Up & Away," loc. cit., 70; "Fashion: The Way of All Flesh," *Time,* May 16, 1969, 62; *Vogue,* May 15, 1965, 21; *Vogue,* April 15, 1965, 106.

26 "Sporting a New Breed of Fashion," *Vogue,* Sept. 1, 1963, 115; "The Girl in the Driver's Seat," *Vogue,* Jan. 1, 1969, 107.

27 *Vogue,* May 1, 1959, 101; "Prediction '65: The Fashion Power of the Body," *Vogue,* Jan. 1, 1965, 71.

28 "A Thin Story," *Mademoiselle,* Sept. 1966, 184.

29 H. Van Horne, "Are We the Last Married Generation?" *McCall's,* May 1969, 69.

30 "Pride of Body," *Vogue,* Oct. 15, 1967, 131.

31 "The Arrival of Twiggy," and "Ad Reinhardt: Honor Comes Late to a Solitary Moralist in Art," *Life,* Feb. 3, 1967, 36, 45.

32 Frank Deford, *There She Is: The Life and Times of Miss America* (New York: Viking Press, 1971). The data on contestants' weights and heights based on my own study of *Miss America Pageant Yearbooks,* which each year describe the contestants, including their weights and heights.

33 *Ladies' Home Journal,* April 1968, 100; "How America Looks," *Ladies' Home Journal,* Sept. 1966, 76.

34 *Vogue,* Feb. 15, 1966, 107—a litany repeated more and more frequently as the sixties moved into the seventies.

35 For a summary of these studies, see Johanna T. Dwyer, Jacob Feldman, and Jean Mayer, "The Social Psychology of Dieting," *Journal of Health and Social Behavior* 11 (1970), 269–87; and another summary in Paul E. Garfinkel and David Garner, *Anorexia Nervosa: A Multidimensional Perspective* (New York: Brunner/Mazel, 1982), chapter 5. The specific studies were R. L. Huenemann, L. R. Shapiro, M. C. Hampton, and B.W. Mitchell, "A Longitudinal Study of Gross Body Composition and Body Conformation and Their Association with Food and Activity in a Teenage Population," in *American Journal of Clinical Nutrition* 18 (1966), 325–38; and J. T. Dwyer, J. J. Feldman, C. C. Seltzer, and J. Mayer, "Body Image in Adolescents: Attitudes Toward Weight and Perception of Appearance," *American Journal of Clinical Nutrition* 20 (1969), 1045–56.

36 Hilde Bruch observed this phenomenon in 1958 and reconfirmed it in 1967. See summary of these studies in Dwyer, Feldman, and Mayer, loc. cit., 1045–56.

37 See USPHS, op. cit., 47; see also Jean Mayer, *Overweight: Causes, Cost and Control* (Englewood Cliffs, N.J.: Prentice-Hall, 1968), especially chapter 6 for a discussion of prevailing attitudes about exercise and weight control.

38 Ibid.

39 Ibid., 82.

40 For an excellent discussion of the exercise/heart disease studies, see Henry A. Solomon, *The Exercise Myth* (San Diego: Harcourt Brace Jovanovich,

1984). The early, classic study was J. N. Morris, J. A. Heady, P. A. Raffle, C. G. Roberts, and J. W. Parks, "Coronary Heart Disease and Physical Activity of Work," *Lancet* 2 (1953), 1053–57, 1111–20, in which they compared London bus drivers and conductors and found the former, whose occupation was more sedentary, had higher rates of heart disease. The authors retracted their conclusions in another article, "A Physique of London Busmen," *Lancet* 2 (1956), 566–70, and eleven years later, R. M. Oliver published his findings regarding the weight and cholesterol levels of men recruited for bus drivers and conductors: He found that significant differences existed *before* the job's activity could have had any effect. He concluded that "it is apparent that British men with certain physical characteristics choose or are chosen to become bus drivers as opposed to conductors," and that his study "supports the view that inherited characteristics, one of which may be susceptibility to heart disease, may predispose to a particular occupation," R. M. Oliver, "Physique and Serum Lipids of Young London Busmen," *British Journal of Industrial Medicine,* (24), 1967, 181–186. Once again, cause and effect had been confused. Despite the retraction, Morris's original study continued to be widely cited. On studies of cholesterol and exercise, see Mayer, op. cit., 1968, 107–9, 111–12.

41 For a good discussion of experts' views, see Peter Wyden, *The Overweight Society* (New York: William Morrow & Company, 1965); Dichter quote on p. 31.

42 Ibid., 299, 305.

43 "Jogging for Health and Heart. It's Catching On," *U.S. News,* Dec. 25, 1967; Jean Mayer, "It's Not Just Overeating That's Killing Us. It's Underexercising, Too," *Forbes,* Oct. 1, 1969, 64; "Why Are They Running, Stretching, Starving?" *Fortune,* Aug. 1970, 132–35.

44 Quoted in Wyden, op. cit., 307, 309.

45 "Why Are They Running . . . ?" loc. cit., 132–35; Lowe quoted in *Time,* May 30, 1969, 80.

46 Bellman quoted in Wyden, op. cit., 304; Ernest Havemann "The Task Ahead: How to Take Life Easy," *Life,* Feb. 21, 1964; Bruce Bliven, "Using Our Leisure Is No Easy Job," *New York Times Magazine,* April 26, 1964, 18–19.

47 Mayer, *Overweight . . . ,* op. cit., 83.

48 For example, "The New Exercise Talk: T'ai Chi," *Vogue,* March 1, 1962, 149, in which *Vogue* said, "The most basic, if slightly embarrassing, truth about exercise is that nobody wants to do the awful stuff," which is why *Vogue* recommended T'ai Chi.

49 For a review of cholesterol studies, see Schwartz, op. cit., 101, 219, 242, 253, 257, 263, 295, 327, and 447, especially for earlier history; Wyden, op. cit., 146; Mayer, *Overweight . . . ,* op. cit., 49, 101, 102, 106–9, 160; and especially the cover story on Ancel Keys in *Time,* Jan. 13, 1961, 48.

50 For a good, simple summary of the opposing opinions and the political-commercial aspects of the diet-heart disease link, see Elizabeth Whelan and Frederick Stare, *The One-Hundred-Percent Natural, Purely Organic, Cholesterol-Free, Megavitamin, Low-Carbohydrate Nutrition Hoax* (New York: Atheneum, 1984), chapter 4; see also the Food and Nutrition Board of the National Academy of Sciences, "Toward Healthful Diets," 1980; and Victor Herbert, *Nutrition Cultism: Facts and Fictions* (Philadelphia: George F. Stickley, 1983), 177–79. A good detailing of the spiraling commercial/scientific controversy about high-cholesterol/high-fat diets can be found in Wyden, op. cit., chapter 8, and in Whelan and Stare, op. cit. Studies comparing cholesterol levels also appear in Mayer, *Overweight . . .*, op. cit., 108. Dr. DeBakey's study appeared in *Journal of the American Medical Association,* Aug. 1, 1974.

51 See Wyden's discussion of this controversy, Wyden, op. cit., chapter 8; *Time,* January 13, 1961, 48.

52 Keys quote in *Time,* Jan. 13, 1961, 48; Wyden, op. cit., 152.

53 For a good discussion of Sylvester Graham, see Stephen Nissenbaum, *Sex, Diet, and Debility in Jacksonian America: Sylvester Graham and Health Reform* (Westport: Greenwood Press, 1980). See also Schwartz, op. cit., chapter 2. A nice summary of the various food systems that had their roots in the sixties can be found in Sam Keen, "Eating Our Way to Enlightenment," *Psychology Today,* Oct. 1978, 62–77, 123.

54 On Buddha and some professional revulsion to these fads, see Hilde Bruch, *Eating Disorders* (New York: Basic Books, 1973), 12; *Newsweek,* April 5, 1965, 92.

55 For a good summary of these studies and their citations, see note 35 above; Dwyer, Feldman, and Mayer, loc. cit., 269–87; and B. J. Kalisch, "The Stigma of Obesity," *American Journal of Nursing* 72 (1972), 1124–27.

56 Quotes from *Time,* Jan. 13, 1961, 149; On historical figures, see Stephen Mennell, *All Manners of Food; Eating and Taste in England and France from the Middle Ages to the Present* (Oxford: Oxford University Press, 1985), chapter 2. Hilde Bruch, one of the few obesity experts with a strong historical awareness, repeatedly made similar observations," see Bruch, op. cit.

57 L. F. Monello, C. C. Seltzer, and J. Mayer, "Hunger and Satiety Sensations in Men, Women, Boys and Girls: A Preliminary Report," *Annals of the New York Academy of Science* 131: (1965), 593. J. Mayer, L. F. Monello, and C. C. Seltzer, "Hunger and Satiety Sensations in Man," *Postgraduate Medicine* 37 (1965), A97; L. F. Monello, and J. Mayer, "Hunger and Satiety Sensations in Men, Women, Boys and Girls," *American Journal of Clinical Nutrition* 20 (1967), 253; For another study and a good review of other relevant studies, see Mark J. Hewitt, "Negative Mood, Hunger and Weight Classification," *Obesity/Bariatric Medicine* 3 (1974), 24–27.

58 Hilde Bruch, op. cit., 384–86.

59 Canning and Mayer study, 1967, cited in Dwyer, Feldman, and Mayer, loc. cit. Interestingly, other studies of the relationship between IQ and obesity have fairly consistently shown that the obese tend to have *higher* IQs and perform better on tests where memory and recall are important: I. P. Bronstein reported these results in 1942; Hilde Bruch reported similarly in her 1973 *Eating Disorders*; and although J. Rodin, D. Elman, and S. Schacter did not actually test IQ, they reported in *Obese Humans and Rats* (Potomac: 1974) that the obese seemed to be better "rememberers" and to process information better than normal-weight people. For a good discussion of these studies, see Anne Scott Beller, *Fat and Thin* (New York: Farrar, Straus & Giroux, 1977), 198–201. Beller's chapter 8, "Psychology: The Brain as Digestive Organ," nicely sums up the efforts and studies to discover a relationship between body weight and other characteristics. There may indeed be some relationship, but a historian cannot help but see these efforts as a modernized continuation of the late nineteenth-century faith in physiognomy as a predictor of behavior, and of early twentieth-century efforts to distinguish traits characteristic of different racial and national groups. Of course, the odd catch in associations between body weight and personality and ability is the question of whether changing body weight also changes these traits. Clearly, in the sixties it seemed to be popularly assumed that they did, which fed the myths of self-transformation. It is also significant that, despite studies that indicated "obesity" (defined in various ways by investigators) generally correlated with higher intellectual abilities, the prejudice remained firmly entrenched that the reverse was always true.

60 See Theodore Isaac Rubin, *Forever Thin* (New York: Bernard Geis, 1970) and "Dietmania," loc. cit., 74–80. Rubin quotes on p. 77; Jean W. on pp. 77–78.

61 Quoted in Wyden, op. cit., 264. Bruch repeated this warning with increasing frequency and firmness as the myth about what weight loss would bring became more inflated and more powerful. In "When *Not* to Diet," *Collier's*, Feb. 5, 1974, 82–84, Bruch warned against the faith that "puffed up ambitions" would be realized with weight loss, against those who "expect reducing to make their dreams come true," and against the promises of "a magic transformation." See also Bruch, *Eating Disorders,* chapter 11, "Thin Fat People."

CHAPTER 8

1 Hilde Bruch, "Psychological Aspects of Obesity," *Medical Insight,* July–Aug. 1973, 24; Albert Stunkard, "The Obese: Background and Programs," *Nutrition Policies in the 70's,* Jean Mayer, ed (San Francisco: Freeman, 1973), 29.

2 Theodore Berland Consumer Guide, *Rating the Diets* (New York: Beekman House, 1983); Don A. Schanche, "Diet Books That Poison Your

Mind . . . and Harm Your Body," *Overweight and Obesity: Causes, Fallacies, Treatment*, Brent Q. Hofen, ed. (Provo: Brigham Young University Press, 1975), 181; On reactions to the Atkins diet book, see "Crash Diet Craze," *Medical World News*, April 1973, 34–40.

3 Exercising statistics in Hillel Schwartz, *Never Satisfied: A Cultural History of Diets, Fantasies and Fat* (New York: The Free Press, 1986), 255.

4 Allan Cott, with Jerome Agel and Eugene Boe, *Fasting as a Way of Life* (New York: Bantam Books, 1977), quoted in Berland, op. cit., 219.

5 U. S. Food and Drug Administration, "Liquid Protein and Sudden Cardiac Deaths," *FDA Drug Bulletin*, May–June 1978, 18.

6 Data on Weight Watchers and Nutri/System Weight Loss Centers in Schwartz, op. cit., 246; on growth of diet food and drink industry, Schwartz, op. cit., 245; Star-Kist ad in Schwartz, op. cit., 253.

7 Data on diet clubs in Schwartz, op. cit., 246; in Berland, op. cit., 143–64; and in Chris Chase, *The Great American Waistline: Putting It On and Taking It Off* (New York: Coward, McCann & Geoghegan, 1981), 314–15.

8 For a good discussion of the religious diet books, see Schwartz, op. cit., 308–10; C. S. Lovett quote in Schwartz, op. cit., 308; Blue Shield ad mentioned in Schwartz, op. cit., 254.

9 Steven Singer, "When They Start Telling You It's Easy to Lose Weight . . . " (from *Today's Health,* 1972) in Hofen (ed.), op. cit., 172; Diet Conscience and diet fork mentioned in Chase, op. cit., 254–55.

10 On the development of surgical interventions, see H. Buchwald, "Jejunoileal Surgery: Which Patients Qualify?" *Medical Opinion,* Aug. 1973; "Intestinal Bypass Operation for Massive Obesity, *Postgraduate Medicine* 55 (1974); and "In Obesity Surgery, Problems Are the Rule," *Medical World News,* Sept. 1973, all in Hofen (ed.) op. cit.; On estimates of numbers of bypass surgery done per year, see Berland, op. cit., 183.

11 An excellent discussion of the developments of these ideas can be found in William Bennett, M.D. and Joel Gurin, *The Dieter's Dilemma: Eating Less and Weighing More* (New York: Basic Books, 1982), 48–59, and in Albert Stunkard, *The Pain of Obesity* (Palo Alto: Bull Publishing Co., 1976); Stuart's work was reported in Richard Stuart, "Behavioral Control of Overeating," *Behavior Research and Therapy* 5 (1967), 357–65 and popularized in R. B. Stuart and Barbara Davis, *Slim Chance in a Fat World* (Champaign: Research Press, 1972). Schachter's work and major studies are nicely summarized in Bennett and Gurin, op. cit., 48–59.

12 Quote on feeding as a form of entertainment from William B. Kannel, "Obesity and Coronary Heart Disease," in *National Nutrition Policy Study Hearings June 19–21: Background Reading Documents,* Select Committee on Nutrition and Human Needs (Washington, D.C.: USGPO, 1974), 79.

13 Mary Catherine and Robert Tyson, *Psychology of Successful Weight Control* (Chicago: Nelson Hall, 1974), quoted in Berland, op. cit., 206.

14 *Obesity and Health: A Sourcebook for Current Information for Professional*

Health Personnel (U.S. Department of Health, Education and Welfare, U.S. Public Health Service, 1966), iv–v; *National Nutrition Policy Study Hearings: June 19–21 . . .,* op. cit., 1.

15 Metropolitan Life Insurance Company, *Statistical Bulletin,* Oct. 1977, 3–4; *Weight by Height and Age for Adults 18–74 Years Old: U.S. 1971–1974,* from the Health and Nutrition Examination Survey (HANES), U.S. Department of Health Education and Welfare, Public Health Service, Office of Health Research (Washington, D.C.: USGPO, 1974), 5.

16 *National Nutrition Policy Study Hearings, June 19–21 . . .,* op. cit., 3, 10, 18.

17 Jules Hirsch and Jerome L. Knittle, "Effect of Early Nutrition on the Development of Rat Epididymal Fat Pads," *Journal of Clinical Investigation* 47 (1968) 2091–98 and "Cellularity of Obese and Nonobese Human Adipose Tissue," *Federation Proceedings* 29 (1970), 1516–21.

18 Jean Mayer, "Fat Babies Grow Into Fat People," *Family Health* 5 (1973), 24–38; "When to Start Dieting? At Birth," *Medical World News,* Sept 1973, 31–33.

19 Daniel W. Schiff, "The Case for Routine Visits," in Daniel H. Smith and Robert A. Hoekelman (eds), *Controversies in Child Health* (New York: McGraw-Hill, 1981), 194; for an excellent discussion of this development, see Schwartz, op. cit., 271–302.

20 Schwartz, op. cit., 301; on Weight Watcher's children's camps, see Chase, op. cit., 204–205; 313.

21 For objections, see Anne Scott Beller, *Fat and Thin: A Natural History of Obesity* (New York: Farrar, Straus & Giroux, 1977), 52–55, 151–54, who quotes Cheek on p. 153; Hilde Bruch, *Eating Disorders* (New York: Basic Books, 1973), 111, 135; and discussion by Myron Winick, "Childhood Obesity," *Nutrition Today,* in Hofen, op. cit., 209–215.

22 Jean Mayer, *Overweight: Causes, Cost, and Control* (Englewood Cliffs, N.J.: Prentice-Hall, 1968), 26–36.

23 "When Is Fat Excessive?" *Ames/Diagnosis* 23 (1972), 15–17, in Hofen, op. cit., 33–36; Covert Bailey, *Fit or Fat* (Boston: Houghton Mifflin Company, 1978), 10–14.

24 Mayer, *Overweight . . .,* op. cit., 35.

25 Joseph A. Califano, Jr., "The Secretary's Foreword," in *Healthy People: The Surgeon General's Report on Health Promotion and Disease Prevention,* U.S. Department of Health, Education, and Welfare, DHEW (PHS) Publication No. 79-55071, (Washington, D.C.: USGPO, 1979), vii.

26 Califano, op. cit., viii; Surgeon General's comment ibid., 9.

27 Ibid., 121, 130.

28 Ibid., 6.

29 "Playboy Interview: Hugh M. Hefner—A Candid Conversation . . . " *Playboy,* Jan. 1974, 70; Gail Sheehy, *Passages: Predictable Crises of Adult Life* (New York: Dutton, 1976); "Vogue Interviews the Experts," *Vogue,*

Jan. 1, 1977, 122. See also Christopher Lasch, *Culture of Narcissism: American Life in an Age of Diminishing Expectations* (New York: Warner Books, 1979), 100, 359–61; and see spoof on the trend in John Leo, "Life Begins at Forty to Fifty," *Time,* May 23, 1977, 91.

30 Robert Lipsyte, "What Price Fitness?" *New York Times Magazine,* Feb. 16, 1986, 33, noted that " . . . so-called natural foods and jogging were a progressive response to an establishment that wanted us passive, blissed out in front of televised sports, too impacted by beer and junk food to prevent the robbery of our health and our country."

31 Califano, op. cit., viii.

32 Gail Sheehy, "Introducing the Postponing Generation," *Esquire,* Oct. 1979, 25–31.

33 Bennett and Gurin, op. cit., 243–72.

34 See discussion in ibid., 3–23, 60–106.

35 Ibid., 142–67.

36 Bailey, op. cit., 18; San Francisco exercise physiologist quoted in Bennett and Gurin, op. cit., 255.

37 J. L. Steinfeld, "Health Conscious Citizens Are a National Asset," *Journal of Physical Education* (March/April 1972), 102; on improving working capacity, Dr. Roy Shephard, *President's Physical Fitness Newsletter* (1973), 5; other quotations in Charles Kuntzleman and Editors of Consumer Guide, *Rating the Exercises,* (New York: Morrow & Co., 1978), 19–22, 31. These ideas were repeated in most weight loss and exercise manuals; see, e.g., Nathan Pritikin, *Permanent Weight Loss Manual* (New York: Bantam Books, 1981), 143–45; for good examples of the different claims and their sources, see Kuntzleman and the Editors of Consumer Guide, op. cit.

38 For a good discussion of this build-up about exercise, see Henry Solomon, M.D., *The Exercise Myth* (San Diego: Harcourt, Brace Jovanovich, 1984), 2, 50–51; Marathon hypothesis in T.J. Bassler, Letter, *Lancet* 2 (1972), 711–12; entrants in NY marathon cited in Bennett and Gurin, op. cit., 244; Whitley exercise ad in Harvey Green, *Fit for America: Health-Fitness-Sport and American Society* (New York: Pantheon Books, 1986), 242.

39 For citations on the studies reported, see Solomon, op. cit., 97–122; and P. D. Thompson, M. P. Stern, M. S. Williams, K. Duncan, W. L. Haskell, and P. D. Wood, "Death During Jogging or Running," *Journal of the American Medical Association* 242 (1979), 1265–67.

CHAPTER 9

1 "Perils of Eating American Style," *Time,* Dec. 18, 1972, 68.

2 Jurgen Schmandt, Rose Ann Shorey, and Lilas Kinch, *Nutrition Policy in Transition* (Lexington: Lexington Books, 1980), 9; Jane Brody, *Jane Brody's Nutrition Book* (New York: Bantam Books, 1981), 5; John and Karen Hess, *The Taste of America* (New York: Grossman Publishers [Div. of Viking Press], 1977), 7.

3 Statistics from United States Department of Agriculture, *Food—From Farm to Table: 1982 Yearbook of Agriculture* (Washington, D.C.: Office of Governmental and Public Affairs, 1982), 253; percentage of fast-food sales, Chris Chase, *The Great American Waistline* (New York: Coward, McCann & Geoghegan, 1981), 93; statistics on family patterns, Andrew Hacker (ed.), *A Statistical Portrait of the American People* (New York: Viking, 1983), 92–93; On women's attitudes, see Hess and Hess, op. cit., 7.

4 Research on snacking based on 1974 Senate nutrition hearings and reported in Hess and Hess, op. cit., 6; but compare Karen J. Morgan and Basile Goungetas, "Snacking and Eating Away From Home," in Food and Nutrition Board, *What Is America Eating?* (Washington, D.C.: National Academy Press, 1986), 91–126 who reported 1980 studies that 59–70% of U.S. children and teenagers had at least one snack per day while adults were less likely to: only 40–64% of them had one snack a day; *Washington Star* editorial cited in Chris Chase, op. cit., 112.

5 Hess and Hess, op. cit., 19.

6 See especially the urgent comments in the *U.S. Congress Senate Select Committee on Nutrition and Human Needs,* Hearings 90th Congress, 2nd Session and 91st Congress, 1st Session, Parts 3–7 (Washington, D.C.: USGPO, 1969); and *National Nutrition Policy Study: Report and Recommendations, V,* Select Committee on Nutrition and Human Needs, June 1974; and introduction in Schmandt, Shorey, and Kinch, op. cit., xxi: "The new policy concerns result from scientific findings linking the dietary consumption patterns of Americans, and of affluent people elsewhere, to the increased incidence of degenerative diseases such as heart disease, diabetes and certain forms of cancer. The impact on productivity, longevity, and enjoyment of life is significant."

7 Quoted in Dr. Elizabeth M. Whelan and Dr. Frederick J. Stare, *Panic in the Pantry: Food Facts, Fads and Fallacies* (New York: Atheneum, 1975), 47.

8 Quoted in Sam Keen, "Food and Consciousness: Eating Our Way to Enlightenment," *Psychology Today,* Oct. 1978, 66.

9 For observations about the effect of Ralph Nader's Study Group report, [James S. Turner, *The Chemical Feast: The Ralph Nader Study Group Report on Food Protection and the Food and Drug Administration* (New York: Grossman Publishers, 1970)], see James Trager, "Health Food: Why and Why Not," *Vogue,* Jan. 1, 1971, 122–36; Keen article, op. cit.; for a list of some of the books which started coming out in the fifties and proliferated in the sixties and seventies, warning about chemicals in our food and with frightening titles, such as *The Hidden Assassins* or *How to Live in a Poisoned World,* see Whelan and Stare, op. cit., 13–15.

10 Whelan and Stare, op. cit., 155.

11 Circulation data from Trager, loc. cit., 134 and Keen, loc. cit., 62; on

Adelle Davis see Whelan and Stare, op. cit., 43–46, and Whelan and Stare, *The 100% Natural, Purely Organic, Cholesterol-Free, Megavitamin, Low-Carbohydrate Nutrition Hoax* (New York: Atheneum, 1984), 13–14, esp. their report, "In 1969, at the White House Conference on Food, Nutrition and Health, the panel on deception and misinformation proclaimed her [Davis] the most damaging single source of false nutritional information in the country." See also Edward H. Rynearson, M.D., "Adelle Davis' Books on Nutrition," *Medical Insight* 5 (1973), 33–34, in which he points out that Davis's references are often misquotes or have nothing to do with points she is making; also see Victor Herbert, M.D., J.D., *Nutrition Cultism* (Philadelphia: George F. Stickley Co., 1983), 91 on law suits brought against Davis's estate for deaths caused by her advice.

12 Statistics reported in Brody, op. cit., 9; see also estimated savings in dollars if Americans change diets and lose weight, in *National Nutrition Policy Study Hearings,* June 19–21, 1974, Background Reading Documents, Select Committee on Nutrition and Human Needs, 1974, 18, and *National Nutrition Policy Study: Report and Recommendations,* June 1974, Part IV, 1–2.

13 On disputes and Eastman's comments, see Keen, loc. cit., 65; see Whelan and Stare, *100% . . . ,* op. cit., 115; see also angry accusations in editorials in the *New York Times,* June 3, 1980 and one by Dr. Samuel Epstein, "Food, Nutrition, and Special Interests," *New York Times,* June 28, 1980; Brody, op. cit., 9.

14 *National Nutrition Policy Study: Report and Recommendations,* Part V, 10.

15 For a good, brief summary of the chronology of the low-cholesterol, low-saturated fat recommendations, see Whelan and Stare, *100% . . . ,* op. cit., 109–32.

16 "The American Diet Shifts and Pays Off," *Psychology Today,* April 1979, 104–105.

17 *Vogue,* Jan. 1979, 148.

18 Comfort quoted in Hess and Hess, op. cit., 276; on Pritikin, see Whelan and Stare, *100% . . . ,* op. cit., 131–32; Patricia Hausman, *Jack Sprat's Legacy: The Science and Politics of Fat and Cholesterol* (New York: Richard Marek, 1981), 15.

19 Harris Poll reported in Keen, loc. cit., 62.

20 For an excellent discussion of the indictments about eating red meat and a very intelligent rebuttal of the false assumptions underlying them, see Dr. G. Alvin Carpenter's statement, representing the American National Cattlemen's Association, to the McGovern committee, in *National Nutrition Policy Study: Report and Recommendations,* op. cit., 69–86, and the presentation about the wastefulness of meat breeding and consumption in ibid., 9–22, especially the concluding comment: "The consumer's growing concern and the increasingly serious problem of world-wide food shortages make it essential that every available communications technique, including

advertising, contribute to the American public's understanding of the relationship between nutrition and health and the entire country's relationship to the food problems of the world." Francis Moore Lappé, *Diet for a Small Planet* (New York: Ballantine Books, 1971).

21 Data on additives in Jane Brody, op. cit., 465 and in Whelan and Stare, *100% . . . ,* op. cit., 159–60.

22 See *National Nutrition Policy Study: Report and Recommendations,* op. cit., Part VII, 4–5; U.S. Senate Select Committee on Nutrition and Human Needs, *Dietary Goals for the United States* (Washington, D.C.: USGPO, 1977); and see Schmandt, Shorey, and Kinch, op. cit. 17–18; and Theodore Berland and the Editors of Consumer Guide, *Rating the Diets* (New York: Beekman House, 1983), 29–30; Whelan and Stare, *100% . . . ,* op. cit., 194.

23 Trager, op. cit., 134; Keen, loc. cit., 68; Jane Fonda repeated these ideas in *Women Coming of Age* (New York: Simon and Schuster, 1984), 196–97; "Harper's Bazaar Reviews the Diet Craze," *Harper's Bazaar,* June 1973, 36.

24 On Yudkin, see Whelan and Stare, *100% . . . ,* op. cit., 207–08, and Berland, op. cit., 82–84, 93.

25 In Keen, loc. cit., 68; Hillel Schwartz, *Never Satisfied: A Cultural History of Diets, Fantasies and Fat* (New York: The Free Press, 1986), 258.

26 William Dufty, *Sugar Blues* (New York: Warner Books, 1976); Dr. Reuben quoted in Whelan and Stare, *100% . . . ,* op. cit., 211–12.

27 Idea of sugar entering amniotic fluid cited in Chris Chase, op. cit., 191.

28 1973 medical statements in Whelan and Stare, *100% . . . ,* op. cit., 204; Brody, op. cit., 128–29; or, for example, see *Mademoiselle,* August 1978, which warns, "But like white, raw, or brown sugar, molasses and corn syrup, honey is rapidly absorbed and can cause hypoglycemia," followed the next month with a retraction, "Hypoglycemia: The Majority of People Who Think They Have It Don't," *Mademoiselle,* Sept. 1978, 69.

29 On sugar and additives affecting childhood behavior, see Dr. Ben Feingold, *Why Your Child is Hyperactive* (New York: Random House, 1975) and Dr. Lendon Smith, *Feed Your Kids Right: Dr. Smith's Program for Your Child's Total Health* (New York: McGraw-Hill, 1979); on Adelle Davis commenting on the Manson murder and on the Twinkie Defense, see Whelan and Stare, *Panic . . . ,* op. cit., 114–15 and *100% . . . ,* op. cit., 258, 268; Twinkie Defense also described in Chris Chase, op. cit., 117; for critiques of all these dietary notions, see Whelan and Stare, *100% . . . ,* op. cit., 258–68.

30 Whittlesay quoted in Whelan and Stare, *100% . . . ,* op. cit., 15; for a good discussion of salt attitudes—and the surprising lack of resistance to them by salt companies—see Daniel P. Puzo, "Salt," *Los Angeles Times,* April 7, 1988, Part VIII, 1, 18.

31 See, for example, Dr. Unglab of Louisiana in *U. S. Congress Senate Select Committee on Nutrition and Human Needs,* Hearings of 90th Congress,

2nd Session and 91st Congress, 1st Session, Parts 3–7, National Nutrition Survey (Washington, D.C.: USGPO, 1969): "There is a tendency, of course, the more affluent they are, that they use more of the convenience foods, the more expensive types of food, TV dinners and things of this sort, which in themselves nutritionally are pretty good." (p. 956.)

32 On the nouvelle cuisine chefs, see Stephen Mennell, op. cit., 163–65; and "Love in the Kitchen," *Time*, Dec. 19, 1977, 54–61.

33 "Love in the Kitchen," loc. cit., 54.

34 For this and the following paragraphs discussing health and nutrition, see Victor Herbert, op. cit., 199–221, which includes the "AMA Concepts of Nutrition and Health," Report of the Council on Scientific Affairs of the AMA and printed in *Journal of the American Medical Association* 242 (1979), 2335; and the Food and Nutrition Board's *Toward Healthful Diets*, 1980.

35 Michael DeBakey, *Journal of the American Medical Association*, Aug. 1, 1974, 124; FNB, *Toward . . .* in Herbert, op. cit., 216.

36 Victor Herbert, "Food Nutrition and a Defamatory Attack on Scientists," *New York Times*, editorial page, July 11, 1980, also reprinted in Herbert, *Nutrition Cultism*, op. cit., 206; also FNB, *Toward Healthful Diets*, in Herbert, op. cit., 216.

37 On milk, see Herbert, *Nutrition Cultism*, op. cit., 92.

38 FNB, *Toward Healthful Diets*, in Herbert, *Nutrition Cultism*, op. cit., 218.

39 Whelan and Stare, *100% . . .*, op. cit., 123–24; National Research Council, *Therapeutic Nutrition*, Publication 234, National Academy of Sciences, (Washington, D.C.: USGPO, 1952), 5.

40 For the discussions on sugar, see Whelan and Stare, *100% . . .*, op. cit., 193–215.

41 International sugar consumption statistics from *United Nations Statistical Yearbook 1983–1984* (United Nations, 1986), 175–78; U.S. consumption from *Statistical Abstract of the U.S.* (U.S. Dept. of Commerce, Bureau of the Census, 1986, No. 198), 121; earlier sugar data from Richard Osborn Cummings, *The American and His Food* (Chicago: University of Chicago Press, 1940, 1941), 114; on percentage of daily calories, see Whelan and Stare, *100% . . .*, op. cit., 195.

42 Whelan and Stare, *100% . . .*, op. cit., 215.

43 FNB, *Toward Healthful Diets*, in Herbert, *Nutrition Cultism*, op. cit., 216–17; Whelan and Stare, *100% . . .*, 132–34.

44 On saga of additives, see Whelan and Stare, *Panic . . .*, op. cit., and *100% . . .*, op. cit., 137–67.

45 Whelan and Stare, *100% . . .*, op. cit., 215.

46 FNB, *Toward Healthful Diets*, in Herbert, *Nutrition Cultism*, op. cit., 220–21.

47 Mennell, op. cit., 163–64

48 FNB, *Toward Healthful Diets*, in Herbert, *Nutrition Cultism*, op. cit.,

215; Whelan and Stare, *100% . . . ,* 136; On sugar, Whelan and Stare, *100% . . . ,* 210–11; ibid., 15; Beauty-diet advice in women's magazines often includes warnings like, "Water retention causes weight gain and the most frequent culprit is excess salt—not excess water," in *Mademoiselle,* Aug. 1978.

49 Sanford Siegal, *Dr. Siegal's Natural Fiber Permanent Weight-Loss Diet* (New York: Dial Press, 1975); Barbara Kraus, *The Barbara Kraus Guide to Fiber in Foods* (New York: Signet, 1975); The Committee on Diet, Nutrition, and Cancer concluded, "The committee found no conclusive evidence to indicate that dietary fiber . . . exerts a protective effect against colorectal cancer in humans . . . . In the only study in which the effects of individual components of fiber were assessed, there was an inverse correlation between the incidence of colon cancer and the consumption of the pentosan fraction of fiber (found in whole-wheat products)," in Committee on Diet, Nutrition, and Cancer, *Diet, Nutrition, and Cancer* (Washington, D.C.: National Research Council, National Academy Press, 1982), 134; Chase, *op. cit.,* 190.

CHAPTER 10

1 Aimee Liu, *Solitaire* (New York: 1979); Christina Probert, *Swimwear in Vogue Since 1910* (New York: Abbeville Press, 1981), photo by Petito Galvez from 1975 *Vogue,* 81; e.g., see Carrie Donovan, "Clothes Designed to Celebrate the Body," in *New York Times Magazine,* Nov. 27, 1977, 123 and photos following.

2 L. M. Vincent, *Competing With the Sylph: Dancers and the Pursuit of Ideal Body Form* (New York: Andrews and McMeel, 1979); Paul E. Garfinkel, M.D. and David M. Garner, Ph.D., *Anorexia Nervosa: A Multidimensional Perspective* (New York: Brunner/Mazel, 1982), 113.

3 Statistics based on my studies of Miss America Pageant Yearbooks, 1972–1983; see also D. M. Garner, P. E. Garfinkel, D. Schwartz and M. Thompson, "Cultural Expectations of Thinness in Women," *Psychological Reports* 47 (1980), 483–91.

4 Garner, Garfinkel, et. al., loc. cit, 108–9.

5 Verushka in "Painted Lady," *Playboy,* Jan. 1974, 122–30; Farrah Fawcett in *Vogue,* April 1977.

6 Kennedy Fraser, *The Fashionable Mind: Reflections on Fashion 1970–1982* (Boston: David Godine, 1985), 13; *Vogue,* May 1974, 125.

7 "The Tuned-Up Body: Exercise," *Mademoiselle,* May 1970, 174–75.

8 Donovan, loc. cit., 123.

9 "The New Young Body—The Young Bosom," *Vogue,* Jan. 1, 1970, 140.

10 "The 1971 Figure—Exercise—Everybody Wants It," *Vogue,* Jan 1, 1971, 97.

11 "Control Cellulite," *Harper's Bazaar,* running theme in Jan. (p.22), Feb. (p.50), and March (p.42), 1971; *Vogue,* April 1973, 100; *Mademoiselle,*

March 1974, 158; In 1979 Blair Sabol made a very telling observation about how emphasis on these details creates concerns about them: "But where was cellulite ten years ago? It seems as if all of us have just noticed that our upper legs or frontal thighs are beginning to break out in dimples," in "Body Talk—Cellulite," *Mademoiselle,* Oct. 1979, 98.

12 Reported in Elizabeth Ewing, *Dress and Undress: A History of Underwear* (New York: Drama Book Specialists, 1978), 171–73.

13 "Beauty Bulletin," *Vogue,* Jan. 15, 1972, 54; *Mademoiselle,* March 1974, 158; *Vogue,* Jan. 1979, 138.

14 Quoted in Fraser, op. cit., 215; "Vogue's Point of View," *Vogue,* Jan. 1, 1972, 37; ads quoted in "Decoding the Styles of the 70's," *New York Times Magazine,* Dec. 30, 1979, 25.

15 "Beauty Is . . . ," *Vogue,* April 1975, 113.

16 *Vogue,* March 1973, 101; *Vogue,* April 1973, 141.

17 Susan Sontag, "On Woman's Beauty," *Vogue,* April 1975, 119; "L-A-D-Y: The New Four Letter Word," *Mademoiselle,* Jan. 1974.

18 See especially Betty Friedan's discussion of various feminist attitudes toward the family and childbearing in *The Second Stage* (New York: Summit Books, 1981), esp. 39–49. Friedan especially faults radical feminists such as Shulamith Firestone who, Friedan justifiably argues, "portrayed motherhood as 'a condition of terminal psychological and social decay, total self-abnegation and physical deterioration.' "

19 Stephen Mennell, *All Manners of Food* (Oxford: Basil Blackwell, 1985), 263–65; on changes in American attitudes toward food and cooking, see "Love in the Kitchen," *Time,* Dec. 19, 1977, 54–61.

20 "Cost of an Affair," *Vogue,* Feb. 15, 1970, 98.

21 "Fitness Is—Seven Experts Tell How To Get It . . . " *Vogue,* Jan. 1977, 121–22.

22 Examples and quotes in Hillel Schwartz, *Never Satisfied: A Cultural History of Diets, Fantasies and Fat* (New York: The Free Press, 1986), 248–50.

23 Marcia Millman, *Such a Pretty Face* (New York: Berkley Books, 1982), 56, 82, 49–64.

24 *Weight, Height and Selected Body Dimensions of Adults,* National Center for Health Statistics, Series 11 No. 8, (U.S. Department of Health, Education and Welfare, Public Health Service, June 1965), 20.

25 "Discrimination: Weighty Problem: Bias Against Overweight Job Seekers," *Newsweek,* March 31, 1975, 64; Robert J. Homant and Daniel B. Kennedy, "Attitudes Toward Ex-offenders: A Comparison of Social Stigmas," *Journal of Criminal Justice* 10 (1982), 383–91; "Better Than Prison," *Time,* June 7, 1971, 39; on stewardess, Chris Chase, *The Great American Waistline* (New York: Coward, McCann & Geoghegan, 1981), 196.

26 Millman, op. cit., 4, 3–27; Mike Wallace quotes in Chris Chase, op. cit., 164–65; Vivian F. Mayer, Foreword, *Shadow on a Tightrope* (Iowa City:

Aunt Lute Book Co., 1983), xii and for history of Fat Liberation, her whole foreword.

27 "Big Can Be Beautiful," *Ebony,* Oct. 1978, 86.

28 On Carol Shaw, see Chris Chase, op. cit., 166–68 and "Spreading the Word That Big Is Beautiful," *Philadelphia Inquirer,* June 16, 1984, C-1, C-8, and issues of *Big Beautiful Woman.*

29 "Dieting to Disaster," *Mademoiselle,* Jan. 1974, 8; "Thin Isn't Always So Beautiful!" *Seventeen,* April 1974, 24; Hilde Bruch, *The Golden Cage* (New York: Basic Books, 1978): "Yet I call it a new disease because for the last 15–20 years, anorexia nervosa is occurring at a rapidly increasing rate. Now it is so common that it represents a real problem in high schools and colleges." (p.viii); Betty-Jane Raphael, "An Opinion: On My Obsession About My Weight," *Mademoiselle,* Sept. 1977, 78, 86; Susie Orbach, *Fat Is a Feminist Issue* (New York: Berkeley Books, 1978).

30 Marlene Boskind-White, Ph.D. and William C. White, Ph.D., *Bulimarexia: The Binge/Purge Cycle* (New York: W. W. Norton & Co., 1983). Their original publications on the subject were Marlene Boskind-Lodahl, "Cinderella's Step-Sisters: A Feminist Perspective on Anorexia Nervosa and Bulimia," *Signs: Journal of Women in Culture and Society,* Spring 1977, and Boskind-Lodahl and Sirlin, "Gorging-Purging Syndrome: Bulimarexia," *Psychology Today,* March 1977, 50–52.

31 Orbach, op. cit., Berkeley Books, 1985 ed., 21; See also the excellent work of Susan C. Wooley and Wayne C. Wooley, e.g., "Should Obesity Be Treated At All?" in A. J. Stunkard and E. Stellar (eds), *Eating and Its Disorders* (New York: Raven Press, 1984), 185–92.

32 Bruch, op. cit., esp. her introductory comments on viii–ix; Boskind-White and White, op. cit; Wooley interviews in Bennett and Gurin, *The Dieter's Dilemma* (New York: Basic Books, 1982); Christopher Lasch, *Culture of Narcissism* (New York: Warner Books, 1979).

CHAPTER 11

1 Robin Marantz Henig, "The High Cost of Thinness," *New York Times Magazine,* Feb. 28, 1988, 41–42.

2 Figures on aerobic exercisers in *Los Angeles Times,* May 6, 1986, V: 1,4; figures on exercise shoe sales in *Los Angeles Times,* May 3, 1987, IV:2, 8.

3 Publishers Note, *American Health,* March 1985, 12; *Ms.,* May 1986, 43.

4 Jane Fonda, *Jane Fonda's Workout Book* (New York: Simon and Schuster, 1981).

5 Data compiled by National Sporting Goods Assn. and National Running Data Center of Tucson, Ariz., and reported in *Los Angeles Times,* Feb. 24, 1987, V:1; see also Henry A. Solomon, M.D., *The Exercise Myth* (San Diego: Harcourt, Brace, Jovanovich, 1984); and William Bennett, M.D. and Joel Gurin, *The Dieter's Dilemma* (New York: Basic Books, 1982), chapter 9.

6 "Hold the Eggs and Butter," *Time,* March 26, 1984, 50–63, quote on p. 62; Food Marketing Institute statistics reported in *American Health,* Oct. 1987, 49.

7 Food Marketing Institute statistics reported in *American Health,* Oct. 1987, 49; Jane Brody, *Jane Brody's Nutrition Book* (New York: Bantam Books, 1981), 298.

8 Michael T. Pugliese et. al., "Fear of Obesity," *New England Journal of Medicine* 309 (1983), 513–17; Joel D. Killen et. al., "Self-Induced Vomiting and Laxative and Diuretic Use Among Teenagers," *Journal of the American Medical Association,* March 21, 1986, 1447–49; On fourth and fifth graders dieting, see Laurel Mellin et. al. of the University of California, San Francisco, studies and other studies reported in *Los Angeles Times,* Oct. 29, 1986, V: 1; see also studies of Drs. M. Pugliese, F. Lifshitz, G. Grad, P. Fort, and M. Marks-Katz, "Fear of Obesity: A Cause of Short Stature and Delayed Puberty," *New England Journal of Medicine,* Sept. 1, 1983, 513–18, and its spread to the lay public in, e.g., "Fear of Obesity Hits Youngsters," *Los Angeles Times,* June 29, 1986, IX: 10.

9 Fonda, op. cit., 24; Jane Fonda, *Women Coming of Age* (New York: Simon and Schuster, 1984), 16.

10 *American Health,* March 1985, 47; *American Health,* cover, June 1982.

11 *Vogue,* Jan. 1979, 146; *Ms.,* May 1986, ad on p. 96.

12 For a good discussion of the development of the futurology ideas, see Christopher Lasch, op. cit., 363–64; Diana Benzia, "Stop the Clock on Aging," *Harper's Bazaar,* Nov. 1979, 182.

13 Frost and Sullivan referred to in David P. Schultz, "Selling the Newest Trendy Pastime: Exercise," *Stores,* Feb. 1983, 5; Jim Seale, "Exercisewear," *Stores,* June 1984, 13.

14 "Body Building for Men," *New York Times Magazine,* June 15, 1980, 58.

15 "Body: Shades of Charles Atlas: Nobody Will Ever Kick Sand in Lisa Lyon's Face," *People,* May 26, 1980, 82; "The New Flex Appeal," *Newsweek,* May 6, 1985, 82–83.

16 "The New Ideal of Beauty," *Time,* Aug. 30, 1982, 72–77, quote on p.75.

17 "The New Ideal Female Body," *Glamour,* July 1981, 60; "The New Flex Appeal," loc. cit., 82.

18 Jane Fonda, *Workout Book,* 16.

19 "Your Shapeup Special," *Harper's Bazaar,* May 1985, 139.

20 Annie Gottlieb, "Getting Strong—Developing Muscle Strength in Women," *Mademoiselle,* March 1981, 198; *Mademoiselle,* Feb. 1986, cover and 148–52.

21 Phyllis Theroux, "The Size-7 Soul," *American Health,* May 1982, 46.

22 Fonda quoted in interview, "The California Workout," *Harper's Bazaar,* Jan. 1980, 82–83.

23 "The New Ideal of Beauty," *Time,* Aug. 30, 1982, 72; Miss America statistics based on *Miss America Pageant* Yearbooks, 1972–1983.

24 "Pumping Iron: Chapter II," *Time,* Nov. 12, 1979, 131; Pat Jordan, "Women of Steel—Behind the Scenes at the Miss Olympia Body Building Championship," *Mademoiselle,* Jan. 1982, 112–13. Jordan observes: "To achieve this look [muscled and veined, devoid of fat], the contestants diet strenuously and work on their weight lifting routines at least 3 or 4 hours a day, 6 days a week."

25 "The New Ideal of Beauty," loc. cit., 74; Reebok ad in *American Health,* Oct. 1987, 34–35.

26 "Your Shapeup Special," *Harper's Bazaar,* May 1985, 139; "Letters," *Ms.,* Aug. 1985, 5.

27 Gottlieb, loc. cit., 239.

28 Colette Dowling, *The Cinderella Complex* (New York: Simon and Schuster, 1981); Fern Schumer, "Life, Liberty, and the Pursuit of Muscle Power," *Forbes,* May 29, 1979, 35.

29 Betty Friedan, *The Second Stage* (New York: Summit Books, 1981), 22; Also see fuller discussion of this theme in American feminism in Karen Offen, "Defining Feminism: A Comparative Historical Approach," *Signs: Journal of Women, Culture and Society,* Fall, 1988, 119–57.

30 Gottlieb, loc. cit., p.47.

31 For a general discussion of prevailing economic conditions, see Christopher Lasch, *Culture of Narcissism: American Life in an Age of Diminishing Expectations* (New York: Warner Books, 1979); other data on decade-long trends in "Growing Pains at 40," *Time,* May 19, 1986, 22–41 (statistic cited on p.37); "Show Me the Way to Go Home," *Time,* May 4, 1987, 106.

32 Robert B. Reich, *Tales of a New America,* Times Books, 1987; also interview with Reich by Gary Abrams, "A Plea to Revamp the National Psyche," *Los Angeles Times,* May 3, 1987, IV, 3.

33 An enormous amount of work has been done on the changes in the American family. I particularly like the work of Sheila M. Rothman, *Woman's Proper Place: A History of Changing Ideals and Practices* (New York: Basic Books, 1978) and Paula Fass, *The Beautiful and the Damned* (Oxford: Oxford University Press, 1977).

34 Robin Norwood, *Women Who Love Too Much* (New York: St. Martin's Press, 1985).

35 Robert Lipsyte, "What Price Fitness?" *New York Times Magazine,* Feb. 16, 1986, 32–33, 71, 75, 84.

36 Norbert Elias, *The Civilizing Process,* tr. Edmund Jephcott, 2 vols; vol. I (Boston: Urizen Books, 1978); vol II (New York: Pantheon Books, 1982).

CHAPTER 12

1 Joan Jacobs Brumberg, *Fasting Girls: The Emergence of Anorexia Nervosa as a Modern Disease* (Cambridge, Harvard University Press, 1988), 12; Paul Garfinkel and David Garner (eds.), *Anorexia Nervosa: A Multidimensional Perspective* (New York: Brunner/Mazel, 1982), 100–104; Jane

Brody recently stated that " . . . the binge-purge syndrome . . . now afflicts up to a quarter of college women," and that, in a recent University of California, San Francisco, study, "all the 18-year-olds said they currently use vomiting, laxatives, fasting or diet pills to help them control their weight," "Personal Health," *New York Times,* March 18, 1987, C3; K. Halmi, J. Falk, and E. Schwartz, "Binge Eating and Vomiting: A Survey of a College Population," *Psychological Medicine,* 11 (1981), 697–706; R. Pyle, E. Mitchell, and E. Eckert, "The Incidence of Bulimia in Freshman College Students," *International Journal of Eating Disorders* 2, (1983), 75–85; "Feeling Fat in a Thin Society," *Glamour,* Feb. 1984, 198–201.

2 "Living—What It Takes Now... The New Discipline," *Vogue,* Jan. 1979, 138.

3 Percentages in Rita Freedman, *Beauty Bound* (Lexington, Mass.: Lexington Books, 1986), 149.

4 *People,* March 26, 1979, 38; "Manufacturing Miss America," *People,* Sept. 19, 1983, 93.

5 Anne Scott Beller, *Fat and Thin* (New York: Farrar, Straus & Giroux, 1977), chapter 3; "When Is Fat Excessive?" *Ames/Diagnosis* 23 (1972), 15–17.

6 Beller, op. cit., 63.

7 "Feeling Fat in a Thin Society," loc. cit; Eugenia Chandler, *The Venus Syndrome* (New York: Doubleday, 1985), preface and 1.

8 Beller, op. cit., chapters 3 and 4.

9 Dr. Barbara Edelstein, *The Woman Doctor's Diet for Women* (Englewood Cliffs, N.J.: Prentice-Hall, 1977); *Mademoiselle,* Feb. 1986, cover and 148–52.

10 Beller, op. cit., chapter 3.

11 A. Keys, J. Brozek, A. Henschel, O. Michelson, and H.L. Taylor, *The Biology of Human Starvation,* 2 vols. (Minneapolis: University of Minnesota Press, 1950); see discussion in William Bennett, M.D. and Joel Gurin, *The Dieter's Dilemma: Eating Less and Weighing More* (New York: Basic Books, 1982), 11–17; Hilde Bruch, *Eating Disorders* (New York: Basic Books, 1973), chapters 1 and 2.

12 Bruch, op. cit., chapters 1, 2, 10, and 11, pp. 122–25; Albert Stunkard, "The 'Dieting Depression,'" *American Journal of Medicine* 23 (1957), 77–86; for other references, see Bennett and Gurin, op. cit., chapter 2.

13 Bruch, op. cit., chapters 1 and 2; Bruch, *The Golden Cage* (New York: Basic Books, 1978), xi; and in James Mitchell (ed.), *Anorexia Nervosa and Bulimia: Diagnoses and Treatment* (Minneapolis: University of Minnesota, 1985), 11.

14 Bruch, *Eating Disorders,* 11, 128.

15 C. Peter Herman and Deborah Mack, "Restrained and Unrestrained Eating," *Journal of Personality* 43 (1975) 647–60; see also the excellent discussion of the studies and growing acceptance of this idea by leading obesity researchers such as Albert Stunkard in Bennett and Gurin, op. cit., 40–48.

16 An excellent discussion of this phenomenon can be found in Bennett and Gurin, op. cit., 40–48; Kim Chernin, *The Obsession: The Tyranny of Slenderness* (New York: Harper & Row, 1981); Susie Orbach, *Fat is a Feminist Issue* (New York: Berkeley Books, 1978).

17 For a discussion of these developments in attitudes toward eating, see Stephen Mennell, *All Manners of Food: Eating and Taste in England and France from the Middle Ages to the Present* (Oxford: Basil Blackwell, 1985).

18 Kim Chernin, *The Hungry Self: Women, Eating and Identity* (New York: Harper & Row, 1985).

19 Brumberg op. cit., 39–40.

20 Bruch, *Eating Disorders,* op. cit., chapter 11; David M. Garner, Paul E. Garfinkel, Donald Schwartz, and Michael Thompson, "Cultural Expectations of Thinness in Women," *Psychological Reports* 47 (1980), 483–91, quotation on 490.

21 This typically new attitude was expressed by Jane Brody in a recent interview about her book, *Good Food Book.* She explained, "The word *diet* is not in my dictionary. Diets don't work." Instead, she described her nutritional regimen as "an eating plan for life"—though it was still based on the McGovern Guidelines and, as such, could be "geared toward general health as well as to the problem of overweight." "To Jane Brody, 'Diet' is a Four-letter Word," *Evening Outlook,* Jan. 27, 1986, C-3.

22 "Instant Swimsuit Makeovers," *Glamour,* June 1986, 200–209.

23 Sir Kenneth Clark, *The Nude: A Study in Ideal Form* (Princeton: Princeton University Press, 1956), 5–6.

24 "Modern Beauty: What's Perfect, What Counts," *Vogue,* Oct. 1985, 484.

25 Christopher Lasch, *The Culture of Narcissism* (New York: Warner Books, 1979), 309.

26 "Feeling Fat in a Thin Society," loc. cit., footnote 1.

CHAPTER 13

1 The best summaries and discussion of weight-mortality statistics are in various publications of Reubin Andres, M.D., "Effect of Obesity on Total Mortality," *International Journal of Obesity* 4 (1980), 381–86; "Aging, Diabetes and Obesity: Standards of Normalcy," *The Mount Sinai Journal of Medicine* 48 (Nov.–Dec. 1981), 489–95; "Mortality and Obesity: The Rationale for Age-Specific Height-Weight Tables," in Reubin Andres, M.D., Edwin L. Bierman, M.D., and William R. Hazzard, M.D. (eds.), *Principles of Geriatric Medicine* (New York: McGraw-Hill, 1985), 311–18; and R. Andres, M.D., D. Elahi, Ph.D., J.D. Tobin, M.D., D.C. Muller, B.A., and L. Brant, Ph.D., "Impact of Age on Weight Goals," *Annals of Internal Medicine* 103 (Dec. 1985), 1030–33. Another excellent discussion is in William Bennett, M.D. and Joel Gurin, *The Dieter's Dilemma: Eating Less and Weighing More* (New York: Basic Books, 1982), especially chap-

ter 5; see also William Kannel and Tavia Gordon, "The Effects of Over-weight on Cardiovascular Disease," in *National Nutrition Policy Study Hearings, June, 1974,* Select Committee on Nutrition and Human Needs, Background Reading Documents (Washington, D.C.: U.S. Government Printing Office, 1974). Other major studies disputing the overweight-mortality links and critiques of the MLIC are, in chronological order:

1955. Ancel Keys, "Obesity and Heart Disease," *Journal of Chronic Diseases* 1 (1955), 456, in which he criticized the statistical validity of the insurance company campaign, questioned the justification of applying the experience of the small number of overweight policyholders—only 2 percent—to the nation at large, calculated that even if all the people who are 20 percent overweight reduced, the rate of heart disease would still be high, and cautioned about the potential dangers of people with circulatory diseases rapidly regaining lost weight.

1962. Acheson, "The Etiology of Coronary Heart Disease: A Review from the Epidemeological Standpoint," *Yale Journal of Biological Medicine* 35, (1962), 143–170.

1963. Pell, S. and D'Alonzo, CA "Acute Myocardial Infarction in Large Industrial Population: Report of a Six Year Study of 1356 Cases," *Journal of the American Medical Association* 185 (1963), 831–38, in which "Autopsy studies have in general failed to show a quantitative relationship between the degree of adiposity and the extent of coronary atherosclerosis found at necropsy, particularly in non-hypertensives and women," quoted by Kannel and Gordon in "The Effects of Overweight on Cardiovascular Disease," op. cit., 31–32.

1963. N. O. Borhani, H. H. Hechter, L. Breslow, "Report of a Ten-year Follow-Up Study of the San Francisco Longshoremen," *Journal of Chronic Diseases* 16 (1963), 1251–66 in which the heaviest subjects, those over 30 percent overweight, had the lowest mortality.

1964. Bjurulf, P. and Lindren, G, "A Preliminary Study on Overweight in the South of Sweden," in ed. G. Blix, *Occurrences, Causes, and Prevention of Overnutrition* (Uppsala, Sweden:, Almqvist & Wisells), in which a survey of the whole population in the south of Sweden indicated body weights were much higher than the MLIC "ideal"—70 percent of the female population over forty years old was 22 pounds "overweight," and 10 percent was 60 pounds or more overweight, yet it did not appear these people were adversely affected by their "overweights."

1964. Ed., G. Blix, op. cit., reported on international symposium on overnutrition held in Sweden in 1963, attended by participants from many different countries in many different disciplines who concurred that "middle aged people with a stable weight excess of 20 to 30 pounds who customarily were rated "overweight" were probably normal for themselves, that this weight excess did not represent a health hazard, except in clearly defined abnormal conditions." quoted in Hilde Bruch, *Eating Disorders* (New York: Basic Books, 1973), 109.

1966. C. C. Seltzer, "Some Re-Evaluations of the Build and Blood Pressure Study, 1959 as Related to Ponderal Index, Somatype, and Mortality," *New England Journal of Medicine* 275 (1966), 254–59, in which reevaluation of the 1959 study demonstrated that there was no significant excess in actual over expected mortality until the level of extreme obesity was reached.

1966. G. W. Comstock, M. A. Kendrick, and V. T. Livesay, "Subcutaneous Fatness and Mortality," *American Journal of Epidemeology* 83 (1966), 548–63. In a large population group in Muscogee County, Georgia, subcutaneous fat thickness was not significantly related to mortality.

1973. N. B. Belloc, "Relationship of Health Practices and Mortality," *Preventive Medicine* 2 (1973), 67–81 in which 6,928 men and women in Alameda County, California, were studied for five-and-a-half years. Only the leanest and the fattest could be associated with premature mortality.

1974. T. J. Cole, J. C. Gilson, and H. C. Olsen, "Bronchitis, Smoking and Obesity in an English and Danish Town: Male Deaths After a 10-Year Follow-Up," *Bulletin Physio. Path. Resp* 10 (1974), 657–79. In the English town, mortality was highest in the lighter subjects, in the Danish town, the men who died had a significantly higher obesity index than the survivors, but the difference was very small.

1975. A. R. Dyer, J. Stamler, D. M. Berkson, H. A. Lindberg, "Relationship of Relative Weight and Body Mass Index to 14 Year Mortality in Chicago People's Gas Company Study," *Journal of Chronic Diseases* 28 (1975), 109–23. Among the 1,233 employees, who were 40–59 when the study started, the best life expectancy correlated with weights 25–32 percent above MLIC desirable weights.

1983. A. L. Stewart and R. H. Brook, "Effects of Being Overweight," *American Journal of Public Health* 73 (Feb. 1983), 171–78. Reviewing all the major weight/health-mortality studies, this Rand Corp. group concluded, "We have extensively reviewed the literature on the relationship of overweight to overall premature mortality, heart disease, diabetes, hypertension and cholesterol. In our review of 21 studies, we found . . . that being severely overweight is clearly associated with premature mortality, although being moderately overweight may not be an important risk factor for this outcome," 171.

2 Paul Sorlie, Tavia Gordon, and William B. Kannel, "Body Build and Mortality," *Journal of the American Medical Association* 243 (1980), 1828–31. W. B. Kannel and Tavia Gordon, "Physiological and Medical Concomitants of Obesity: The Framingham Study," in George A. Bray, M.D. (ed.) *Obesity in America* (Washington, D.C.: National Institutes of Health Publication No. 79–359, Nov. 1979), 141.

3 Ancel Keys, "Overweight, Obesity, Coronary Heart Disease and Mortality," *Nutrition Reviews* 38 (1980), 297–307; Ancel Keys et. al., *Seven Countries: A Multivariate Analysis of Death and Coronary Heart Disease* (Cambridge: Harvard University Press, 1980), 194.

4 Andres, *Principles of Geriatric Medicine,* op. cit., 316.

5 Kannel and Gordon in Bray, op. cit., 138. The graph they present suggests worst life expectancy for men is at or below MLIC "desirable weight" and that it improves most precipitously from 15 percent above ideal weight to 30 percent above, and begins to increase, slightly, again after 40 percent above "desirable" weight. Andres, *International Journal of Obesity,* op. cit., 382.

6 Andres raises this question in his articles, and Bennett and Gurin, op. cit., 109 and 113–22.

7 Bennett and Gurin, op. cit., chapter 5.

8 Andres, "Aging, Diabetes and Obesity: Standards of Normality," op. cit., 495; and Andres, *International Journal of Obesity,* op. cit., 382. Ten percent overweight is thus equivalent to 25 and 31 percent over desirable weight for men and women respectively.

9 Andres, "Effect of Obesity on Total Mortality," op. cit., 385 and "Mortality and Obesity: The Rationale for Age-Specific Height-Weight Tables," op. cit.

10 Metropolitan Life Foundation, "1983 Metropolitan Height and Weight Tables," *Statistical Bulletin* 64, No. 1, (Jan.–June 1983), 3–8. When the *Build Study 1979* was published, there were several articles in the popular press, among them, "Weight and Mortality: Skinny Isn't Best," *Science News,* May 1980; "Thinner May Not Mean Healthier," *Business Week,* July 1981; "Overblown Reports Distort Obesity Risks," in *Science,* Jan. 1981; and "As 70 Million Americans Try to Shed Weight," *US News,* Dec. 1980. The number now not fat is a minimum estimate, Bennett and Gurin report, announced by the Society of Actuaries, April 12, 1979 in a press release and applied only to people aged forty to sixty-nine; Bennett and Gurin, op. cit., footnote #1, 304.

11 "1983 Metropolitan Height and Weight Tables," op. cit., 9–12.

12 Ibid.

13 Ibid. 12

14 Andres, "Mortality and Obesity: The Rationale for Age-Specific Height-Weight Tables," op. cit., 315; Hillel Schwartz, *Never Satisfied: A Cultural*

History of Diets, Fantasies and Fat (New York: The Free Press, 1986), 337–38.

15 Bennett and Gurin, op. cit., chapters 1–3; C. S. Chlouverakis, "Nature and Nurture in Human Obesity," *Obesity/Bariatric Medicine* 3 (1974), 28–31; H. A. Jordan, "In Defense of Body Weight," *Journal American Dietetic Assn* 62 (1973), 17–21; Jules Hirsch and Rudolph L. Leibel, "New Light on Obesity," *New England Journal of Medicine* 318 (Feb. 25, 1988), 509–11; Hilde Bruch, *Eating Disorders* (New York: Basic Books, 1973).

16 Ethan A. H. Sims, "Studies in Human Hyperphagia," in George Bray and John Bethune, *Treatment and Management of Obesity* New York, 1974, 29 and "Experimental Obesity in Man," *Transactions of the Assoc. of American Physicians* 81 (1968), 153–70. For a nice summary of Sims work, see Bennett and Gurin, op. cit., 17–21.

17 See physical anthropologist, Anne Scott Beller, *Fat and Thin* (New York: Farrar, Straus and Giroux, 1977), chapter 2, in which she concluded from national and international studies that "like farm animals and laboratory mice, different genetic strains of human beings metabolize their food in individually idiosyncratic ways . . . ." with variations as great, possibly, as a lean person needing 6,000 calories to gain a kilo (2.2 pounds) and a fat-inclined one needing only 2,500 calories, 39–41.

18 See Bennett and Gurin's summary of the data including their interviews in op. cit., chapters 2–3; UC Berkeley study reported in "Dieting: The Losing Game," in *Time,* Jan 20, 1986, 56; see similar data reported in Bennett and Gurin of studies on humans and rats, op. cit., 71–73; Hirsch and Leibel, op. cit., 510.

19 Eric Ravussin et. al., "Reduced Rate of Energy Expenditure as a Risk Factor for Body-Weight Gain," in *New England Journal of Medicine* 318, Feb. 25, 1988, 467–72 and Susan B. Roberts, et. al., "Energy Expenditure and Intake in Infants Born to Lean and Overweight Mothers," in ibid., 461–72; Theresa A. Spiegel, "Caloric Regulation of Food Intake in Man," *Journal of Comparative and Physiological Psychology* 84 (1973), 24–37.

20 J. Leray, *Embonpoint et obesité, conceptions et therapeutiques actuelles,* (Paris: Masson et Cie., 1931), quoted in Bruch, op. cit., 113, and also Bruch's discussion, 109–11, and her summary of the 1963 conference, 110.

21 The obesity authority was Geheimrath Leyden, quoted in Bruch, op. cit., 311; Studies at Rockefeller Institute by Jules Hirsch, Rudolph Leibel and Irving Faust, described by Gina Kolata, "Weight Regulation May Start in Our Cells, Not Our Psyches," *Smithsonian,* Jan. 1986, 93–94.

22 "Dieting: The Losing Game," *Time,* op. cit., 58; Albert Stunkard, "Presidential Address—1974," *Psychosomatic Medicine* 37 (1975), 195–236.

23 Bennett and Gurin, op. cit., esp. 84–87 and their interview with Susan Wooley, 87; on these effects of yoyo dieting, see studies of M.R.C. Greenwood of Vassar and George Blackburn of Harvard in Gina Kolata, op. cit., 96–97; and it has now entered popular culture through "Dieting: The

Losing Game," op. cit., which reports the work of Psychologist Richard Keesey and of international obesity expert, Dr. T. Van Itallie, 58.

24 "Whatever the handicaps and dangers associated with overweight, they are negligible in comparison to the suffering and invalidism that excessive reducing and self-starvation create. The fact that among the many hundreds of fat youngsters there was only one whose death . . . appeared to be related to his superobese state in contrast to 5 deaths among 70 anorexics, is a sign of the disparity in suffering and illness created by over- as compared to under-nutrition," Bruch, op. cit., 384; recent estimates of 19 percent from Joan Jacobs Brumberg, *Fasting Girls: The Emergence of Anorexia Nervosa as a Modern Disease* (Cambridge: Harvard University Press, 1988), 13.

25 For a good summary of some of the psychoanalytic data, see Bennett and Gurin, op. cit., 24–36.

26 Bruch, op. cit., 109–11; Robert Simon, "Obesity as a Depressive Equivalent," *Journal of the American Medical Association* 183 (1963), 208–10.

27 Bennett and Gurin, op. cit., 34; Stewart and Brooks, "Effects of Being Overweight," loc. cit., footnote 1, observed that "No association was observed between weight-for-height and positive well-being," though among those who perceived themselves to be overweight (only 12 percent were severely overweight, 10 percent moderately so, but 41 percent perceived themselves to be overweight) "pain, worry and restricted activities all increase as weight increases and were all greater in women . . . ," 176.

28 Beller, op. cit, 198–99; H. Canning and J. Mayer, "Obesity: An Influence on High School Performance," *American Journal of Clinical Nutrition* 20 (April 1967), 352–54.

29 "Heavy Duty for Heavyweights," *Newsweek,* May 11, 1981, 21 Bennett and Gurin, op. cit., 254; Beller, op. cit., 46; Bruch, op. cit., 135; Marjorie Waxman and Albert Stunkard, "Caloric Intake and Expenditure of Obese Boys," *Journal of Pediatrics* 2 (1980), 187–93.

30 Bennett and Gurin provide a nice discussion of this in op. cit., 24–34; Stanley Conrad, "The Problem of Weight Reduction in the Obese Woman," *American Practitioner and Digest of Treatment* 5 (1954), 38–47.

31 Kim Chernin, *The Hungry Self: Women, Eating & Identity* (New York: Harper & Row, 1985); Susie Orbach, *Fat is a Feminist Issue: The Anti-Diet Guide to Permanent Weight Loss* (New York: Berkley Books, 1978), 60

32 Bennett and Gurin, op. cit., 25–34; Colleen Rand, "Obesity and Human Sexuality," *Medical Aspects of Human Sexuality* Jan. 1979, 140–52; Henry Jordan and Leonard Levitz, "Sex and Obesity," *Medical Aspects of Human Sexuality* Oct. 1979, 104–17; Bruch, op. cit., 118.

33 Cited in Beller, op. cit., 74–75.

34 See Bennett and Gurin's discussion of Keys's experiment, esp p. 14; Ancel Keys et. al., *Biology of Human Starvation,* op. cit.; see also Bruch's more general description of effects of starvation, op. cit., 9–13; Phyllis Mensing

(AP writer), "Eating Disorders Have Severe Effect on Sexual Function," *Evening Outlook,* April 6, 1987, D6.

35 Beller cites deWaard's work in op. cit., 76–79.

36 Hirsch quoted in "Dieting: The Losing Game," op. cit., 60.

37 Hilde Bruch remarked that "Fat people are apt to blame all their difficulties on being fat and they hope for a new lease on life after they get thin. Many begin reducing confident of finding the pot of gold at the end of the rainbow . . . . From my observations there are three outcomes for people who reduce with the unrealistic goal of expecting a changed life before they have experienced the inner emotional changes which make these new adjustments possible. The great majority will try . . . . will lose some weight and then, suddenly they will give up and regain and often overshoot their former weight. For others the stress of starving themselves, the loss of their size, the new real or imagined expectations may prove too much, and serious emotional disturbances, even frank psychotic behavior, may break through . . . . " op. cit., 194–45.

38 C. Branach and L. Eurman, "Social Attitudes Toward Patients with Anorexia Nervosa," *American Journal of Psychiatry* 137 (1980), 631–32; Ann Landers column, *Los Angeles Times,* April 5, 1988, V, 6.

39 Jean Mayer, *Overweight: Causes, Costs, and Control* (Englewood Cliffs: Prentice-Hall, 1968), 72–73; Covert Bailey, *Fit or Fat?* (Boston: Houghton Mifflin Co., 1978), 10–13; Bennett and Gurin reported that "Exercise alone is typically a slow route to weight loss," op. cit., 253, and "The effects of exercise on the production of metabolic heat are still not entirely clear," op. cit., 248; and *Time* also reported that "experts did not agree about whether exercise has long-term effects on metabolic rates, that is, the body's use of fat for fuel," *Time,* "Dieting . . . ," op. cit., 58; Greenwood quote in Gina Kolata, op. cit., 92.

40 Grant Gwinup, Reg Chelvam, and Terry Steinberg, "Thickness of Subcutaneous Fat and Activity of Underlying Muscles," *Annals of Internal Medicine* 74 (1971), 408–11; Covert Bailey, op. cit., 55.

41 Henry A. Solomon, M.D., *The Exercise Myth* (San Diego: Harcourt Brace Jovanovich, 1984), chapter 4; Bennett and Gurin, "The hypothesis that physical activity is a major means of preventing heart attacks has not been proved, but a great deal of suggestive evidence makes it seem very likely . . . . Even the most impressive of recent research, that conducted by Stanford's Paffenbarger, has not completely resolved the quandry," Bennett and Gurin, op. cit., 264.

42 See especially Solomon's description of the differences between fitness and health, and especially, his example of a superbly fit astronaut, killed in a space capsule fire, who, on autopsy, was found to have extensive coronary artery disease, Solomon, op. cit., chapter 7, and 110.

43 M. Moser, "Nonpharmacologic Therapy for Hypertension: Is It Effective?" *Primary Cardiology* 6 (April 1980), 11; H. Erlick, "Distance Run-

ners as Models of Optimal Health," *Physician and Sportsmedicine* 9 (Jan. 1981), 64–68. Other studies listed in Solomon, op. cit., chapter 5, and for details of studies indicating exercise can cause death, see 116–21.

44 Solomon, op. cit., 21–23, 116–20.

45 Blair Sabol, *The Body of America* (New York: Arbor House, 1986) or see, for example, Patricia Locerock, "Portrait of a Dropout," *Los Angeles Times* Magazine, Jan. 17, 1988, 19–20.

46 See Solomon, op. cit., chapter 7; Bennet and Gurin cite Stanford physicians' report of 18 people who died during or just after jogging. "They found that the victims were inclined to be fanatic exerciser and had ignored clear symptoms in order to continue with a scheduled run," Bennett and Gurin, op. cit., 263.

47 Dr. William P. Morgan, "Negative Addiction in Runners," *Physician and Sports Medicine* 7 (Feb. 1979), 57–60; for the ongoing debate in the medical literature about the behavior patterns of obligatory runners, see Alayne Yatres, Kevin Leehy and Catherine Shisslak, "Running—An Analogue of Anorexia?" *New England Journal of Medicine* 308 (Feb. 3, 1983), 251–55 and the less convincing counter-argument, J. Blumenthal, L. O'Toole, and J. Chang, "Is Running an Analogue of Anorexia Nervosa?" *Journal of the American Medical Association* 252 (July 27, 1984), 520–23; a good summary of the controversy is in Solomon, op. cit., 101–05; see also how these ideas are expressed in the popular press, for example, Stanton Peele, "Tough Talk on Obsession: Bust Loose from that Ball and Chain," *Fitness,* Oct. 1986, 12.

48 Iris F. Litt, M.D., "Amenorrhea in The Adolescent Athlete: Exploration of a Growing Phenomenon," *Postgraduate Medicine* 80 (1986), 245–53; see also Solomon's discussion of the evidence in Solomon, op. cit., 105–06.

49 See Dr. Elizabeth M. Whelan and Dr. Frederick Stare, *The 100% Natural, Purely Organic, Cholesterol-Free, Megavitamin, Low-Carbohydrate Nutrition Hoax* (New York: Atheneum, 1984), 45–55, in which they discuss the results of the 1971–1974 Health and Nutrition Examination Survey, conducted by the Department of Health, Education and Welfare, and published in *Vital and Health Statistics*; the Human Nutrition Center of the U.S. Department of Agriculture (USDA) conducted these surveys in 1965 and 1977. The figures are cited in Bennett and Gurin, op. cit., 244; USDA disappearance data estimated average caloric consumption in 1909–1913 was 3,490 calories a day, in 1976 it was 3,160, reported in Jurgen Schmandt, Rose Ann Shorey, and Lilas Kinch, *Nutrition Policy in Transition* (Lexington: Lexington Books, 1980), 202. See also Benjamin Senauer, "Economics and Nutrition," in *What is America Eating? Proceedings of a Symposium* of the National Research Council (Washington, DC.: National Academy Press, 1986), 47, in which he reports that the highest level of caloric intake in typical American households was 86 percent of recommended daily caloric intake. He observed, "This finding does not agree

with the generally accepted observation that overconsumption of calories is far more widespread than underconsumption in the United States."

50 Daniel P. Puzo, "Salt," *Los Angeles Times,* April 7, 1988, VIII, 1, 18, observes that " . . . medical researchers have repeatedly confirmed earlier studies, originally conducted in the 1950s, indicating that only 10 percent of the U.S. population is salt-sensitive," and he quotes Norman Kaplan, M.D., who chairs a policy committee for American Society of Hypertension who "concedes that the campaign to reduce sodium in the diet may have been 'over enthusastic," p. 18. Recently, the *Los Angeles Times* also reported that "A coalition of health and consumer groups led by the American Dietetic Assn. charged . . . that the nation's $2.6 billion-a-year vitamin supplement industry peddles products most adults and children don't need to maintain good health and warned that toxic reactions can result from vitamin overuse," *Los Angeles Times,* April 9, 1987, V, 1.

51 A recent effort to dispell dietary myths is *U.S. News & World Report, Health and Nutrition* (a supplementary guide) (Washington, D.C.: U.S. News & World Report, 1988), especially 4–14.

52 Marshall H. Becker, "The Cholesterol Saga: Whither Health Promotion?" *Annals of Internal Medicine* 106 (April, 1987), 623–25; Robert Steinbrook, "Soviet-US Study Rebuts Idea of 'Good' Cholesterol," *Los Angeles Times,* Nov. 18, 1987, 1, 22.

53 Becker, loc. cit., 623–25.

54 Becker, loc. cit., 625; Food and Nutrition Board, *Toward Healthful Diets,* 1980, reprinted in Victor Herbert, M.D., J.D., *Nutrition Cultism* (Philadelphia: George F. Stickley Co, 1983), 214.

55 Becker, loc. cit., 625.

56 A. Fallon and P. Rozin, "Sex Differences in Perception of Desirable Body Shape," *Journal of Abnormal Psychology* 94, (1985), 102–05; see also expanded discussion of this study and others in Daniel Coleman, "Dislike of Own Body Found Common Among Women," *New York Times,* March 19, 1985, C1 and C5.

CHAPTER 14

1 "Thin Model Ban," *Advertising Age,* Aug. 3, 1981, 2, 63; *Glamour* decision cited in Hillel Schwartz, *Never Satisfied: A Cultural History of Diets, Fantasies and Fat* (New York: Free Press, 1986), 450, footnote 38; Mallen De Santis, "Beauty: Whatever Happened to the Voluptuous Girl," *Cosmopolitan,* Feb. 1987, 210.

2 "The 'Weight Shrinks' Dig In," *Time,* Jan. 12, 1987, 64.

3 "A Rousing No to Mini-pulation," *Time,* April 25, 1988, 91–94.

4 On the peculiar hypochondriacism of contemporary Americans, and on the fact that while American health and well-being have steadily improved over the past 30 years, the general public tends to regard itself as less healthy than in the past and is more preoccupied with health and medical

issues, see Arthur J. Barsky who attributes this change to four factors: "First, advances in medical care have lowered the mortality rate of acute infectious diseases, resulting in a comparatively increased prevalence of chronic and degenerative disorders. Second, society's heightened consciousness of health has led to greater self-scrutiny and an amplified awareness of bodily symptoms and feelings of illness. Third, the widespread commercialization of health and the increasing focus on health issues in the media have created a climate of apprehension, insecurity and alarm about disease. Finally, the progressive medicalization of daily life has brought unrealistic expectations of cure that make untreatable infirmities and unavoidable ailments seem even worse;" Arthur J. Barsky, M.D., "The Paradox of Health," *New England Journal of Medicine,* Feb. 18, 1988, 414–18.

5 Information about children suffering from diets is based on the studies of Fima Lifshitz and his colleagues and was publicized in the *Los Angeles Times,* June 29, 1986, IX: 10, and, in the same issue, "Nutritionists Express Worries About Children Following Adult Diets," 6.

6 Norbert Elias, tr. Edmund Jephcott, *The Civilizing Process,* 2 vols; vol. I (Boston: Urizen Books, 1978); vol. II (New York: Pantheon Books, 1982).

7 David Hume, *An Enquiry Concerning Human Understanding and Other Essays,* E. Mossner, ed. (New York: Washington Square Press, Inc., 1963), 360–66.

8 John Rechy, *The Sexual Outlaw* (New York: Grove Press, orig. publication 1977, 1984 edition), 112.

9 On fasting and its elevation to a virtue, and its use as a form of political protest, see Schwartz, op. cit., 115–24; and Hilde Bruch, *Eating Disorders* (New York: Basic Books, 1973); 9-15.

10 On this ongoing controversy about excessive individualism in American Culture, see especially Robert Bellah, *Habits of the Heart: Individualism and Commitment in American Life* (Berkeley and Los Angeles: University of California Press, 1985), Carol Gilligan, *In a Different Voice* (Cambridge: Harvard University Press, 1982); Christopher Lasch, *The Culture of Narcissism: American Life in an Age of Diminishing Expectations* (New York: Warner Books, 1979) and Lasch, "Why the Left Has No Future," *Tikkun,* Vol. 1, No. 2, 92–7; Karen Offen, "A Comparative Historical Approach," *Signs: Journal of Women in Culture and Society,* Fall, 1988, 119–57; Shella M. Rothman, *Woman's Proper Place: A History of Changing Ideals and Practices,* 1870 to the Present (New York: Basic Books, 1978).

11 Susan Sontag, *Illness as Metaphor* (New York: Farrar, Straus & Giroux, 1978).

12 Robin Marantz Henig, "The High Cost of Thinness," *New York Times Magazine,* Feb. 28, 1988, 41–42.

Index

DATE DUE

SEP 2 0 1993	
NOV 2 0 1996	
DEC 0 8 1996	
NOV 2 6 1997	
DEC 0 6 1997	
MAR 3 0 1998	
MAR 0 7 1999	
MAY 0 9 2002	
OCT 2 8 2010	

GAYLORD   PRINTED IN U.S.A.